Cambridge Monographs on Cancer Research

Sulfur analogues of polycyclic aromatic hydrocarbons (thiaarenes)

Cambridge Monographs on Cancer Research

Scientific Editors
M. M. Coombs, Imperial Cancer Research Fund Laboratories, London
J. Ashby, Imperial Chemical Industries, Macclesfield, Cheshire
M. Hicks, Science Director, United Biscuits UK Ltd, Maidenhead

Executive Editor
H. Baxter, formerly at the Laboratory of the Government Chemist, London

Books in this Series
Martin R. Osborne and Neil T. Crosby *Benzopyrenes*
Maurice M. Coombs and Tarlochan S. Bhatt
Cyclopenta[a]phenanthrenes
M. S. Newman, B. Tierney and S. Veeraraghavan
The chemistry and biology of benz[a]anthracenes

Sulfur analogues of polycyclic aromatic hydrocarbons (thiaarenes)

Environmental occurrence, chemical and biological properties

JÜRGEN JACOB

Professor at the University of Hamburg, FRG

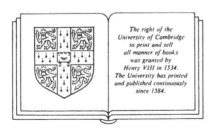

The right of the
University of Cambridge
to print and sell
all manner of books
was granted by
Henry VIII in 1534.
The University has printed
and published continuously
since 1584.

CAMBRIDGE UNIVERSITY PRESS

Cambridge

New York   Port Chester

Melbourne   Sydney

CAMBRIDGE UNIVERSITY PRESS
Cambridge, New York, Melbourne, Madrid, Cape Town, Singapore, São Paulo, Delhi

Cambridge University Press
The Edinburgh Building, Cambridge CB2 8RU, UK

Published in the United States of America by Cambridge University Press, New York

www.cambridge.org
Information on this title: www.cambridge.org/9780521103565

First published 1990
This digitally printed version 2009

A catalogue record for this publication is available from the British Library

Library of Congress Cataloguing in Publication data
Jacob Jürgen.
Sulfur analogues of polycyclic aromatic hydrocarbons (thiaarenes):
environmental occurrence, chemical and biological properties/
Jürgen Jacob.
    p.   cm. – (Cambridge monographs on cancer research)
Includes bibliographical references.
ISBN 0–521–30120–3
1. Thiaarenes – Toxicology.   2. Thiaarenes – Environmental aspects.
I. Title.   II. Series.
[DNLM: 1. Air Pollutants, Environmental.   2. Carcinogens,
Environmental.   3. Polycyclic Hydrocarbons.   4. Structure-Activity
Relationship.   5. Sulfur.   QV 633 J15s]
RA1242. T53J33
615.9'5 – dc20   89–22084   CIP

ISBN 978-0-521-30120-6 hardback
ISBN 978-0-521-10356-5 paperback

To my parents

Contents

Abbreviations employed in this book

In addition to lists of abbreviations given in previous books of this series, the usages outlined below will be found useful.

Journal titles

ACS Symp. Ser.   ACS Symposium Series
Acta Chem. Scand.   Acta Chemica Scandinavica
Acta Med. Okayama   Acta Medica Okayama
Actes Colloqu. Int.   Actes du Colloque International
Adv. Heterocycl. Chemistry   Advances in Heterocyclic Chemistry
Adv. Mass Spectrom.   Advances in Mass Spectrometry
Agr. Biol. Chem.   Agricultural and Biological Chemistry
Am. Assoc. Petr. Geol. Bull.   American Association of Petrologists and
  Geologists Bulletin
Am. Ind. Hyg. Assoc. J.   American Industrial Hygiene Association Journal
Anal. Chem.   Analytical Chemistry
Ang. Chem.   Angewandte Chemie
Ang. Chem. Int. Ed. Engl.   Angewandte Chemie, International Edition in
  English
Ann. Chim.   Annali di Chimica
Ann. Fac. Agrar.   Annali Facolta di Agraria
Arch. Environ. Contam. Toxicol.   Archives of Environmental Contamination
  and Toxicology
Biotechnol. Bioeng.   Biotechnology and Bioengineering
Bol. Sci. Fac. Chim. Ind. Bologna.   Bollettino di Sciencia Faculta Chimica
  Industria Bologna
Brennstoff-Chem.   Brennstoff-Chemie
Bull. Environ. Contam. Toxicol.   Bulletin of Environmental Contamination
  Control and Toxicology
Bull. Soc. Chim. Belges.   Bulletin de la Société de la Chimique Belges
Can. Mines Res. Rep.   Canadian Mines Research Report
Carcinogen. Compr. Survey.   Carcinogenesis Comprehensive Survey
Chem. Pharm. Bull. (Tokyo)   Chemical and Pharmacological Bulletin
  (Tokyo)

Chem. Scr.   Chemica Scripta
Chem. Ser.   Chemometrics Series
Chem. Tech.   Chemistry and Technology
Chem. Ztg.   Chemiker Zeitung
Chromatogr. Newsletter.   Chromatography Newsletter
Compend. Dtsch. Ges. Mineralölwiss. Kohlechem.   Compendium-Deutsche
  Gesellschaft für Mineralölwissenschaft und Kohlechemie
Corsi-Semin. Chim.   Corsi e Seminari di Chimica
Cryst. Struct. Commun.   Crystalline Structure Communications
Electrochim. Acta.   Electrochimica Acta
Environ. Health Persp.   Environmental Health Perspectives
Environ. Meas. Lab. Environ. Q.   Environmental Measurement Laboratory for
  Environmental Quality
Environ. Pollut.   Environmental Pollution
Environ. Sci. Res.   Environmental Science Research
Environ. Sci. Technol.   Environmental Science and Technology
Erdöl und Kohle-Erdgas-Petrochem.   Erdöl und Kohle-Erdgas-Petrochemie
Fortschr. Chem. Forsch.   Fortschritte der Chemischen Forschung
Fresenius Z. Anal. Chem.   Fresenius Zeitschrift Analytische Chemie
Funkt. Biol. Med.   Funktionelle Biologie und Medizin
Gazz. Chim. Ital.   Gazzetta Chimica Italiana
Geochim. Cosmochim. Acta.   Geochimica et Cosmochimica Acta
Gig. Sanit.   Gigicna i Sanitariya
Godoshnik Khim.-Technol. Inst.   Godoshnik Khimiiya-Technologia Institut
High Resolut. Chromatogr. Commun.   High Resolution Chromatography
  Communication
Ind. Eng. Chem. Process. Des. Dev.   Industrial Engineering and Chemical
  Processing Design Development
Indian J. Med. Res.   Indian Journal of Medical Research
Instr. Anal. Toxicol (Haupt. Vortr. Symp.)   Instrumentelle Analytik in der
  Toxikologie [Hauptteil der Vorträge des Symposiums "Instrumentelle
  Analytik in der Toxikologie"]
Int. Arch. Occup. Environ. Health.   International Archives of Occupational and
  Environmental Health
Int. J. Anal. Environ. Chem.   International Journal of Analytical
  Environmental Health Chemistry
Int. J. Mass Spectrometr. Ion Phys.   International Journal of Mass
  Spectrometry and Ion Physics
Istanbul Tek. Univ. Bult.   Istanbul Teknik Universitesi Bulteni
Izv. Akad. Nauk SSR.   Izvestiya Akademii Nauk SSSR
Izv. Akad. Nauk Gruz. SSR.   Izvestia Akademiia Nauk Gruzinskoi SSR
Izv. Vyssh. Ucheb. Zaved. Khim. Tekhnol.   Izvestiia Vysshie Uchebnye
  Zavedeniia Khimiia Khimicheskaia Tekhnologiia
J. Am. Ind. Hyg. Assoc.   Journal of the American Industrial Hygiene
  Association

J. Chem. Eng. Data.   Journal of Chemical Engineering Data

J. Chromatogr.   Journal of Chromatography

J. Ecol. Entomol.   Journal of Ecological Entomology

J. Fish. Res. Board Can.   Journal of the Fisheries Research Board of Canada

J. Gas Chromatogr.   Journal of Gas Chromatography

J. Hydrol. (Amsterdam).   Journal of Hydrology (Amsterdam)

J. Inst. Petrol.   Journal of the Institute of Petrology

J. Mol. Spectr.   Journal of Molecular Spectroscopy

J. Polymer Sci.   Journal of Polymer Science

J. Prakt. Chem.   Journal für Praktische Chemie

J. Phys. Chem. Ref. Data.   Journal of Physics and Chemistry Reference Data

J. Sci. Ind. Res. (India).   Journal of Scientific and Industrial Research (India)

J. Soc. Dyers Colour.   Journal of the Society of Dyers and Colour

Jpn. J. Antibiot.   Japanese Journal of Antibiotics

Khig. Zdraveopaz.   Khigiena i Zdraveopozvane

Khim. Farm. Zh.   Khimia i Farmakologiia Zhurnal

Khim. Geterosikl. Soedin.   Khimiia i Geterosiklicheskikh Soedinenii-Akademiia Nauk Latviiskoi SSR

Khim. Ind. (Sofia).   Khimiia i Industriia (Sofia)

Khim. Sera. Azotorg. Soedin., Soderzh. Neftyakh Neft.   Khimiya Sera-i Azotorganicheskikh Soedinenii, Soderzhashchikhsyav Neftyakh i Nefteproduktake

Khim. Tekhnol. Topl. Masel.   Khimia i Tekhnologiia Topliv i Masel

Koks Khim.   Koks i Khimiia

Liebigs Ann. Chem.   Liebigs Annalen der Chemie

Makromol. Chem.   Makromolekulare Chemie

Mar. Biol.   Marine Biology

Mar. Environ. Res.   Marine Environmental Research

Mar. Pollut. Bull.   Marine Pollution Bulletin

Materialov., Sb. Voronezh.   Materialovy Sbornik Voronezh

Mem. Fac. Eng., Osaka City Univ.   Memoirs of Faculty of Engineering, Osaka City University

Mikrochim. Acta.   Mikrochimica Acta

Monatschr. Chem.   Monatschrift für Chemie

Mutat. Res.   Mutation Research

Neftek Khim.   Neftek Khimii

Oesterr. Chemiker-Ztg.   Oesterreichische Chemiker Zeitung

Opt. i Spectroskopya   Optika i Spectroskopiia

Org. Magn. Resonance.   Organic Magnetic Resonance

Org. Mass Spectrom.   Organic Mass Spectrometry

Org. Prep. Proced. Int.   Organic Preparations and Procedures International

Org. Synth. Coll.   Organic Syntheses Collection

Otkrytiya, Izobret., Prom. Obraztsy Tovarnye Znaki.   Otkrytiia, Izobreteniia, Promyshlennye Obraztsy, Tovarnye Znaki

Petrol. Refiner.   Petroleum Refiner

Phytopathol. Z.   Phytopathologische Zeitschrift

Pol. J. Chem.   Polish Journal of Chemistry

Prep. Pap.-Am. Chem. Soc. Div. Fuel Chem.   Preparation Papers – American Chemical Society Division of Fuel Chemistry

Progr. Food Nutr. Sci.   Progress in Food and Nutrition Science

Rec. Trav. Chim.   Recueil des Travaux Chimiques

Rec. Trav. Chim. Pays-Bas.   Recueil des Travaux Chimiques des Pays-Bas

Rep. Nord. PAH Proj.   Report Nordic PAH Project

Repr. Chem. Soc. Rev.   Reproductive Chemical Society Revue

Rev. Inst. Fr. Petr.   Revue de l'Institute Française pour Petroléum

Riv. Combust.   Rivista dei Combustibili

Sb. Vyssh. Sk. Chem.-Technol. Praze, Technol. Paliv.   Sbornik Vysoke Skoly Chemicko-Technologicke v Praze Technologie Paliv

Scand. J. Work Environ. Health.   Scandinavian Journal of Work Environment and Health

Sci. Total Environ.   Science of the Total Environment

Soobshch. Akad. Nauk Nauk Gruz. SSR.   Soobshcheniia Akademiia Nauk Nauk Gruz SSR

Staub-Reinhalt. Luft.   Staub Reinhaltung der Luft

Tezisy Dokl.-Vses. Soveshch. Lyumin.   Tezisy Dokladov-Vsesoyuznogo Soveshehanic polyuminestsentsii.

Toxicol. Lett.   Toxicology Letters

Vestn. Mosk. Univ.   Vestnik-Moskovskii Universitet

Water Res.   Water Research

Wiad. Chem.   Wiadomosci Chemiczne

Z. Allg. Mikrobiol.   Zeitschrift für Allgemeine Mikrobiologie

Z. Chem.   Zeitschrift für Chemie

Z. Krebsforsch.   Zeitschrift für Krebsforschung

Z. Naturforsch.   Zeitschrift für Naturforschung

Zavod. Lab.   Zavodskaia Laboratoriia

Zbl. Bakt. Hyg.   Zentralblatt für Bakteriologie und Hygiene

Zh. Fiz. Khim.   Zhurnal Fizicheskoi Khimii

Zh. Org. Khim.   Zhurnal Organicheskoi Khimii

Zh. Prike. Spektrosk.   Zhurnal Prikeladnoi Spektroskopii

Some other common abbreviations

b.p.   boiling point

h/v one quantum of energy

m.p.   melting point

m.w.   molecular weight

NMR   nuclear magnetic resonance

Preface

The intention of this monograph is to give practical information on some selected sulfur-containing polycyclic aromatic compounds with regard to analytical, synthetic, metabolic and toxicological aspects to chemists, biologists and other scientists who are particularly interested in environmental problems. This class of compounds has been neglected by the ecological chemists until it became evident that at least some individuals exhibit potent mutagenic activities and more recent investigations showed that there are also carcinogenic compounds among them. Initially it was planned to include also the oxygen analogues of polycyclic aromatic hydrocarbons in this book; however, during the literature search it became obvious that this would extend the length of the monograph too much and that it would require another book. In total, about 400 compounds were found in the search covered by more than 1000 references in Chemical Abstracts since 1948. Accordingly, the only compounds discussed in this monograph are those which have been detected or which are likely to be found in the environment, as well as compounds related to them and on which substantial information was obtainable. This is necessarily a subjective selection resulting in omissions which will not find every reader's consent. For instance, the monocyclic system thiophene together with all its derivatives or the various thiapyranes were deleted.

Although only a comparatively few sulfur-containing polycyclic aromatic compounds (thiaarenes) have been definitely identified in environmental matter it may be expected that more will be found with modern analytical methods, especially in the higher boiling fractions of fossil fuels, in their derivatives and, accordingly, in their combustion exhausts. Since hitherto no biological fractionation of these matrices with regard to sulfur-containing polycyclic aromatic compounds has been carried out, their contribution to the carcinogenic potential of environmental matter is still an open question. This should encourage scientists to undertake appropriate experiments because legislation must be based on scientific cognition.

It will be noted that all formulas have been drawn in the conventional way in accordance with the IUPAC nomenclature monograph and most of the literature. As a consequence of the bond lengths in the thiophene ring, the actual shape of the various thiaarene molecules, however, differs significantly from this formal description. In cases where comparisons are made on isosterism between arenes and thiaarenes the more precise formulas have been preferred. Italicized figures in parentheses [e.g. (*29*)] in Part 1 refer to individual compounds described in detail in Part 2.

The author thankfully acknowledges the valuable contribution made by Dr W. Schmidt and the assistance on the data collection by Dr A. Glaser and Mr G. Raab. He would like to express also his gratitude to Professor Dr G. Grimmer for many fruitful discussions and Mrs C. Röhler for her assistance in typewriting the manuscript. Thanks go also to the editor and the publisher for their patience and the appreciation that the preparation of the manuscript took longer than expected.

Hamburg, 1986   J. Jacob

1

General chapter on thiaarenes

1.1   Introduction

Based on their wide distribution in the environment and considering their carcinogenic and mutagenic potential, polycyclic aromatic hydrocarbons have been thoroughly investigated as far as their occurrence, formation, identification, monitoring, metabolic pathways and toxicological effects in various species are concerned. However, the closely related heterocyclic analogues such as thiaarenes, azaarenes and oxaarenes have not found the interest of scientists to the same extent, perhaps because (a) they occur in smaller concentration – sometimes only as traces – in environmental matter, and (b) nothing was, and only little still is, known about their biological activities.

This monograph summarizes in condensed form our knowledge on thiaarenes, one of the above classes, restricted to those compounds which have been detected in environmental matter or which are closely related to them by structure and which may be found as contaminants in future investigations.

In view of the revived interest in coal as an energy source, the various attempts at coal liquification and the temporarily increased interest in shale oils, more intense investigations on thiaarenes are indicated and justified. Accordingly numerous publications on the identification and syntheses of thiaarenes appeared during the past seven years following the modern rule that sponsorship is more readily to be obtained if relevance can be proven. But there are still many open questions and uncertainties on the various subjects of thiaarene chemistry.

Many investigators still have obvious difficulties with the nomenclature of this class of compounds. For instance, for the very common and abundant benzo[*b*]naphtho[2,1-*d*]thiophene at least four other terms have been – and unfortunately sometimes still are – used (naphtho[2,1-

b]benzothiophene, 1,2-benzo-9-thiofluorene, 9-thia-1,2-benzofluorene, 11-thiabenzo[*a*]fluorene); and benzo[*kl*]thioxanthene has also been named as benzothioxanthene, 1,10-benzothiaxanthene, 1,10-benzo-5-thiaxanthene, and 7-thiabenzanthracene. In section 1.2 (Nomenclature) this topic, therefore is briefly discussed. It refers to terms as used in Chemical Abstracts and recommended by the International Union of Pure and Applied Chemistry (IUPAC).

For characterization and identification various analytical methods have recently been improved and specifically modified. Today, detectors in gas chromatography are available which specifically respond to sulfur. Ligand-exchange chromatography on palladium II chloride-impregnated supports has been successfully applied to the separation of thiaarenes from complex mixtures and this technique perhaps will replace the traditional method consisting of oxidation of thiaarenes to the corresponding sulfones, separation of the latter by silica chromatography and subsequent reduction to the original thiaarenes. Capillary gas chromatography and high-performance liquid-chromatography methods have been substantially improved and have achieved better resolution of thiaarene isomers, and the applications of high-resolution and tandem mass spectrometry to thiaarene identification allow a discrimination of these compounds from carbocyclic systems together with which they are often co-eluted. The various methods are summarized in Section 1.4 (Analytical aspects in thiaarene chemistry) and technical preconditions for these methods, such as the spectral data are briefly reviewed in Section 1.3 (Spectral and physical data).

Studies on the occurrence of thiaarenes are still ongoing and we have only limited ideas on their formation (see Section 1.5 Occurrence and formation). The main sources of thiaarenes are fossil fuels such as coal, petroleum and shale oils from which they are released to our environment, directly and by combustion processes. Thiaarenes are often considerably enriched by refining processes (tar, pitch and also coal liquids).

For identification and also for biological testing, the pure compounds are required. Since separation and purification from natural sources (coal tar) is an almost hopeless or at least an extremely time-consuming task, synthetic efforts have been undertaken to provide reference compounds. Especially, Tilak, Klemm and more recently Lee *et al.* have synthesized a large number of thiaarenes, and their efforts have considerably stimulated further investigations on thiaarenes by other working groups and have encouraged chemists and biologists to study the distribution, biochemistry and toxicology of this chemical class. General methods applied to the synthesis of thiaarenes are briefly summarized in Section 1.6 (Synthesis) and specific routes for the various compounds in Chapter 2, Sections 2.1–2.7.

There are still many gaps to be filled in our knowledge and understanding of the biological activities of thiaarenes. Actually, only very limited and insufficient information is available on the specific contribution of thiaarenes to the mutagenic and/or carcinogenic potencies of environmental matter. Even for coal-combustion emissions it is not yet known to what extent or whether at all thiaarenes play a role as carcinogenic hazards to man. Biological balances with various environmental matrices with regard to thiaarenes therefore are strongly required. Our limited knowledge on the mutagenic and carcinogenic activities of thiaarenes is summarized in Section 1.7 (Biological activity). As is known for polycyclic aromatic hydrocarbons, these activities are based on the *in vivo* metabolic conversion to proximate and ultimate carcinogens. However, no systematic investigations on the metabolism of thiaarenes hitherto have been carried out and the few studies which have been performed seem to indicate that the main biological pathways of thiaarenes differ from those observed with their carbocyclic analogues (see Section 1.8, Metabolism).

The second part of the monograph (Chapter 2, Compounds) summarizes information on the various thiaarene systems, compound by compound including some 250 compounds.

1.2   Nomenclature

Since many scientists feel uncertain about the nomenclature of aromatic compounds, a fact which often has resulted in serious misunderstandings, the nomenclature of the compounds mentioned in this monograph will be briefly discussed in this chapter. For more complete information the reader is referred to the IUPAC-monograph (1979) and a number of reviews (McNaught, 1976; Jacob and Grimmer, 1979; Loening and Merritt, 1983; Later *et al.*, 1984).

The names shown in Table 1 are used as a basis for condensed systems The term 'thenyl' is used as radical name for methylthiophene.

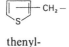

thenyl-

The nomenclature of higher fused compounds derives from the parent compounds listed in Table 1. Ring systems attached to the base structure are indicated by lettering (following the numbering, so that the bond between C-1 and C-2 becomes side 'a', etc.) using a letter (roman, in italics

Table 1. *Trivial names on which the nomenclature of thiaarenes is based*

Parent compound	Name	Radical name	Prefix in composed structures
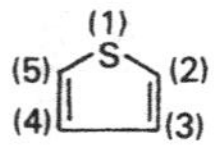	thiophene	thienyl-	thieno-
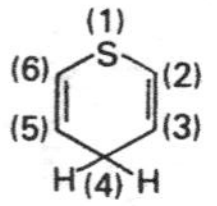	4H-thiopyran	thiopyranyl	thiopyrano-
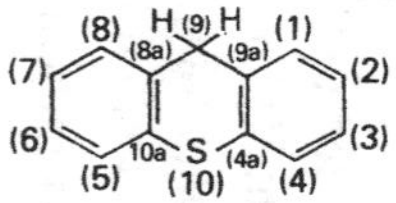	thioxanthene	thioxanthenyl-	thioxantheno-
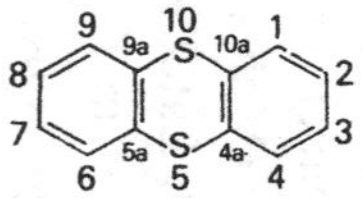	thianthrene	thianthrenyl-	thianthreno-

and in square brackets) as early in the alphabet as possible (example: benzo[*b*]thiophene *not* benzo[*d*]thiophene:

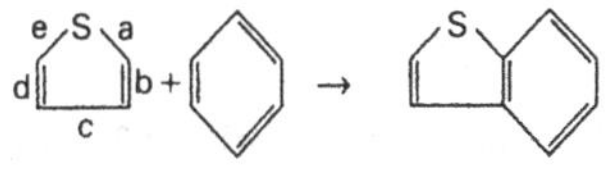

benzo[*b*]thiophene

When there is a choice in attaching a system to the sulfur-containing base structure, both partial structures participating in the fusion have to be indicated: (i) the side(s) of the base S-PAC structure is indicated by italic(s) (*not* interrupted by a comma when more than one side is involved) and (ii) the side(s) of the attached partial structure are indicated by numbers of the participating carbon atoms being as low as possible in accordance with the numbering of the attached component (example: benzo[*b*]naphtho[1,2-*d*]thiophene; benzo[*b*]naphtho[2,1-*d*]thiophene; benzo[*b*]naphtho[2,3-*d*]thiophene):

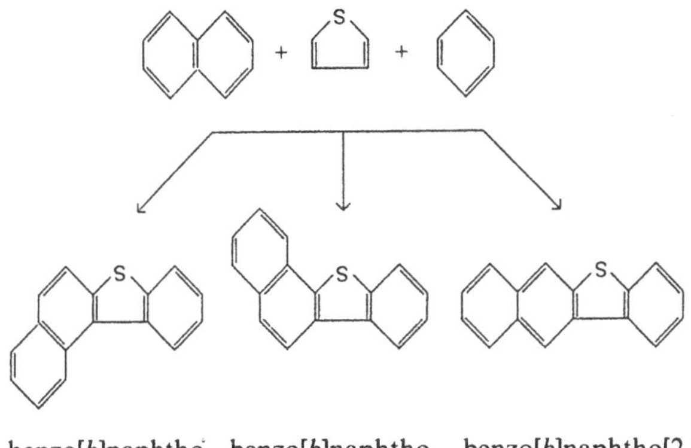

benzo[*b*]naphtho   benzo[*b*]naphtho   benzo[*b*]naphtho[2,3-*d*]thiophene
[1,2-*d*]thiophene   [2,1-*d*]thiophene

When there is more than one system attached, this has to be alphabetically arranged so that the prefixes appear in alphabetical order (benzo[*b*]naphtho[2,1-*d*]thiophene *not* naphtho[2,1-*b*]benzo[*d*]thiophene).

The *orientation* of the final system is arranged so that (1) the greatest number of rings appear in a horizontal row, (2) a maximum number of rings appear in the upper right-hand quadrant, and (3) as few as possible in the lower left-hand quadrant. If there remains a choice after having given preference to the orientation, the structure has to be arranged so that the hetero atom receives the lowest number possible. Hence, the aforementioned benzonaphthothiophenes have to be orientated as follows:

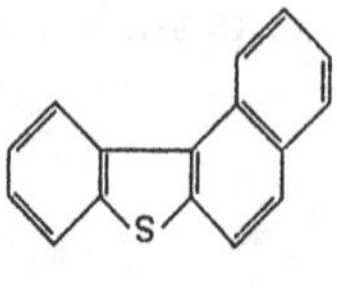

benzo[*b*]naphtho   benzo[*b*]naphtho   benzo[*b*]naphtho[2,3-*d*]thiophene
[1,2-*d*]thiophene   [2,1-*d*]thiophene

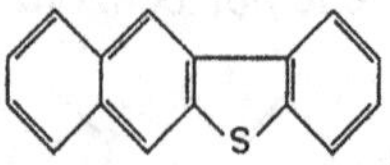

Numbering begins in the upper right-hand ring with the first carbon atom not engaged in a ring fusion and continues in a clockwise direction around the molecule. Atoms common to two or more rings are designated by adding roman letters (a, b, c . . .) to the number of the position immediately preceding. Interior atoms follow the highest number taking a clockwise sequence wherever there is a choice. (See first example below.)

Example:

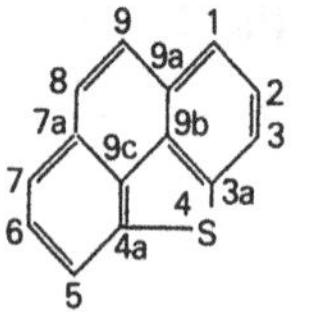

phenanthro[4,5-*bcd*]thiophene

When there is still a choice after having obeyed these rules, carbon atoms common to two or more rings receive the lowest possible numbers.

Example:

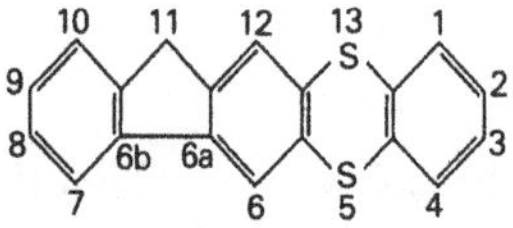

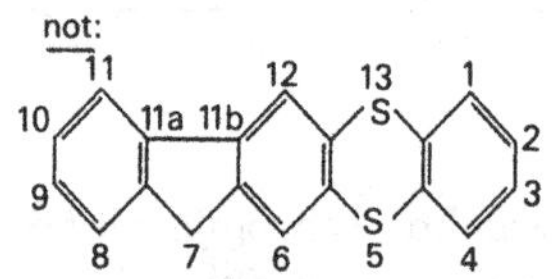

indeno[2,3-*b*]thianthrene

Hydrogenated compounds are designated by prefixes such as 'dihydro-' 'tetrahydro-', 'octahydro-', etc. followed by the name of the corresponding unhydrogenated hydrocarbon. The location of the hydrogenated carbon atoms are indicated by the position number.

Example:

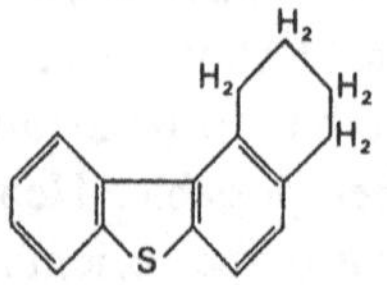

1,2,3,4-tetrahydrobenzo[*b*]naphtho[1,2-*d*]thiophene

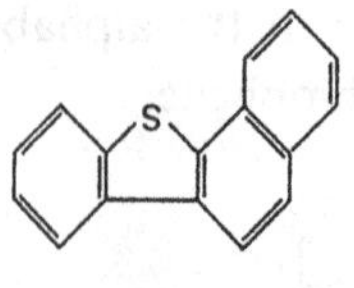

The prefix 'perhydro' signifies full hydrogenation. Where there is a choice for a H which is used for the indicated hydrogen, the lowest available number has to be used.

Apart from the aforementioned nomenclature a second so-called replacement or 'a'-nomenclature exists in which heterocyclic systems are derived from a carbocyclic one by replacing one or more carbon atoms with hetero atoms. In case of sulfur-containing polycyclic compounds this is indicated by the prefix 'thia' to which the position number of the substituted carbon atom in the parent carbocycle is added.

Example:

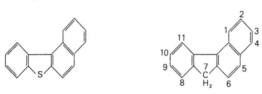

7-thiabenzo[*c*]fluorene   benzo[*c*]fluorene

derived from

or:

1,4-dithianaphthalene   naphthalene

Nomenclature is more intricate in cases of compounds possessing more than one sulfur-containing ring such as dithiophenes, trithiophenes, etc. For practical reasons the nomenclature used in Chemical Abstracts is followed here. Systems with two peripheral thiophene rings are designated as dithiophenes. Sides of the attached thiophene are indicated by roman letters and with prime-bearing roman letters for additional thiophene rings, whereas sides of the base compound participating in the fusion are indicated by the position numbers. Designations belonging to two different attached rings are separated by a colon.

Example:

benzo[1,2-*b*:3,4-*b'*]dithiophene

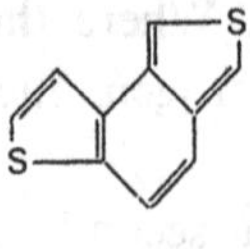

benzo[1,2-*b*:3,4-*c'*]dithiophene

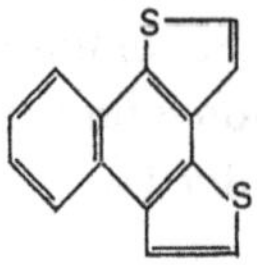

naphtho[1,2-*b*:3,4-*b'*]dithiophene

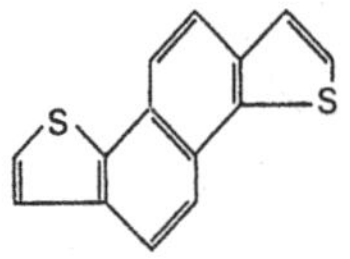

naphtho[1,2-*b*:5,6-*b'*]dithiophene

Some examples for the nomenclature of higher systems with internal thiophene rings are given below.

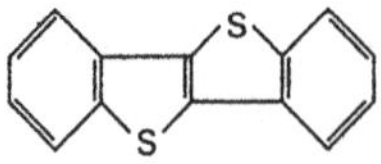

[1]benzothieno[3,2-*b*][1]benzothiophene

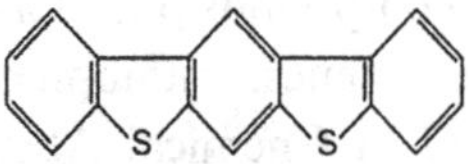

benzo[1,2-*b*:5,4-*b'*]bis[*1*]benzothiophene

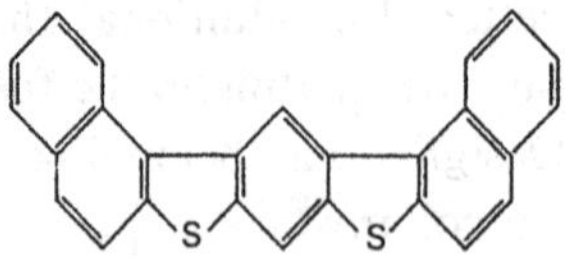

dinaphtho[1,2-*d*:1',2'-*d'*]benzo[1,2-*b*:5,4-*b'*]dithiophene

To minimize possible confusion names including numbering of all compounds described in Chapter 2, Sections 2.1–2.7, as used in *Chemical Abstracts*, are given.

1.3   Spectral and physical data of thiaarenes

1.3.1   *UV spectra*

Polycyclic aromatic compounds possess characteristic, richly banded UV spectra which are uniquely suited for characterization purposes. This holds true also for isomers which are not readily distinguished by other techniques, e.g. mass spectrometry. Alkyl substituents and hydroaromatic rings usually lower the extinction coefficients, blur the vibrational structure and cause small shifts – in most cases to the red – in the band positions; the basic chromophore can still be recognized, however. Due to spectral overlap, identification of individuals in PAC mixtures is rendered difficult if they contain more than two or three components. This underlines the need for an efficient class separation procedure, followed by fractionation (TLC, HPLC, preparative GC) into pure individual components.

The UV spectra of some 250 parent PAH synthesized up to 1963 have been compiled and discussed by Clar (1964) in the context of the annelation principle (Clar, 1972). This concept relates in a general fashion the positions of the α-, p-, β- and β'-bands (Platt synonyms: ^1L_b, ^1L_a, ^1B_b, ^1B_a) to the number of aromatic sextets which in turn depend on the molecular graph. A more recent compilation, in which special emphasis is laid upon environmental PAH, has been published by Karcher *et al.* (1985) who also present the UV spectra of five thiaarenes.

In comparing the UV-spectra of arenes and their isosteric thiaarenes, three major effects are apparent. First, the α-band has gained in intensity at the expense of the β-band. This can be traced to the breakdown of the pairing theorem (Platt, 1964) when a sulfur atom replaces an ethylenic double bond. Consequently, the transition moments of the two one-electron excitations which give rise to the α-state do no longer cancel, resulting in a non-vanishing, yet small, oscillator strength. Published thiaarene spectra show significantly enhanced α-bands whose extinction coefficients, in cyclohexane, exceed those of the corresponding arenes by a factor ranging from 4 to 30. Conversely, the β-bands of the thiaarenes are, in most cases, slightly weaker than those of the arenes. The effect is not so pronounced as with the α-bands because the oscillator strength of the β-bands is very high from the outset and is hence not dramatically altered by substituting a sulfur atom for an ethylenic double bond. The extinction coefficients of the p-bands, being relatively constant between 8000 and about 24 000, show much less variation than those of the arenes which range from 5000 to 56 000.

Secondly, the vibrational structure in the p- and β-bands of the thiaarene spectra is less pronounced. This seems to be due to the combined effects of the lowered molecular symmetry and the different vibrational frequency of the C-S vs. the C–C bond. In the arene spectra, the uniform 1400 cm^{-1} progression seen in the p- and β-bands is due to an alternate lengthening and shortening of successive C–C bonds. Replacing one of these bonds by a sulfur atom modulates this vibrational motion to some extent, resulting in a blurring and broadening of the vibrational components. However, there is also one counter example: benzo[*b*]naphtho[1,2-*d*]thiophene shows a better resolved structure than its arene counterpart, benzo[*c*]phenanthrene, where this is also smeared out because of overcrowding. In the thiaarene, this overcrowding is relaxed for simple geometrical reasons.

A third difference, which is important to the practising analytical chemist, is illustrated in Table 2 with some representative examples. Corresponding bands in the thiaarenes are systematically blue-shifted by typically 10–20 nm relative to those of the arenes. For newly isolated thiaarenes of unknown structure, this rule is useful in eliminating certain structures from an otherwise fairly large pool of alternatives. However, we note one exception in the Table for which no explanation can be offered: the β-band of benzo[2,3]phenanthro[4,5-*bcd*]thiophene is at definitely longer wavelength than that of benzo[*a*]pyrene namely 303 vs. 297 nm. As the assignment of the p- and β-bands in the thiaarene spectra is not always straightforward, further exceptions to this rule may exist. Clearly, better resolved spectra, preferably recorded at cryogenic temperature, and specimens of proven purity are needed before the limits of this rule can be fully appreciated. For example, the thiaarene spectrum presented by Karcher *et al.* (1983) (stated sample purity 99.0%) contains impurity bands at 403 and 397 nm because the fluorescence excitation spectrum does not match the UV spectrum and because there is no mirror symmetry between absorption and emission.

1.3.2   Fluorescence spectroscopy

Fluorescence is as useful a tool for the identification of PAC as UV spectroscopy and offers at the same time higher sensitivity and selectivity. This higher selectivity stems from the fact that bands are usually narrower and extend over a limited wavelength region, typically 100 nm, so that band overlap is less severe than with UV-spectra. Using selective excitation, fairly complex PAC mixtures comprising up to 6 or 8 PAC have been successfully analysed.

Quantitation is somewhat of a problem because the response factors of individual PAC vary widely as a result of the different fluorescence quantum yields and the different absorptivities at the excitation wavelength. Several compounds, prime among them acenaphthylene and cyclopenta[*cd*]pyrene, are known to be non-fluorescent and hence escape detection. Also, energy transfer between individual components and quenching due to impurities may occur. To eliminate these error sources, clean-up and fractionation by TLC or HPLC should precede fluorescence analysis.

Selectivity and sensitivity may both be enhanced by lowering the temperature. The change from continuous (broad-band) to quasi-linear (phonon-less) spectra which occurs under specific experimental conditions is known as the Shpol'skii effect. Solvent, temperature, cooling rate and concentration are crucial parameters which must be carefully selected by trial and error. Cyclohexane, tetrahydrofuran and dioxan occasionally give good results, but the solvents of choice are *n*-alkanes. A golden rule states that the length of the longest axis of the PAC must match the length of the *n*-alkane for correct embedding in the solvent matrix to occur. Cooling must be rapid, and the temperature as low as possible. Spectroscopists prefer solid or liquid helium (1.36 or 4.2 K, respectively) as cooling medium, while the practising analytical chemists are usually satisfied with solid or liquid nitrogen (63 or 77 K, respectively). At these conventional temperatures, one of the basic advantages of Shpol'skii spectroscopy – the identification of the 0–0 transition at the expense of the higher vibrational components – is lost, however.

Ordinary room-temperature spectra (*n*-hexane, cyclohexane) as well as low-resolution Shpol'skii spectra (63 or 15 K, *n*-hexane or *n*-octane) of thiaarenes have been reported by Colmsjö and coworkers (Colmsjö and Östman, 1982; Colmsjö *et al.*, 1982, 1984) and Karcher *et al.* (1985). Where sample purity was satisfactory, good mirror symmetry between absorption and emission is noted, and the Stokes shifts match those found with the arenes. In other words, the fluoresence spectra of the thiaarenes correspond to blue-shifted arene spectra, the shifts being (with one exception) in the 10–20 nm range. The Shpol'skii spectrum of dibenzothiophene in *n*-heptane at 10 K has been presented and discussed by Vial *et al.* (1986).

1.3.3 *Phosphorescence spectroscopy*

The phosphorescence of arenes is rarely intense enough for this technique to be of practical value. With thiaarenes, the situation is different in that the sulfur atom provides for efficient spin-orbit coupling and hence increases the intersystem crossing rate from the S_1 state to the triplet manifold. Consequently, phosphorescence quantum yields are expected to be higher than with arenes.

Table 2. *Comparison of the α-, p- and β-band maxima (0–0 transitions, in nm, cyclohexane solution) in the UV spectra of arenes and their isosteric thiaarenes; uncertain assignments are in parentheses*

Arene	α	p	β	Isosteric thiaarene	α	p	β
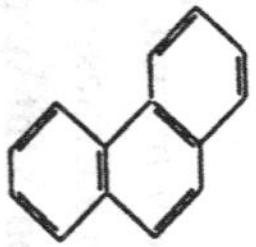	346	292	251	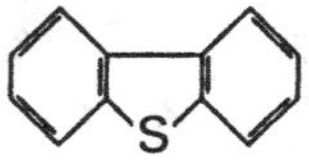	326	286	236
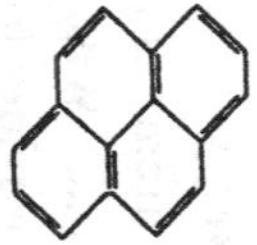	372	335.5	273	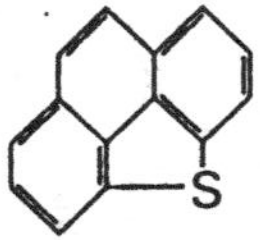	357	331	274
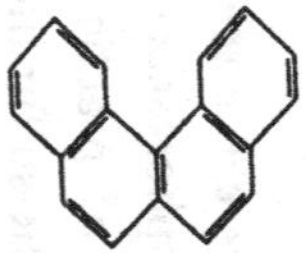	372	(327)	283	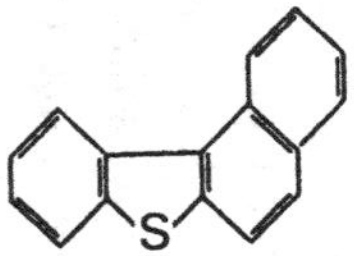	351	321	264.5
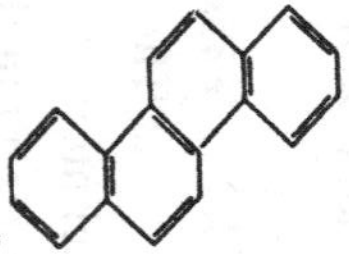	361.5	320.5	269	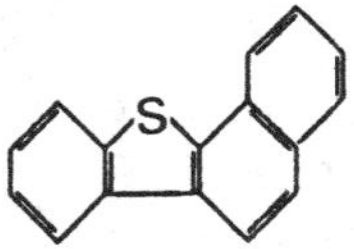	348	(303)	(253.5)

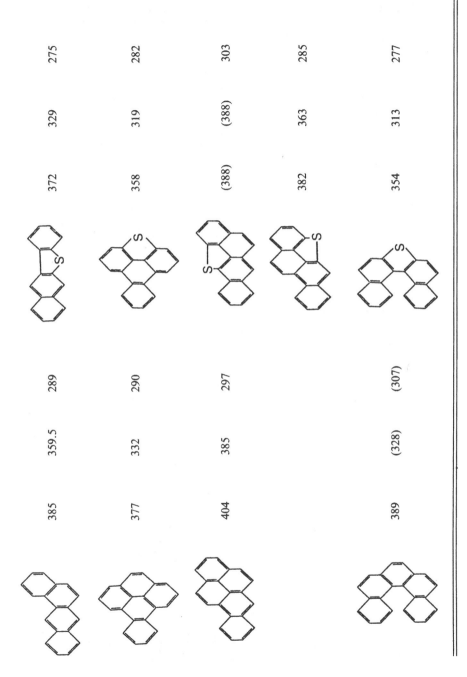

275	282	303	285	277
329	319	(388)	363	313
372	358	(388)	382	354

289	290	297		(307)
359.5	332	385		(328)
385	377	404		389

Table 3. *Comparison of the phosphorescence maxima (0–0 transitions, in nm, frozen* n-*alkanes) for arenes and their isosteric thiaarenes; uncertain identifications are in parentheses*

Arene		Isosteric thiaarene	
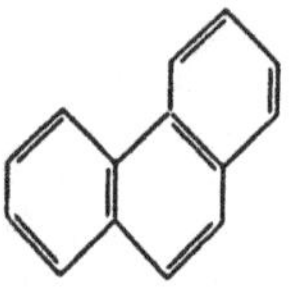	462	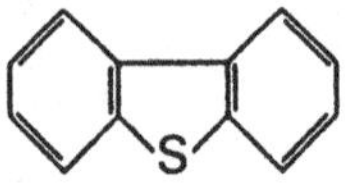	409.5
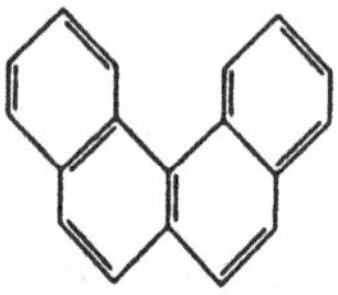	499.5	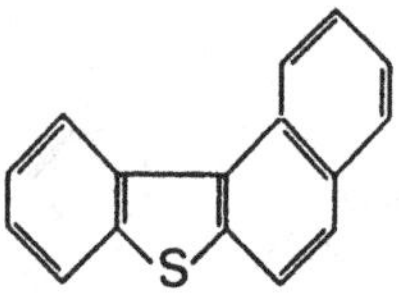	489.1
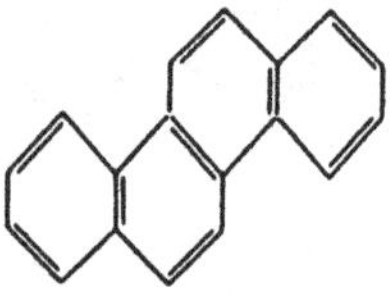	499	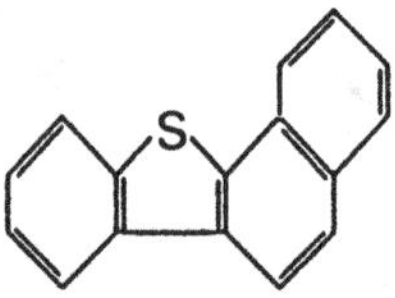	477.5
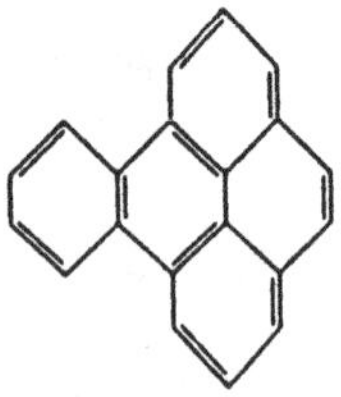	537	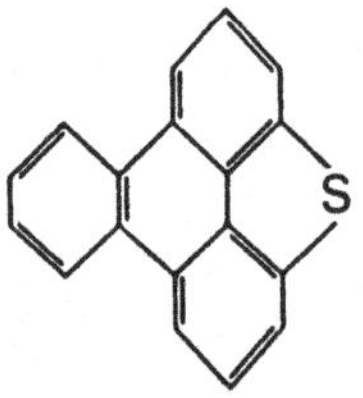	455.3
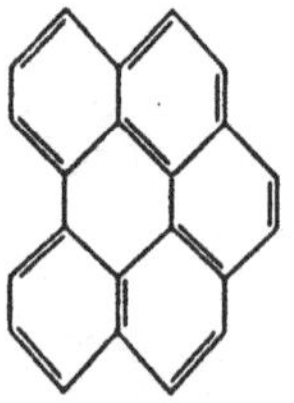	618	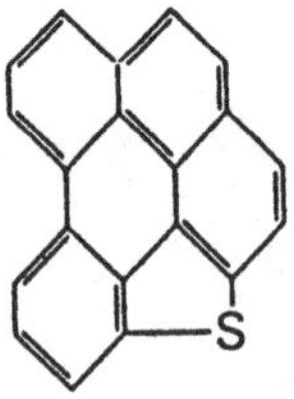	548.9
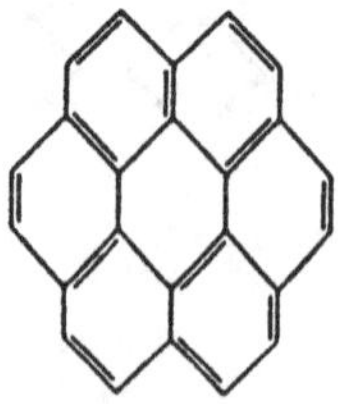	515.5	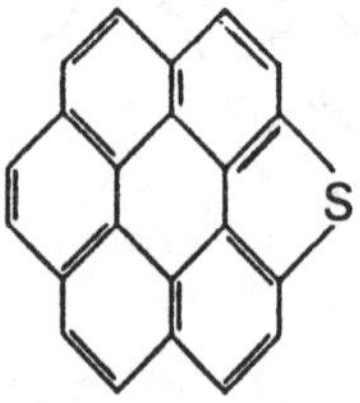	(542.3)

Table 4. *Phosphorescence data on some thiaarenes and their isosteric carbazoles (from Zander, 1976)*

Compound	$\bar{\nu}_{phos}$ cm^{-1} (ethanol)	τ_{phos}(s)		ϕ_P/ϕ_F	
		(ethanol)	(ethanol/ethyl-bromide (1:1; v/v))	(ethanol)	(ethanol/ethyl-bromide (1:1; v/v))
Carbazol	24510	6.8	1.5	0.46	3.3
Dibenzothiophene	24100	1.5	0.65	12.6	16.2
7H-Dibenzo[a,g]carbazol	20660	3.4	0.85	0.05	0.31
Dinaphtho[1,2-b:1',2'-d]thiophene	20040	0.74	0.50	5.6	10.0
7H-Dibenzo[c,g]carbazol	19610	2.1	0.63	0.14	0.72
Dinaphtho[2,1-b:1',2'-d]thiophene	18350	0.19	0.10	2.2	3.9
7H-Dibenzo[a,i]carbazol	21460	5.4	1.1	0.10	1.5
Dinaphtho[1,2-b:2,1'-d]thiophene	20660	1.6	0.76	10.2	12.0

τ_{phos} = phosphorescence lifetime.
ϕ_P/ϕ_F = phosphorescence/fluorescence quantum yield ratio.

So far, few authors appear to have utilized this feature. However, Vial *et al.* (1986) explicitly mention that the phosphorescence of dibenzothiophene (*n*-heptane, 10 K) is many times more intense than the fluorescence. In Table 3 the 0–0 phosphorescence transitions of some thiaarenes, from the literature (Colmsjö and Östman, 1982; Colmsjö *et al.*, 1982, 1984; Karcher *et al.*, 1985; Vial *et al.*, 1986) are compared with those of the arenes. With the possible exception of benzoperylothiophene, all thiaarenes show blue-shifted phosphorescence relative to the arenes, as was the case with fluorescence. The shifts are larger, however, and show considerable variation across the series.

Zander (1976) has published data on the phosphorescence spectra, lifetimes and quantum yield ratios of phosphorescence and fluorescence for dibenzothiophene, dinaphtho[1,2-*b*:1',2'-*d*]thiophene, dinaphtho[2,1-*b*:1',2'-*d*]thiophene and dinaptho[1,2-*b*:2'1'-*d*]thiophene at 77 K and compared them with isosteric carbazoles. Data are collected in Table 4 which show that (a) the energy of the lowest triplet state is structure dependent, (b) the life-times are significantly shorter, and (c) the quantum yield ratios are higher in thiaarenes than in isosteric carbazoles. Some phosphorescence spectra are given in Fig. 1. More recently, Zander *et al.* (1987) have studied empirical quantitative models that relate phosphorescence transition energies of thiaarenes and carbocyclic systems on the basis of 20 compounds. They also reported phosphorescence 0–0 bands, phosphorescence/fluorescence quantum yield ratios, and phosphorescence lifetimes of the following thiaarene systems: naphtho[2,1-*b*]thiophene, naphtho[1,2-*b*]thiophene, phenanthro[9,10-*b*]thiophene, benzo[*b*]naphtho[2,3-*d*]thiophene, anthra[1,2-*b*]benzo[*d*]thiophene, benzo[*b*]phenanthro[1,2-*d*]thiophene, dinaphtho[2,3-*b*:2',3'-*d*]thiophene, dinaphtho[1,2-*b*:2',3'-*d*]thiophene, phenanthro[4,5-*bcd*]thiophene, triphenyleno[1,12-*bcd*]thiophene, chryseno[4,5-*bcd*]thiophene, and benzo[2,3]phenanthro[4,5-*bcd*]thiophene.

1.3.4   IR- and NMR-spectra

Infrared spectra of thiaarenes have not been found to be very helpful in their definite identification although in some cases the position of the substituent in various methyl-substituted derivatives may be recognized and hence allow isomers to be distinguished. As in the IR-spectra of arenes, thiaarenes exhibit CH stretching bands in the region 2960–3120 cm^{-1}, CH out-of-plane bands between 700 and 890 $^{-1}$, as well as less intense bands arising from combination vibrations found between 1650 and 2000 cm^{-1}. Some infra-red spectral data recently have been reported by Karcher *et al.* (1985) including full spectra of

Fig. 1. Phosphorescence spectra (77K) in ethanol (———) and ethanol/ethyl bromide (1:1; v/v). All spectra have been adjusted to equal intensities using the most intense band (from Zander, 1976).

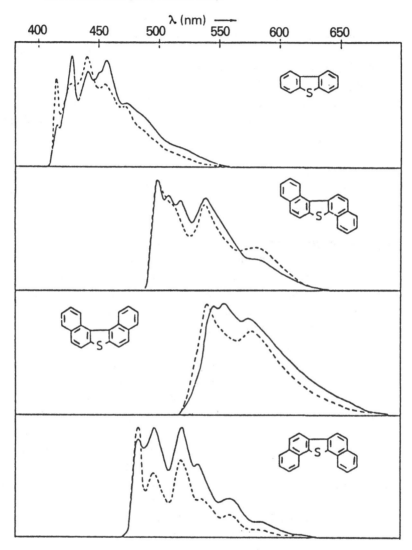

benzo[*b*]naphtho[1,2-*d*]thiophene, benzo[*b*]naphtho[2,1-*d*]thiophene, benzo[*b*]naphtho[2,3-*d*]thiophene, benzo[2,3]phenanthro[4,5-*bcd*]thiophene, and phenanthro[4,5-*bcd*]thiophene.

Sulfones exhibit intense bands at about 1300 cm^{-1} (asymmetric $\nu_{S=O}$) and at 1155–1170 cm^{-1} (symmetric $\nu_{S=O}$) which may be used for their characterization in mixtures (Drushel and Sommers, 1967).

NMR-spectroscopy has been widely used for the characterization and identification of thiaarenes (for references see Chapter 3; data have been reviewed by Klemm, 1982). More recently Karcher *et al.* (1985) published ^{1}H- and ^{13}C-NMR spectral data of some highly purified thiaarenes such as phenanthro[4,5-*bcd*]thiophene, benzo[*b*]naphtho[1,2-*d*]thiophene, benzo[*b*]naphtho[2,1-*d*]thiophene, benzo[*b*]naphtho[2,3-*d*]thiophene and benzo[2,3]phenanthro[4,5-*bcd*]thiophene.

Two-dimensional NMR spectroscopy has been applied to structure confirmation and elucidation of various thiaarenes. The technique recently has been reviewed by Castle *et al.* (1984) who demonstrated the advantages in comparison to conventional ^{1}H- and ^{13}C-NMR spectroscopy with a series of examples presenting two-dimensional homonuclear chemical shift correlation spectra (COSY-spectra) recorded with benzo-[2,3]phenanthro[4,5-*bcd*]thiophene, phenanthro[1,2-*b*]thiophene and phenanthro[3,4-*b*]thiophene.

1.3.5   Mass spectrometry

The most commonly used mass spectrometric technique in thiaarene characterization and identification is electron impact mass spectrometry recording preferentially at 60–80 eV (high voltage technique). Although sulfur-containing compounds generally may be recognized from the natural isotope distribution of $^{32}S/^{34}S$ (which is about 25:1) by comparing the intensities of doublets differing by two mass units, the evaluation of specific fragments is more recommended, since overlapping with other fragments often complicates the method based on isotope comparison. Mass spectrometric fragmentation of thiaarenes yields prominent peaks at the mass (M-45) according to the loss of a (CH = S)-unit. The charge also may remain on the fragment itself so that an ion $HC^+ = S$ ($m/z = 45$) is observed. Gallegos (1975) reported on the relative intensities of this and the following ions m/z 33 (SH), m/z 34 (H_2S), m/z 46 (CH_2S), and m/z 47 (CH_3S) appearing in the mass spectra of various thiaarenes, a selection of which is given in Table 5. He also provided mass spectra of variously alkyl-substituted thiophenes showing that intense ions with m/z 97 may arise from ring enlargement by radical elimination according to (Hanuš and Čermák, 1959):

$$\text{(structure)} \xrightarrow[-R^\cdot]{e^-} \text{(structure)} \quad m/z\ 97$$

Apart from the intense (M-45)-ion a (M-32)-fragment is observed in parent thiaarenes caused by elimination of the sulfur heteroatom. As in

Table 5. Relative abundance of some low mass fragments in the spectra of various thiaarenes (Gallegos, 1975)

Compound	m/z 33(SH)	m/z 34(H_2S)	m/z 45(CHS)	m/z 46(CH_2S)	m/z 47(CH_3S)
			% of total ionization		
2-Methylthiophene	0.21	0.10	7.68	0.54	0.84
Thiacyclohexane	0.13	0.17	6.25	5.87	3.16
2,3-Dihydrobenzo[b]thiophene	0.11	0.09	2.74	0.27	0.18
3-Methylbenzo[b]thiophene	—	—	4.50	0.19	0.23
1,2,3,4,6,7,8,9-Octahydrodi-benzothiophene	0.02	0.04	1.25	0.05	0.17
4-Methyldibenzothiophene	—	—	1.24	0.12	0.18
4,9-Dimethylnaphtho[2,3-b]-thiophene	0.02	0.02	0.84	0.04	0.04
Benzo[b]naphtho[2,1-d]thiophene	—	—	0.85	0.03	0.04
7,8,9,10-Tetrahydrobenzo[b]-naphtho[2,3-d]thiophene	0.01	0.02	0.38	0.01	0.04

the mass spectra of PAH, in unsubstituted thiaarenes intense molecular ions (M$^+$), (M-2)- and (M-26)-fragments are observed, due to ionisation and elimination of two hydrogen atoms or a (CH=CH)-moiety. (M-2) generally is more intense than (M-1) in parent thiaarenes. Doubly charged ions such as (M$^+$/2e) and (M-45)/2e and sometimes (M-26)/2e are also common in these spectra. In the spectra of monomethyl-substituted thiaarenes for most of the above fragments there is a shift by one mass unit so that (M-26) becomes (M-27), (M-32) becomes (M-33), and (M-45) becomes (M-46). As in the mass-spectra of methyl-substituted PAH, (M-1) is more intense than (M-2) in methyl-thiaarenes. The key fragments of

Table 6. *Key ions for characterization of unsubstituted and monomethyl-substituted PAH, thiaarenes and oxaarenes (furans) (from Grimmer et al., 1981a)*

	PAH	Me-PAH	S-PAC	Me-S-PAC	O-PAC	Me-O-PAC
M	+	+	+	+	+	+
M-1	<M-2	>M-2	<M-2	>M-2	<M-2	>M-2
M-2	>M-1	<M-1	>M-1	<M-1	>M-1	<M-1
M-16	−	−	−	−	(+)	−
M-17	−	−	−	−	−	+
M-26	+	−	−	−	−	−
M-27	−	+	−	+	−	−
M-29	−	(+)	−	−	+	−
M-30	−	−	−	−	−	+
M-32	−	−	+	−	−	−
M-33	−	−	−	+	−	−
M-45	−	−	+	−	−	−
M-46	−	−	−	+	−	−
M-55	−	−	−	−	+	−
M$^+$/2e	+	+	+	+	+	+
(M-1)/2e	−	+	−	+	−	−
(M-16)/2e	−	−	−	−	+	−
(M-17)/2e	−	−	−	−	−	+
(M-26)/2e	+	(+)	+	−	−	−
(M-27)/2e	−	+	−	+	−	−
(M-29)/2e	−	−	−	−	+	−
(M-30)/2e	−	−	−	−	−	+
(M-33)/2e	−	−	−	+	−	−
(M-45)/2e	−	−	+	−	−	−
(M-46)/2e	−	−	−	+	−	−
(M-55)/2e	−	−	−	−	+	−

parent and monomethyl-substituted PAH, thiaarenes and oxaarenes(furans) are listed in Table 6 (taken from Grimmer *et al.*, 1981*a*). The typical mass spectra for parent and monomethyl-substituted thiaarenes are presented in Figs. 2 and 3 (benzo[*b*]naphtho[2,1-*d*]thiophene and its monomethyl derivative; position of the methyl group unknown).

Arenes which possess a 'fjord'-structure and which, as a consequence, may undergo further cyclization by the loss of a hydrogen atom, exhibit intense (M-1)- and (M-2)-fragments which can become as intense as their molecular ions. This ratio $M^+ \approx (M-1) \approx (M-2)$ is also obtained in similarly structured thiaarenes. Riepe and Zander (1979) have postulated a two-step mechanism for the ring-closure in case of dinaphtho[2,1-*b*:1′,2′-*d*]thiophene to give perylo[1,12-*bcd*]thiophene:

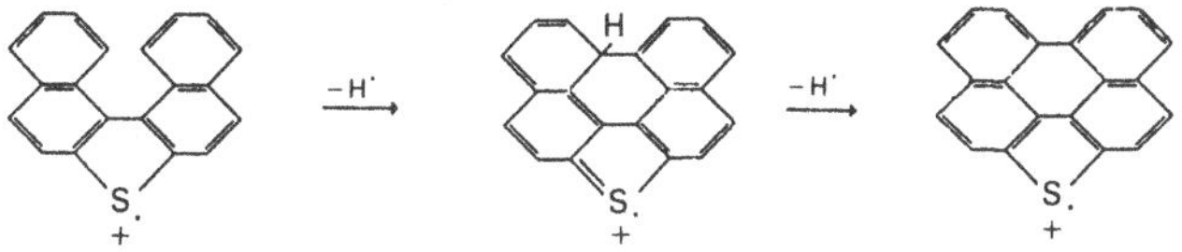

Riepe and Zander (1979) also postulated a ring-contraction of thiaarenes to biphenylenes when this is possible from topological reasons as an explanation to sulfur elimination (M-32):

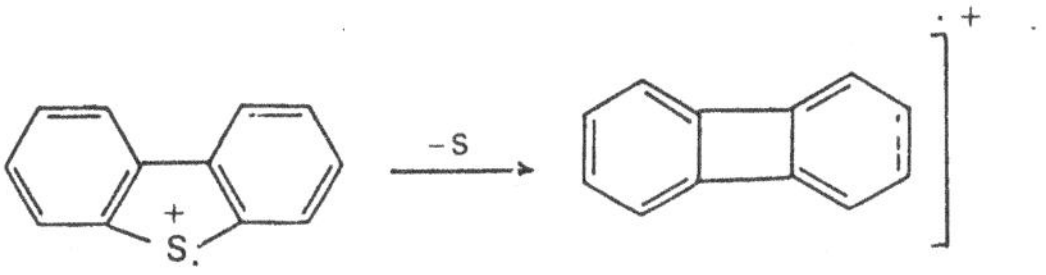

The same authors also presented mass spectral data of nine parent thiaarene systems (dibenzothiophene, benzo[*b*]naphtho[2,1-*d*]thiophene, dinaphtho[2,1-*b*:1′2′-*d*]thiophene, dinaphtho[1,2-*b*:2′1′-*d*]thiophene, dinaphtho[1,2-*b*:1′2′-*d*]thiophene, dibenzo[2,3:10,11]perylo[1,12-*bcd*]thiophene, diacenaphtho[1,2-*b*:1′2′-*d*]thiophene, benzo[1,2-*b*:4,3-*b*′]bis[1]-benzothiophene and benzo[1,2-*b*:3,4-*b*′]bis[1]benzothiophene) which are listed in Table 7. Mass spectra of many thiaarenes have been recorded by various authors and references referring to single compounds may be found in Chapter 2.

High-resolution low-voltage mass spectrometry (at 8–10 eV) during which spectra are obtained in which only molecular ions are formed, have been applied to the identification of thiaarenes in petroleum fractions (Reid *et al.*, 1966) and in emissions of oil- and gas-fired furnaces (Herlan, 1974, 1978; Herlan and Mayer, 1979). The poor reproducibility of signal

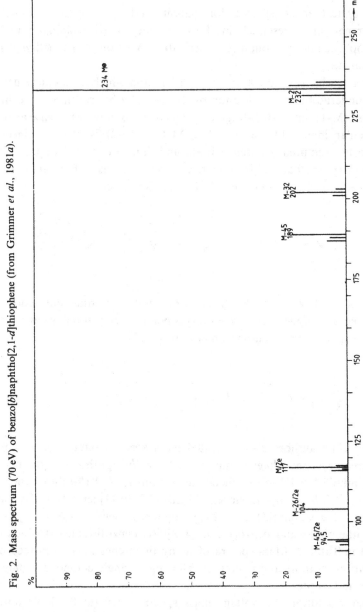

Fig. 2. Mass spectrum (70 eV) of benzo[*b*]naphtho[2,1-*d*]thiophene (from Grimmer *et al.*, 1981*a*).

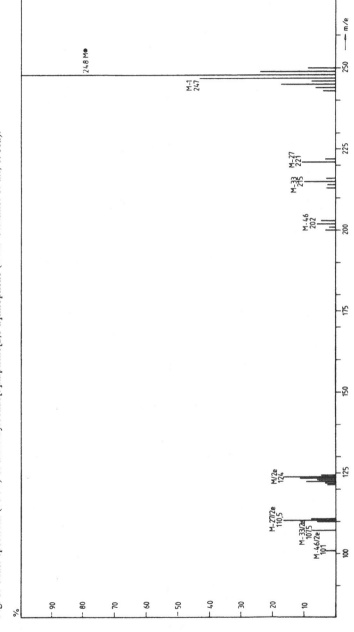

Fig. 3. Mass spectrum (70 eV) of a methylbenzo[*b*]naphtho[2,1-*d*]thiophene (from Grimmer *et al.*, 1981*a*).

Table 7. *Masses and intensities of the main fragments in the mass spectra of various thiaarenes (recorded at 70 eV) (from Riepe and Zander, 1979)*

Compound		M^+	$(M-H)^+$	$(M-2H)^{+\cdot}$	$(M-S)^{+\cdot}$	$(M-SH)^+$	$(M-H_2S)^{+\cdot}$	$(M-CS)^{+\cdot}$	$(M-HCS)^+$	$(M-H_2CS)^{+\cdot}$
						Fragment				
Dibenzothiophene	m/z	184	183	182	152	151	150	140	139	138
	intensity*	100	4.8	—	3.4	—	—	13.7	14.4	—
Benzo[b]naphtho-[2,1-d]thiophene	m/z	234	233	232	202	201	200	190	189	188
	intensity	100	5.3	9.5	8.3	1.5	2.6	1.9	9.6	3.1
Dinaphtho[2,1-b:1',2'-d]thiophene	m/z	284	283	282	252	251	250	240	239	238
	intensity	100	91.3	85.1	—	—	2.7	—	3.2	2.8
Dinaphtho[1,2-b:2',1'-d]thiophene	m/z	284	283	282	252	251	250	240	239	238
	intensity	100	5.1	14.7	5.0	1.3	3.3	1.1	4.5	1.8
Dinaphtho[1,2-b:1'2'-d]thiophene	m/z	284	283	282	252	251	250	240	239	238
	intensity	100	7.3	19.0	5.4	1.2	3.2	1.3	4.4	1.7
Dibenzo[2,3:10,11]-perylo[1,12-bcd]-thiophene	m/z	382	381	380	350	349	348	338	337	336
	intensity	100	6.5	16.1	1.1	—	1.1	—	—	—
Diacenaphtho[1,2-b:1',2'-d]thiophene	m/z	332	331	330	300	299	298	288	287	286
	intensity	100	5.9	12.7	2.5	1.4	3.0	0.9	2.8	2.4
Benzo[1,2-b:4,3-b']-bis[1]benzothiophene	m/z	290	289	288	258	257	256	246	245	244
	intensity	100	3.6	5.5	8.6	1.1	1.6	1.5	7.6	1.8
Benzo[1,2-b:3,4-b']-bis[1]benzothiophene	m/z	290	289	288	258	257	256	246	245	244
	intensity	100	4.2	9.2	7.4	0.9	1.9	1.5	7.4	2.2

* In % related to the base peak (= 100%).

responses (Hastings *et al.*, 1956) in this technique, encountered in earlier investigations, has been overcome by optimizing instrumental conditions (Reid *et al.*, 1966).

Other more recently developed mass spectrometric techniques such as chemical ionization using methane/argon mixtures and negative ion mass spectrometry using argon as collision gas as well as field-ionization, field desorption, and photoionization mass spectrometry have not or only sporadically applied to the identification of thiaarenes (e.g. Greinke and Lewis, 1979*a*; Albers, 1980; Wood *et al.*, 1985).

1.4   Analytical aspects in thiaarene chemistry

Great efforts have been made to improve methods for isolation, separation and identification of polycyclic aromatic hydrocarbons from various matrices and several analytical schemes have been published. The state of the art has been summarized in various monographs (e.g. by Lee *et al.*, 1981; Grimmer, 1983; IARC, 1979: and Bjørseth, 1983; Bjørseth and Ramdahl, 1986). A very comprehensive review has been presented by Bartle *et al.* (1981). Until recently little attention has been devoted to the problem of separating thiaarenes from the above class of compounds to which they actually are very similar in behaviour. Physico-chemically the thiophene ring resembles very much the benzene ring so that it is difficult to take advantage of this structural difference for analytical procedures without derivatization. Thin layer chromatographic attempts to separate thiaarenes from polycyclic aromatic hydrocarbons on inorganic adsorbents (alumina or silica) failed, even when elution with very flat gradients of polarity was applied (Snook, 1978). Poirier and Smiley (1984), however, more recently described the enrichment of lower molecular weight thiaarenes by dual-packed silica-alumina columns. Accordingly, no selective separation of thiaarenes and PAH could be achieved by HPLC or GC, although both techniques have been successfully used in separating complex mixtures of purified thiaarene fractions (see below).

At present four methods are available for a selective analysis of thiaarenes in two of which they are separated from other chemical classes (Methods 1 and 2, below).

Method 1. This method makes use of the fact that thiaarenes can be converted into polar sulfones by oxidation. The sulfones can then be readily separated from polycyclic aromatic hydrocarbons by column chromatography on silica according to their greater polarity.

Method 2. Thiaarenes may be separated from PAH also by ligand exchange chromatography on $PdCl_2$-impregnated silica gel (Nishioka *et al.*, 1986*a*; Gundermann *et al.*, 1983).

Method 3. By means of a sulfur-selective flame photometric (Adlard *et al.*, 1972; Wenzel and Aiken, 1979; Bates and Carpenter, 1979*a*; Lee *et al.*, 1980; Burchill *et al.*, 1982*a,b*; Nishioka *et al.*, 1985*a*), microcoulometric (Martin and Grant, 1965*a,b*; Drushel and Sommers, 1967) or an electrolytic conductivity detector (McCarthy *et al.*, 1981), thiaarenes may be distinguished from other compounds. Especially the first detector system has been successfully applied to thiaarene detection.

Method 4. Recently, tandem mass spectrometry (MS/MS) combined with a calcium/mixed amines reduction system has been successfully used for the characterization of thiaarenes by Wood *et al.* (1985).

1.4.1   Separation of thiaarenes from other chemical classes especially from PAH

1.4.1.1   The oxidation/reduction procedure

The separation of thiaarenes from other polycyclic aromatic compounds in asphalt by converting them into sulfones by oxidation and subsequent chromatography on silica was first reported by O'Donnell (1951). Drushel and Miller (1958) and Drushel and Sommers (1967) applied the procedure to petroleum fractions and various other groups studied and modified this method (Nikolaeva *et al.*, 1959; Prinzler, 1964; Thompson *et al.*, 1964; Gal'pern *et al.*, 1965; Karaulova *et al.*, 1965). Drushel and Sommers (1967) performed the oxidation of thiaarenes to sulfones by refluxing them for 2 h in acetic acid/benzene solution while adding hydrogen peroxide (3 mol to 1 mol of sulfur). The sulfones then were separated from non-oxidized hydrocarbons by silica chromatography, thereby eluting unconverted hydrocarbons with benzene and sulfones with dioxane. They also reported on conditions to obtain sulfoxides. The uses of potassium hydrogenpersulfate (Kennedy and Stock, 1960; Trost and Curran, 1981) or iodobenzene dichloride in tetrahydrofuran/pyridine/water (Lucas and Kennedy, 1955; Klemm and Hsin, 1976) for the preparation of sulfones and sulfoxides were also described.

Andersson (1987*d*) applied meta-chloroperbenzoic acid to obtain sulfones from the corresponding thiaarenes and observed that some systems possessing terminal thiophene rings cannot be oxidized under these conditions. He stated that in the case of methyldibenzothiophenes the sulfones are better resolved by HPLC than the corresponding thiaarenes.

Reductions of the sulfones and/or sulfoxides were carried out with zinc/hydrochloric acid or sodium bis(2-methoxyethoxy)aluminium-hydride in benzene (Ho and Wong, 1975). An improved procedure in which sulfones are reduced with LiAlH₄ in ether was presented by Willey *et al.* (1981*b*) which later was modified by King *et al.* (1984). Many studies on thiaarenes in various environmental matrices refer to this method. Unfortunately, the oxidation procedure does not affect thiaarenes exclusively, but also some more-sensitive polycyclic aromatic hydrocarbons are converted to quinones under these conditions. They cannot easily be re-converted to the original compounds and yield hydroquinones upon the above reduction. Thus, balancing the biological activity of environmental samples is not possible when one follows this procedure.

Schematic presentations for (1) obtaining an aromatic fraction, and (2) isolating thiaarenes from an aromatic fraction as published by Grimmer *et al.* (1985) and by Willey *et al.* (1981*b*) are given in Figs. 4 and 5.

Fig. 4. Scheme of enrichment of PAH, S-PAC, O-PAC and N-PAC (from Grimmer *et al.*, 1985).

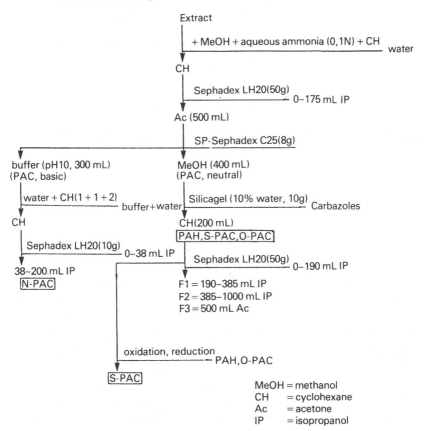

Fig. 5. Scheme for isolation of the sulfur heterocyclic fraction (from Willey *et al.*, 1981*b*).

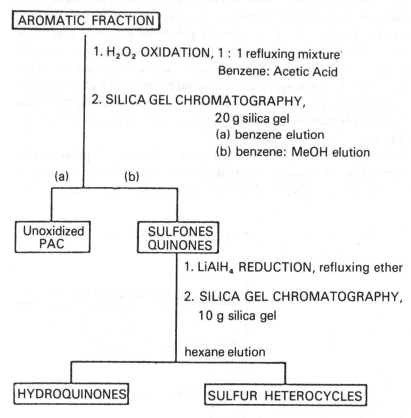

1.4.1.2 The ligand-exchange chromatography

Gundermann *et al.* (1983) separated phenanthrene from dibenzo-thiophene on $PdCl_2$-impregnated silica and Nishioka *et al.* (1986*a*) elaborated a method which has been tested with various thiaarenes giving satisfactory results. For the preparation of the ligand exchange silica column, 100 g of silica gel (type H, 60–200 mesh) are mixed with 5 g $PdCl_2$ in aqueous solution. The mixture is predried at 95°C overnight and then activated at 160°C for 24 h before use. Five grams of this material are mixed with chloroform/*n*-hexane (1:1) to give the gel bed; 0.05–0.2 g of a sample to be separated are dissolved in a few ml of dichloromethane and adsorbed onto 0.3 g $PdCl_2$-impregnated silica and added to the top of the column. With 30 mL chloroform/*n*-hexane (1:1), polycyclic aromatic hydrocarbons are eluted, whereas another 50 mL elute the thiaarenes. The latter fraction is evaporated and 250 μL of the Lewis base diethylamine are added to destroy Pd-thiaarene-complexes. It has been observed that during this ligand-exchange chromatography some sensitive PAH such as cyclopenta(*cd*)pyrene and anthanthrene may be partially destroyed on the silica, and this has to be taken into account when fractions are prepared for biological testing experiments (Jacob, 1986). Nishioka *et al.* (1986*a,b*) applied this method successfully to the separation of thiaarenes from coal liquids. They also described analytical procedures for the detection and isolation of thiaarene-related compounds such as azathiaarenes (Nishioka *et al.*, 1985*b*, 1986*c*), hydroxythiaarenes (Nishioka *et al.*, 1985*c*) and aminothiaarenes (Nishioka *et al.*, 1985*b,d*) from the same source. Some of these compounds have been synthesized by Kudo *et al.* (1985).

Recently Andersson (1987*c*) presented data for HPLC retention times of PAH and thiaarenes on 5% PdCl$_2$/silica columns. He also noticed that thiaarenes with a terminal thiophene ring are more rapidly eluted than those with internal thiophene rings.

For the separation of thiaarenes containing one and two rings from hydrocarbons chromatography on silver nitrate-impregnated silica columns has also been proven to be effective (Joyce and Uden, 1983). Although successfully used for the separation of organic sulfides, ligand-exchange chromatography using zinc (Orr, 1967), mercury (Orr, 1966; Kaimai and Matsunaga, 1978) and copper salts (Vogh and Dooley, 1975) failed to separate thiaarenes selectively. Andersson (1987*a,b*) tested mercuri acetate substituted phenylsilica phases and found that thiaarenes were not selectively separated from PAH.

1.4.2   High-performance liquid chromatography (HPLC)

Neither normal nor reversed-phase high-performance liquid chromatography is successful in the preparation of pure thiaarene fractions from complex mixtures. Even combinations of both procedures as used e.g. by Lucke *et al.* (1985) distributed the various thiaarenes into distinct fractions. The application of organo-mercury phases introduced by Ray and Frei (1972) seems to be more promising. However, HPLC may be very efficient in separating thiaarene impurities from the isosteric hydrocarbons. Depaus (1979) separated benzo[2,3]phenanthro[4,5-*bcd*]thiophene and chryseno[4,5-*bcd*]thiophene as well as tetrahydrobenzo[*a*]pyrene from a commercial batch of benzo[*a*]pyrene using a Partisil 5 column (25 cm × 0.9 cm) which was eluted with *n*-hexane (7 mL/min). Karcher *et al.* (1979, 1981) separated phenanthro[4,5-*bcd*]thiophene, dinaphtho[2,1-*b*:1′,2′-*d*]thiophene, and a compound tentatively identified as perylo[1,12-*bcd*]thiophene, from commercial samples of pyrene, benzo[*j*]fluoranthene and benzo[*ghi*]perylene, respectively.

The HLPC technique and its applicability to thiaarene separation and identification have their limits (for review see Lee *et al.*, 1981; Bartle *et al.*, 1981; Wise, 1983). The general advantages of HPLC reside in the facts (a) that it is a substance-saving technique, (b) that it may be applied even to temperature-sensitive and to high-boiling and non-volatile compounds, and (c) that the detector may give considerable information on the structure of the compounds separated (UV- and/or fluorescence spectra). On the other hand, there are also inherent disadvantages: (a) the separation efficiency is limited and is generally less than in GC so that isomers often are not resolved, (b) there is no carbon content-dependent response for the compound detected and response factors have to be measured prior to quantification which often is impossible since reference materials are not available, and (c) coupling to a mass spectrometer, although described and presently commercially offered, is not yet a common technique as it is in GC. However, improvement of HPLC and HPLC/MS is in rapid progress. More recently Wise *et al.* (1983) demonstrated that isomeric thiaarenes may be well separated when appropriate columns are used. For instance, the authors obtained excellent separations for a series of five-membered peri-condensed thiaarenes with molecular weight 258 and also for a series of five-membered cata-condensed thiaarenes molecular weight 284 by reversed-phase HPLC (see Figs. 6 and 7).

The HPLC resolution of various thiaarenes can be calculated from Table 8 which lists their retention times in normal- and reversed-phase HPLC as measured by Wise *et al.* (1983).

As a consequence of the above facts, HPLC is a preferred technique for subfractionation prior to GC or GC/MS identification in order to obtain less complex mixtures. For this purpose it has been used e.g. for analyzing coal liquids (Wise *et al.*, 1980), tobacco smoke condensate (Schmid *et al.*, 1985), marine samples (Berthou and Vignier, 1986), Shale oils (Willey, 1981a), minerals containing organic matter (Wise *et al.*, 1986), etc. Colmsjö and Östman have used HPLC for fractionating thiaarenes-containing mixtures from carbon black and from soil prior to their characterization by their Shpol'skii spectra (Colmsjö and Östman, 1982; Colmsjö *et al.*, 1982).

Since GC presently seems to have reached its limits with thiaarenes of molecular weights of about 340 daltons, HPLC will be the most promising method for the separation of the higher molecular weight homologues as occurring e.g. in emissions from coal combustion and other coal-derived products.

Fig. 6. Reversed-phase HPLC of selected five-ring peri-condensed thiaarenes of molecular weight 258. Conditions: Vydac 201 TP 5μ column; mobile phase: linear gradient of 80–100% acetonitrile in water at 1%/min at 1.5 mL/min; UV detection at 254 nm (from Wise *et al.*, 1983).

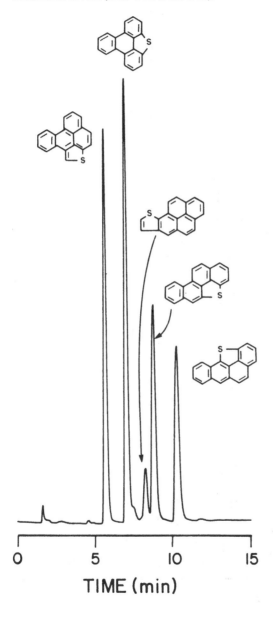

Fig. 7. Reversed-phase HPLC of selected five-ring cata-condensed thiaarenes of molecular weight 284. Conditions same as in Fig. 6, except linear gradient of 90–100% acetonitrile in water at 1%/min; imp = impurity (from Wise *et al.*, 1983).

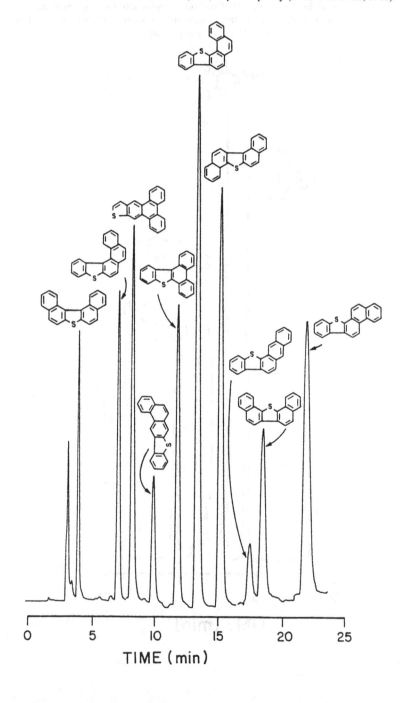

Table 8. *HPLC retention data for various thiaarenes of molecular weight 234, 258 and 284* (from Wise et al., 1983)*

Compound	Normal-phase**	Reversed-phase*** I	II
Benzo[b]naphtho[1,2-d]thiophene	3.65	3.79	4.02
Benzo[b]naphtho[2,3-d]thiophene	3.78	4.05	4.05
Benzo[b]naphtho[2,1-d]thiophene	3.59	4.20	4.24
Anthra[2,3-b]thiophene	4.19	3.41	2.97
Phenanthro[3,4-b]thiophene	3.89	3.57	3.70
Phenanthro[2,3-b]thiophene	4.26	3.65	3.70
Phenanthro[3,2-b]thiophene	4.24	3.67	3.67
Phenanthro[9,10-b]thiophene	3.89	3.77	3.86
Anthra[2,1-b]thiophene	4.14	3.78	3.74
Phenanthro[4,3-b]thiophene	3.94	3.79	3.86
Phenanthro[2,1-b]thiophene	4.13	3.80	3.71
Anthra[1,2-b]thiophene	3.94	3.99	3.93
Phenanthro[1,2-b]thiophene	3.98	4.08	3.93
Triphenyleno[1,12-bcd]thiophene	4.09	4.30	4.61
Chryseno[4,5-bcd]thiophene	4.04	4.51	4.77
Benzo[2,3]phenanthro[4,5-bcd]thiophene	3.83	4.65	4.98
Benzo[1,2]phenaleno[4,3-bc]thiophene	—	4.16	4.81
Pyreno[4,5-b]thiophene	4.32	4.31	4.55
Benzo[1,2]phenaleno[3,4-bc]thiophene	—	4.35	4.62
Pyreno[2,1-b]thiophene	4.55	4.35	4.44
Benzo[4,5]phenaleno[9,1-bc]thiophene	—	4.36	4.51
Benzo[4,5]phenaleno[1,9-bc]thiophene	—	4.37	4.48
Pyreno[1,2-b]thiophene	4.32	4.45	4.62
Benzo[b]phenanthro[4,3-d]thiophene	4.00	4.18	4.80
Benzo[b]phenanthro[3,2-b]thiophene	4.91	4.52	4.84
Benzo[b]phenanthro[9,10-d]thiophene	4.49	4.68	5.17
Benzo[b]phenanthro[2,3-d]thiophene	4.81	4.74	4.91
Benzo[b]phenanthro[3,4-b]thiophene	4.49	4.81	5.21
Dinaphtho[2,3-b:2',3'-d]dithiophene	4.77	4.84	5.12
Dinaphtho[1,2-b:1',2'-d]thiophene	4.33	4.95	5.27
Anthra[1,2-b]benzo[d]thiophene	4.52	>5	5.25
Dinaphtho[1,2-b:2',1'-d]dithiophene	4.40	>5	5.51
Benzo[b]phenanthro[2,1-d]thiophene	4.58	>5	5.32
Dinaphtho[1,2-b:2',3'-d]thiophene	4.55	>5	5.38
Triphenyleno[2,1-b]thiophene	4.81	4.21	4.53
Triphenyleno[2,3-b]thiophene	4.16	4.30	4.61
Triphenyleno[1,2-b]thiophene	4.98	4.40	4.68

* Retention data are given as log *I* related to log *I* of benzene (1.00), naphthalene (2.00), phenanthrene (3.00), benz[a]anthracene (4.00), and benzo[b]chrysene (5.00) (from Wise *et al.*, 1980).
** μBondapak NH$_2$ column, *n*-hexane as the mobile phase.
*** I = Vydac 201 TP 5 μm and II = Zorbax ODS column, 85/15 (v/v) acetonitrile/water as the mobile phase.

1.4.3   Gas-liquid chromatography (GC)

Capillary gas-liquid chromatography, often in combination with mass spectrometry, is the technique most widely applied to separation, identification and characterization of thiaarenes. According to their relative high abundance in environmental matter, inventories of thiaarenes have been made for carbon black (Lee and Hites, 1976), crude oil (Nishioka *et al.*, 1985*a*; Grimmer *et al.*, 1983*a*; Damsté and de Leeuw, 1986; Snook *et al.*, 1979), shale oil (Nishioka *et al.*, 1985*a*), fresh and used motor oil (Grimmer *et al.*, 1981*b*; Peake and Parker, 1980; Grimmer *et al.*, 1981*a*), coal tar (Nishioka *et al.*, 1985*a*), coal liquids (Nishioka *et al.*, 1985*a*; Kong *et al.*, 1982; Lee and Hites, 1976; Lee *et al.*, 1980), marine organisms (Ogata *et al.*, 1980*a*; Berthou *et al.*, 1981; Vassilaros, 1982*a,b*; West *et al.*, 1985), sediments (West *et al.*, 1985), and for water (West *et al.*, 1985; Olufsen, 1980).

The subject has been reviewed by Lee and Wright (1980) and by Lee *et al.* (1982). As stationary phase, mostly methyl silicone (SE 30, OV 1, OV 101, or SP 2100) as well as mixed phenyl/methyl silicones (SE 52, SE 54, OV 3, OV 7, OV 17) have been used. Also carborane/methyl silicone (Dexsil 300) or carborane/methyl phenyl silicone (Dexsil 400) have been applied. More recently, Lee *et al.* (1984) and Kuei *et al.* (1984) reported on 25% biphenyl–/1% vinyl–/74% methylpolysiloxane and 88% cyanopropyl–/10% tolyl–/2% methylpolysiloxane as stationary phases for the separation of thiaarenes. For resolving various dimethyldibenzothiophenes (2,6-, 2,8-, 3,4-, 3,6-, 3,7-, 3,8- and 4,6-dimethyldibenzothiophene) they found 50% phenyl–/1% vinyl–/49% methylpolysiloxane and 25% biphenyl–/1% vinyl–/74% methylsiloxane to be the suitable phases. A 25% biphenyl–/75% methyl–polysiloxane (0.25 μm film thickness) has been used as a highly selective stationary phase for the separation of thiaarenes from heavy oils and tars (Nishioka *et al.*, 1985*a*). Liquid crystal (BBBT = N,N'-bis(*p*-butoxybenzilidine)-α,α'-bi-*p*-toluidine;   BMBT = N,N'-bis(*p*-methoxybenzilidine)-α,α'-bi-*p*-toluidine   and   BH $\times$ BT = N,N'-bis(*p*-hexoxybenzylidene)-α,α'-bi-*p*-toluidine),   non-polar [SE 52 (5% phenyl–/95% methylsilicone)] and polar stationary phases [Superox 20 M (polyethylene glycol)] and mixtures thereof have been evaluated for the separation of thiaarenes. None of the columns tested succeeded in separating all the individuals of a complex mixture of 3–5 rings-containing thiaarenes. However, they were resolved by using columns in combination (Kong *et al.*, 1982).

In a systematic investigation, a linear retention index system for temperature-programmed capillary gas chromatography of thiaarenes has been introduced by Vassilaros *et al.* (1982*c*) which is very valuable for their preliminary identification. Retention times were evaluated relative to naphthalene (2 rings), phenanthrene (3 rings), chrysene (4 rings) and picene (5 rings) which were set to 200.00, 300.00, 400.00, and 500.00, respectively. Table 9 presents the relative retention times of 114 different thiaarenes as measured by the above authors using a SE 52 coated fused-silica column (15–20 m in length, either 0.3 mm inner diameter and 0.25 μm film thickness or 0.2 mm inner diameter and 0.17 μm film thickness, with hydrogen as carrier gas (100 cm/s) and a temperature program 40°–265°C at 4°C/min with a 2-min initial isothermal period).

Generally speaking, thiaarenes exhibit shorter retention times than their carbocyclic isosters; mostly RRTs of about 0.980–0.993 are found (e.g. for the pairs: phenanthro[4,5-*bcd*]thiophene/pyrene (9.992); benzo[*b*]-naphtho[2,3-*d*]thiophene/benz[*a*]anthracene (0.993); triphenyleno-(1,12-*bcd*)thiophene/benzo[*e*]pyrene (0.991); chryseno[4,5-*bcd*]thiophene/benzo[*a*]pyrene (0.993); dibenzo[1,2-*b*:2′,3′-*d*]thiophene/benzo[*b*]chrysene (0.980).

1.4.4 Sulfur-specific detectors

Various sulfur-specific detectors have been developed and used for the characterization of thiaarenes in combination with GC. A microcoulometric sulfur detector (MCD) based on titration of SO_2 with potassium triiodide and the anodic reconversion of the iodide to triiodide (Martin and Grant, 1965*a,b;* Fredericks and Harlow, 1964) using a Dohrmann microcoulometric cell in combination with GC has been applied to thiaarenes by Drushel and Sommers (1967). The use of an electrolytic conductivity detector has been reported by McCarthy *et al.* (1981). In modern constructions such as the Hall electrolytic conductivity detector (HECD), its sensitivity and selectivity against carbon are superior to all other sulfur-selective detectors (Cox and Anderson, 1980). The most widely applied sulfur-selective detector system is the flame photometric detector (FPD) (Brody and Chaney, 1966; Dressler, 1983) in which sulfur-containing compounds are combusted in an excess of hydrogen; under these conditions S_2-molecules are formed, the light emissions of which at 365 nm may be measured. The non-linearity and the quenching of the sulfur-response when hydrocarbons are co-eluted are the main disadvantages of this detector (Burnett *et al.*, 1978; Grice *et al.*, 1970; Wenzel and Aiken, 1979; Patterson, 1978; Schultz *et al.*, 1979). They have been partially overcome by modifying the geometry of the detector (Patterson, 1978; Patterson *et al.*, 1978; Frederiksson and Cedergreen, 1981). By optimizing the FPD flame conditions, Burchill *et al.* (1982*a*) achieved a linear response over two decades (0.1–10 ng) for dibenzothiophene, an

36   *General chapter on thiaarenes*

Table 9. *Relative retention times of various thiaarenes related to naphthalene (= 200.00), phenanthrene (= 300.00), chrysene (= 400.00) and
picene (= 500.00), for GC conditions see text (from Vassilaros et al.,
1982c)*

Compound	Mole weight	Retention time
Benzo[*b*]thiophene	134	201.57
7-Methylbenzo[*b*]thiophene	148	219.16
2-Methylbenzo[*b*]thiophene	148	220.76
5-Methylbenzo[*b*]thiophene	148	222.09
6-Methylbenzo[*b*]thiophene	148	222.11
3-Methylbenzo[*b*]thiophene	148	223.08
4-Methylbenzo[*b*]thiophene	148	223.15
5-Ethylbenzo[*b*]thiophene	162	236.14
3,5-Dimethylbenzo[*b*]thiophene	162	243.56
1,2,3,4,4a,4b-Hexahydrodibenzothiophene	190	271.69
Naphtho[1,2-*b*]thiophene	184	295.80
Dibenzothiophene	184	296.01
Naphtho[2,1-*b*]thiophene	184	300.00
Naphtho[2,3-*b*]thiophene	184	304.47
5-Methylnaphtho[2,1-*b*]thiophene	198	306.53
2-Methylnaphtho[2,1-*b*]thiophene	198	311.77
4-Methyldibenzothiophene	198	312.72
8-Methylnaphtho[1,2-*b*]thiophene	198	315.61
2-Methyldibenzothiophene	198	316.19
3-Methyldibenzothiophene	198	316.32
4-Methylnaphtho[1,2-*b*]thiophene	198	317.19
4-Methylnaphtho[2,1-*b*]thiophene	198	318.12
6-Methylnaphtho[1,2-*b*]thiophene	198	319.55
1-Methyldibenzothiophene	198	319.69
8-Methylnaphtho[2,1-*b*]thiophene	198	319.86
7-Methylnaphtho[2,1-*b*]thiophene	198	320.26
6-Methylnaphtho[2,1-*b*]thiophene	198	323.57
1-Methylnaphtho[2,1-*b*]thiophene	198	323.58
9-Methylnaphtho[2,1-*b*]thiophene	198	325.25
3-Ethyldibenzothiophene	212	328.34
4,6-Dimethyldibenzothiophene	212	329.17
2,6-Dimethyldibenzothiophene	212	332.42
2-Ethyldibenzothiophene	212	332.65
3,6-Dimethyldibenzothiophene	212	332.88
2,8-Dimethyldibenzothiophene	212	335.90
3,7-Dimethyldibenzothiophene	212	336.02
3,8-Dimethyldibenzothiophene	212	336.09
1,7-Dimethyldibenzothiophene	212	339.36
Phenanthro[4,5-*bcd*]thiophene	208	348.75
Phenaleno[6,7-*bc*]thiophene	208	353.45

Table 9 *cont.*

Compound	Mole weight	Retention time
Benzo[*b*]naphtho[2,1-*d*]thiophene	234	389.37
Benzo[*b*]naphtho[1,2-*d*]thiophene	234	392.92
Phenanthro[9,10-*b*]thiophene	234	394.96
Phenanthro[4,3-*b*]thiophene	234	395.03
Anthra[1,2-*b*]thiophene	234	395.39
Benzo[*b*]naphtho[2,3-*d*]thiophene	234	395.97
Phenanthro[1,2-*b*]thiophene	234	396.01
Phenanthro[3,4-*b*]thiophene	234	396.43
Anthra[2,1-*b*]thiophene	234	399.31
Phenanthro[2,1-*b*]thiophene	234	400.59
Phenanthro[3,2-*b*]thiophene	234	401.89
Phenanthro[2,3-*b*]thiophene	234	402.19
1-Methylbenzo[*b*]naphtho[1,2-*d*]thiophene	248	402.59
11-Methylbenzo[*b*]naphtho[1,2-*d*]thiophene	248	404.15
10-Methylbenzo[*b*]naphtho[2,1-*d*]thiophene	248	404.28
3-Methylbenzo[*b*]naphtho[2,1-*d*]thiophene	248	407.55
Anthra[2,3-*b*]thiophene	234	407.57
2-Methylbenzo[*b*]naphtho[2,1-*d*]thiophene	248	407.63
8-Methylbenzo[*b*]naphtho[2,1-*d*]thiophene	248	407.69
9-Methylbenzo[*b*]naphtho[2,1-*d*]thiophene	248	407.93
2-Methylbenzo[*b*]naphtho[1,2-*d*]thiophene	248	408.00
8-Methylbenzo[*b*]naphtho[1,2-*d*]thiophene	248	409.04
10-Methylbenzo[*b*]naphtho[1,2-*d*]thiophene	248	409.04
6-Methylbenzo[*b*]naphtho[1,2-*d*]thiophene	248	409.48
5-Methylbenzo[*b*]naphtho[2,1-*d*]thiophene	248	410.58
3-Methylbenzo[*b*]naphtho[1,2-*d*]thiophene	248	411.48
4-Methylbenzo[*b*]naphtho[2,3-*d*]thiophene	248	411.60
4-Methylbenzo[*b*]naphtho[2,1-*d*]thiophene	248	411.65
6-Methylbenzo[*b*]naphtho[2,1-*d*]thiophene	248	411.71
9-Methylbenzo[*b*]naphtho[1,2-*d*]thiophene	248	411.81
7-Methylbenzo[*b*]naphtho[2,1-*d*]thiophene	248	412.08
10-Methylbenzo[*b*]naphtho[2,3-*d*]thiophene	248	414.26
9-Methylbenzo[*b*]naphtho[2,3-*d*]thiophene	248	414.62
1-Methylbenzo[*b*]naphtho[2,1-*d*]thiophene	248	414.62
8-Methylbenzo[*b*]naphtho[2,3-*d*]thiophene	248	414.68
2-Methylbenzo[*b*]naphtho[2,3-*d*]thiophene	248	414.69
6-Methylbenzo[*b*]naphtho[2,3-*d*]thiophene	248	415.02
3-Methylbenzo[*b*]naphtho[2,3-*d*]thiophene	248	415.11
4-Methylbenzo[*b*]naphtho[1,2-*d*]thiophene	248	415.41
1-Methylbenzo[*b*]naphtho[2,3-*d*]thiophene	248	415.54
7-Methylbenzo[*b*]naphtho[2,3-*d*]thiophene	248	417.07
3-Methylphenanthro[9,10-*b*]thiophene	248	417.70
1-Methylanthra[2,1-*b*]thiophene	248	418.22

Table 9 *cont.*

Compound	Mole weight	Retention time
10-Methylphenanthro[2,1-*b*]thiophene	248	422.14
11-Methylbenzo[*b*]naphtho[2,3-*d*]thiophene	248	422.85
3-Methylphenanthro[2,1-*b*]thiophene	248	423.48
2-(2'-Naphthyl)benzo[*b*]thiophene	260	430.65
Benzo[2,3]phenanthro[4,5-*bcd*]thiophene	258	443.29
Pyreno[4,5-*b*]thiophene	258	446.51
Benzo[1,2]phenaleno[3,4-*bc*]thiophene	258	447.66
Triphenyleno[1,12-*bcd*]thiophene	258	448.45
Pyreno[1,2-*b*]thiophene	258	449.30
Chryseno[4,5-*bcd*]thiophene	258	450.62
Pyreno[2,1-*b*]thiophene	258	455.01
Benzo[4,5]phenaleno[1,9-*bc*]thiophene	258	455.99
Benzo[4,5]phenaleno[9,1-*bc*]thiophene	258	457.30
Benzo[*b*]phenanthro[4,3-*d*]thiophene	284	470.47
Dinaphtho[2,1-*b*:1',2'-*d*]thiophene	284	472.62
Dinaphtho[1,2-*b*:2',1'-*d*]thiophene	284	482.60
Benzo[1,2]phenaleno[4,3-*bc*]thiophene	284	482.99
Dinaphtho[1,2-*b*:1',2'-*d*]thiophene	284	486.58
Benzo[*b*]phenanthro[9,10-*d*]thiophene	284	487.32
Benzo[*b*]phenanthro[3,4-*d*]thiophene	484	487.76
Anthra[1,2-*b*]benzo[*d*]thiophene	284	488.45
Benzo[*b*]phenanthro[2,1-*d*]thiophene	284	488.89
Dinaphtho[1,2-*b*:2',3'-*d*]thiophene	284	489.14
9,13-*H*-Triphenyleno[2,3-*b*]thiophene	286	489.81
Benzo[*b*]phenanthro[3,2-*d*]thiophene	284	491.02
Benzo[*b*]phenanthro[1,2-*d*]thiophene	284	492.31
Benzo[*b*]phenanthro[2,3-*d*]thiophene	284	493.31
Triphenyleno[2,1-*b*]thiophene	284	493.90
Triphenyleno[1,2-*b*]thiophene	284	494.41
Dinaphtho[2,3-*b*:2',3'-*d*]thiophene	284	495.17
Triphenyleno[2,3-*b*]thiophene	284	500.00
13-Methylbenzo[*b*]phenanthro[3,2-*d*]thiophene	298	511.19

elimination of hydrogen-caused quenching and disappearance of negative peaks. By means of this detector they determined and identified a large number of thiaarenes and azathiaarenes occurring in coal tar (Burchill *et al.*, 1982*a*) and anthracene oil (Burchill *et al.*, 1982*b*). This detector has also been applied to the analysis of thiaarenes and their derivatives in sediments and oils (Vassilaros *et al.*, 1982*a*; Lee *et al.*, 1982), shale oil (Willey *et al.*, 1981*b*), petroleum fractions (Nishioka *et al.*, 1986*a*), synfuels (Later *et al.*, 1981), coal tar and coal liquids (Willey *et al.*, 1981*b*; Nishioka *et al.*, 1985*a,c*; 1986*b,c*; White and Lee, 1980), coal-derived products (Lee *et al.*, 1980; Lee and Hites, 1976), air particulate matter (Lee *et al.*, 1982), cigarette smoke condensate (Schmid *et al.*, 1985), fish (Lee *et al.*, 1982; Vassilaros *et al.*, 1982*a*), and in minerals (Wise *et al.*, 1986). Attempts have also been made to adapt electrochemical detector cells and microwave-induced plasma detectors to GC (reviewed in Oehme, 1982). These systems, however, are not routinely used. A comparison of the various sulfur-selective detectors, their limits of detection, their range of measurements, and their selectivity against carbon is given in Table 10.

1.4.5   Mass spectrometry

The specific masses (e.g. M-32, M-45 and related fragments) occurring in the mass spectrometric fragmentation patterns of thiaarenes as well as the isotope ratio $^{32}S/^{34}S$ have been used for identification of thiaarenes and related compounds in petroleum and petroleum-related products (Reid *et al.*, 1966; Nishioka *et al.*, 1986*a*; Drushel and Summers, 1967; Albers, 1980), in oils (Damsté and de Leeuw, 1986; Nishioka *et al.*, 1985*a*; Grimmer and Glaser, 1975; Gallegos, 1975; Grimmer *et al.*, 1981*a,b*; Peake and Parker, 1980), shale oil (Willey *et al.*, 1981*b*; Chiu *et al.*, 1983), synfuel (Later *et al.*, 1981; Kong *et al.*, 1984), coal (Chiu *et al.*, 1983), coal combustion emission (Grimmer *et al.*, 1985; Olufsen, 1980), tars (Nishioka *et al.*, 1985*a*, 1986*b,c*; Borwitzky *et al.*, 1977; Burchill *et al.*, 1982*a*), coal liquids (Sharkey, 1976; Nishioka, 1985*a,b,c*, 1986*a,b,c*; Kong *et al.*, 1982; Willey *et al.*, 1981*b*; Lucke *et al.*, 1985; White and Lee, 1980; Lee *et al.*, 1980), anthracene oil (Burchill *et al.*, 1982*b*), oil- and gas-combustion emissions (Herlan and Mayer, 1979), carbon black (Lee and Hites, 1976), tobacco smoke condensate (Schmid *et al.*, 1985), fish (Vassilaros *et al.*, 1982*a,b*); sediments (Damsté and de Leeuw, 1986), minerals (Wise *et al.*, 1986), and in commercial polycyclic aromatic hydrocarbons (Depaus, 1979; Karcher *et al.*, 1979, 1981), using low as well as high voltage ionization.

An improvement of this technique has recently been described by Wood *et al.* (1985) using a combination of chemical reduction of thiaarenes with calcium/mixed amines and tandem mass spectrometry. Reduction of thiaarenes (dibenzothiophene, benzo[*b*]thiophene and alkylated derivatives) forms substituted thiophenols which after negative ion chemical ionization (NICI) lead to characteristic daughter spectra. For instance, the above thiaarenes result in the formation of *o*-cyclohexylthiophenol (M = 192) and *o*-ethylthiophenol (M = 138) upon reduction with Ca/mixed amines. In the NICI daughter spectra of their anions *m/z* 191 and *m/z* 137

Table 10. *Sulfur-selective detectors and their properties (from Oehme, 1982, and Grob, 1985)*

Detector	Limit of detection (g/s)	Range of measurement (decade potencies)	Selectivity against carbon
Microcoulometric detector (MCD)	10^{-9}–10^{-10}	3	10^3
Electrolytic conductivity detector (HECD)	10^{-11}–10^{-12}	4	10^4–10^5
Flame photometric detector (FPD)	10^{-10}–10^{-11}	2–3	10^4–10^5
Electrochemical cell detector (ECCD)	10^{-10}–10^{-11}	3	10^3
Microwave-induced plasma detector (MIPD)	10^{-10}–10^{-11}	3–4	10^2–10^3

Fig. 8. Scheme for characterization of benzo[*b*]thiophene, dibenzothiophene and alkylated derivatives after chemical reduction by tandem-mass spectrometry (from Wood *et al.*, 1985).

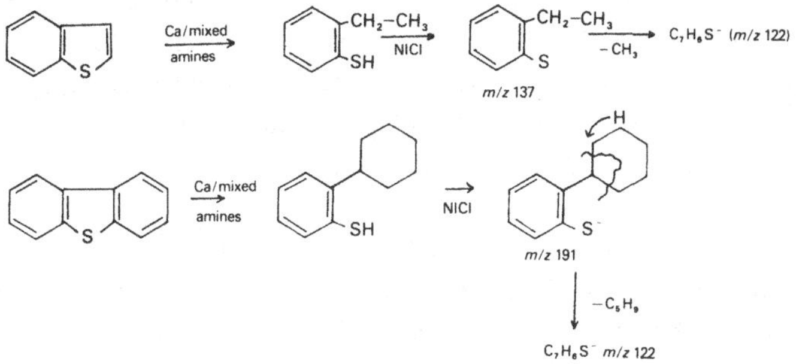

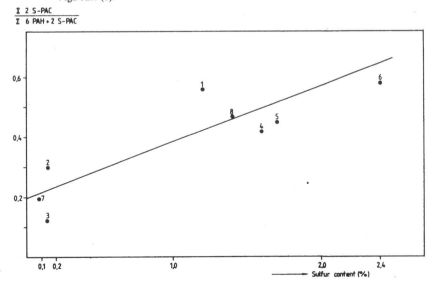

the thiatropylium radical anion $C_7H_6S^-$ (*m/z* 122) is observed which can be considered as a key ion for the above structures as demonstrated in Fig. 8.

1.5 Occurrence and formation of thiaarenes

The most likely origin of thiaarenes is degradation of biomass during the process of fossilation. Hydrogen sulfide and elemental sulfur,

Fig. 9. Linear correlation* between the relative concentration of thiaarenes of various crude oils** and their total sulfur content (from Grimmer *et al.*, 1983*a*). * Calculated from concentration of two thiaarenes benzo[*b*]naphtho[1,2-*d*]- and -[2,1-*d*]thiophene and six polycyclic aromatic hydrocarbons pyrene, benz[*a*]anthracene, chrysene + triphenylene, benzo[*e*]pyrene, benzo[*a*]pyrene, and benzo[*ghi*]perylene, ** Origins: Qatar (1), Nigeria (2), Sarir (3), Gach Saran (4), Dubai (5), Arabia (6), Sahara (7), and Aga Jari (8).

both formed by microorganisms, and sulfur-containing amino acids may be the main sources of sulfur in geochemically formed thiaarenes. Accordingly, this class of compounds occurs in crude oils, shale and in coal in higher concentrations. For instance, concentrations of >0.1% of thiaarenes have been found in Qatar crude oil (Grimmer *et al.*, 1983*a*) and a linear correlation between the relative concentration of thiaarenes of various crude oils and their total sulfur content has been reported by Grimmer *et al.*, 1983*a* (Figure 9).

Douglas and Mair (1965) reported on the incorporation of elemental sulfur into terpenoids and steroids which may play a role in the natural formation of thiaarenes. Damsté *et al.* (1986*a,b*, 1987) and Ten Haven *et al.* (1986) also suggested that during early stages of diagenesis hydrogen sulfide reacts with isoprenoid structures like phytol and farnesol resulting in organic sulfur compounds. They found C_{20}-isoprenoidal thiophenes (a) in young sediment, and related dithiophenes (b) in oil samples. They also detected homologues series of alkylated thiophenes (c), thiolanes (d), and thiacyclohexanes (e).

(a)

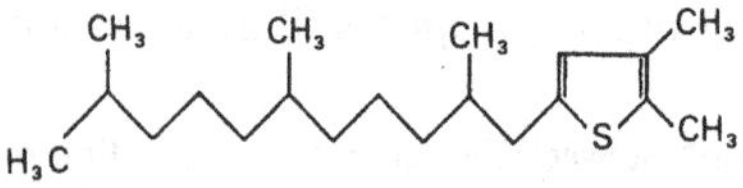

2,3-dimethyl-5-[2,6,10-trimethyl-undecyl]thiophene

(b)

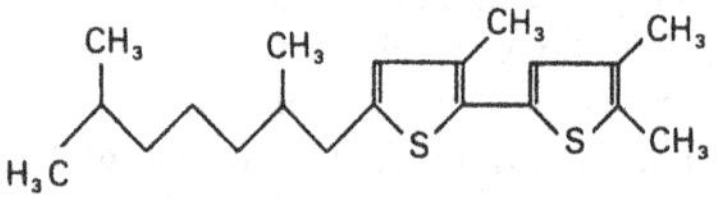

2',3,3'-trimethyl-5-[2,6-dimethyl-heptyl]-2,2'-bis-thiophene

(c)

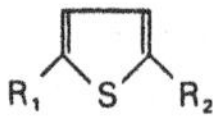

2,5-dialkylthiophenes

(d)

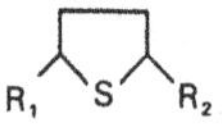

2,5-dialkylthiolanes

(e)

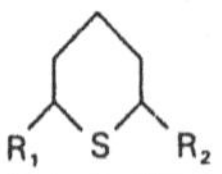

2,6-dialkylthiacyclohexanes

The same authors also reported on the occurrence of substituted benzothiophenes in crude oil.

Sulfur insertion into polycyclic aromatic hydrocarbons during the formation of petroleum also may be suggested from the structural resemblance of thiaarenes and their tentative precursors, e.g. phenanthrene/phenanthro[4,5-*bcd*]thiophene, 1-phenylnaphthalene/ben-zo[*b*]naphtho[1,2-*d*]thiophene, or triphenylene/triphenyleno[1,12-*bcd*]-thiophene etc.

Coal is associated with the occurrence of considerable concentration of elemental sulfur, and organic sulfur compounds in coal can reach 10%. Reactions of hydrocarbons with elemental sulfur or with pyrite have been suggested to play an important role in the formation of thiophenes during coalification (White and Lee, 1980). Model experiments at moderate temperatures (130–200°C) have been carried out with toluene or ethylben-zene and sulfur by Horton (1949) and by DeRoo and Hodgson (1978) and yielded, e.g., 2-phenylbenzo[*b*]thiophene and 2,4-diphenylthiophene, respectively:

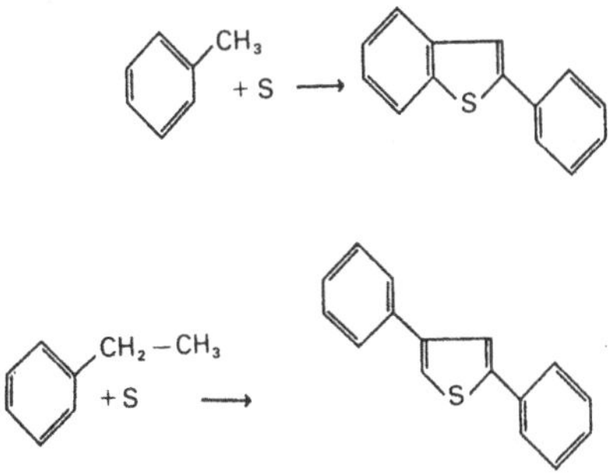

Further reactions of thiaarenes to more complex thiaarene systems during the pyrolysis of diacenaphtho[1,2-*b*:1′,2′-*d*]thiophene, dibenzyl-disulfide and dibenzothiophene as model compounds have been studied by Greinke and Lewis (1979*a*,*b*) who found a large number of thiaarenes with masses between 198 and 930 dalton using field desorption mass spec-trometry. Similar carbonization experiments have been described by other authors (Madison and Roberts, 1958; Edstrom and Lewis, 1969; Lentz *et al.*, 1962; Aitken *et al.*, 1968; Masciantonio and Walter, 1964).

Although thiophenes are thermodynamically stable, and hence favoured structures, it is doubtful whether they are formed *de novo* during combustion processes such as gasoline-, oil- or coal-combustion. The occurrence of thiaarenes in vehicle exhaust (Otto engine less than in diesel) and in oil- or coal-fired furnaces possibly may be attributed to their presence in the original fuels rather than to combustion processes. This is confirmed by the fact that thiaarene concentration decreases significantly in comparison to polycyclic aromatic hydrocarbons when the combustion process is optimized.

Table 11. *Occurrence of thiaarenes in fossil fuels, technical products and in environmental matter*

Compound	Mole weight	Occurrence
2H-Cyclopenta[b]thiophene (*1*)	122	Crude oil/petroleum: Birch, 1953
4H-Cyclopenta[c]thiophene (*2*)	122	Crude oil/petroleum: Birch, 1953
Benzo[b]thiophene (*3*)	134	Crude oil/petroleum: Kuras et al., 1982; Nesterenko et al., 1983; Poirier and Smiley, 1984; Johansen, 1977; Parfenova et al., 1977; Mel'nikova et al., 1980; Vol'tsov and Lyapina 1980; Mel'nikova et al., 1979, 1981; Numanov, 1977; Drushel and Sommers, 1967; Nishioka et al., 1985a; Potolovskii et al., 1977; Brodskii et al., 1977; Lyapina et al., 1980a,b; Mostecky, 1982
		Coal tar/pitch: Van Graas et al., 1981; Nishioka et al., 1985a; Weissgerber and Kruber, 1920; Weissgerber and Moehrle, 1921; Burchill et al., 1982a
		Coal/coal products: Burchill et al., 1982b; Nishioka et al., 1985a; Kong et al., 1984; Navivach et al., 1982; 1982; McKague and Meier, 1984; Kazarova et al., 1979; White and Lee, 1980; Lee et al., 1980
		Shale oil: Van Graas et al., 1981; Willey et al., 1981a; Kong et al., 1984; Willey et al., 1981b
		Sediment/soil: Bates and Carpenter, 1979b
		Air: Dimitriev et al., 1984; Hanson et al., 1980; Chiu et al., 1983
		Water: Warner, 1975; Winters and Parker, 1977
		Fish/marine organisms: Ogata et al., 1980b, 1981a,b; Ogata and Miyake, 1978, 1979
Perhydro-1-benzothiopyran (*6*)	156	Crude oil: Lyapina et al., 1982
Dicyclopenta[b,d]thiophene (*7*)	158	Crude oil: Mel'nikova et al, 1981

5H-Indeno[5,6-b]thiophene (9)

2H-Naphtho[1,8-bc]thiophene (35)
Dibenzothiophene (29)

172

172
184

Crude oil: Lyapina et al., 1980b, 1982; Mel'nikova et al., 1981

Crude oil: Kuras et al., 1982; Mostecky, 1982

Crude/oil petroleum: Kuras et al., 1982; Nesterenko et al., 1983; Poirier and Smiley, 1984; Mel'nikova et al., 1979; Brodskii et al., 1977; Lyapina et al., 1980a; Mostecky, 1982; Clugston et al., 1972, 1974, 1976; Nuzzi and Casalini, 1978; Choudhury and Bush, 1981; Rebbert et al., 1984; Baig et al., 1982; Yu and Hites, 1981; Howard and Mills, 1983; Castex et al., 1983; Poirier and Das, 1984; Speight and Pancirov, 1983; Grimmer and Böhnke, 1978; Grimmer et al., 1983a; Drushel and Sommers, 1967; Lohinska-Gasowska et al., 1979

Coal tar/pitch: Burchill et al., 1982a; Borwitzky and Schomburg, 1979; Gerasimenko et al., 1981; Burchill et al., 1982b; Nishioka et al., 1985a, 1986b; Kruber and Raeithel, 1954; Kruber, 1927

Coal/coal products: Lee et al., 1980; White and Lee, 1980; Kong et al., 1984; Willey et al., 1981b; Burchill et al., 1982b; Nakamura, 1983; Ozdemir, 1971; Hayatsu et al., 1975; Kekin et al., 1978; Fitch and Smith, 1979; Vo-dingh and Martinez, 1981; Stadelhofer and Gerhards, 1981; Wise et al., 1983; Later et al., 1981; Holstein and Severin, 1982; Kong et al., 1982; Chiu et al., 1983; Miki and Sugimoto, 1983; Grimmer et al., 1983b, 1985; Nishioka et al., 1986b; Kong et al., 1984

Shale oil: Kong et al., 1984; Willey et al., 1981a,b

Table 11 *cont.*

Compound	Mole weight	Occurrence
		Sediment/oil: Bates and Carpenter, 1979*b*; Lee *et al.*, 1982; Teal *et al.*, 1978; Nakamura and Kashimoto, 1979*a*; Imanaka *et al.*, 1980; Heit and Tan, 1979; Eganhouse and Kaplan, 1982; Sporstøl *et al.*, 1983; West *et al.*, 1985
		Air: Lee *et al.*, 1982; Bjørseth and Lunde, 1977; Bjørseth *et al.*, 1978*a,b*, 1981; Tong *et al.*, 1984; Moehnle *et al.*, 1984; Hanson *et al.*, 1977; Katz *et al.*, 1978; Bjørseth *et al.*, 1980; Murayama and Moriyama, 1982; Lunden *et al.*, 1982; Hung and Bernier, 1983; Hasanen *et al.*, 1984; York Res. Corp., 1979; Grimmer *et al.*, 1983*b*, 1985; Chiu *et al.*, 1983; *Hanson et al.*, 1980
		Water: Berthou *et al.*, 1981; Calder and Boehm, 1979; Hutchins and Ward, 1984; Gjessing *et al.*, 1984; Lygren *et al.*, 1984; Eganhouse and Kaplan, 1982; Kveseth *et al.*, 1982; Berglind, 1982; Mattox and Humenick, 1979; Hoffman *et al.*, 1984; Pearlman *et al.*, 1984; West *et al.*, 1985; Olufsen, 1980
		Fish/marine organisms: Warner, 1975; Ogata and Miyake, 1978, 1979; Ogata *et al.*, 1980*b*; Ogata and Miyake, 1980; Lee *et al.*, 1982; Fukushima *et al.*, 1983; Nakamura and Kashimoto, 1977; Bjørseth, 1978; Grahl-Nielsen *et al.*, 1978; Ogata *et al.*, 1979; Nakamura *et al.*, 1979; Clarke and Law, 1981; Paasivirta *et al.*, 1981; West *et al.*, 1985; Vassilaros *et al.*, 1982*b*; Oudot *et al.*, 1981; Friocourt *et al.*,

1981; Herzschuh and Paasivirta, 1983; Kira et al., 1983; Murray et al., 1983; Mackie et al., 1980; Ibe et al., 1978; Clement et al., 1980; Miranov and Shchekaturina, 1981; Ogata and Miyake, 1981; Ogata and Fujisawa, 1980; Eastmond et al., 1984; Vassilaros et al., 1982a

Foodstuffs: Beck and Stoebet, 1982

Sewage: Kveseth et al., 1982

Tobacco smoke: Schmid et al., 1985

Technical products/oils: Frycka, 1979; Kipot et al., 1980; Arsic et al., 1983; Grimmer et al., 1981a; Peake and Parker, 1980

Carbon black: Lee and Hites, 1976; Serth and Hughes, 1980

Naphtho[1,2-b]thiophene (*30*)	184	Crude oil/petroleum: Nishioka et al., 1985a; Carruthers and Douglas, 1959 Coal tar/pitch: Nishioka et al., 1985a; Borwitzky and Schomburg, 1979; Kruber and Raeithel, 1953. Coal/coal products: Lee et al., 1980; Kruber and Raeithel, 1953; Proksch, 1966; Nakamura, 1983 Shale oil: Nishioka et al., 1985a
Naphtho[2,1-b]thiophene (*32*)	184	Coal tar/pitch: Nishioka et al., 1985a; Kruber and Raeithel, 1953 Coal products: Nishioka et al., 1985a; Kruber and Raeithel, 1953; Proksch, 1966; Nakamura, 1983; Kong et al., 1984; Lee et al., 1980; Willey et al., 1981b Shale oil: Willey et al., 1981b
Naphtho[2,3-b]thiophene (*33*)	184	Crude oil/petroleum: Nishioka et al., 1985a Coal tar/pitch: Nishioka et al., 1985a, 1986b; Kruber and Raeithel, 1953

Table 11 cont.

Compound	Mole weight	Occurrence
		Coal products: Proksch, 1966; Kong et al., 1984
		Shale oil: Willey et al., 1981b; Pailer and Berner-Fenz, 1973
		Sediments/soil: Vassilaros et al., 1982c; Lee et al., 1982
		Fish/marine organisms: Lee et al., 1982; Vassilaros et al., 1982a,b
Dimethyl-8H-indeno[2,1-b]thiophene see: (8)	200	Technical products: Frycka, 1979
1-Methylbenzo[1,2-b:4,3-b']dithiophene see: (16)	204	Shale oil: Pailer and Berner-Fenz, 1973
Phenanthro[4,5-bcd]thiophene (80)	208	Crude oil: Pailer and Berner-Fenz, 1973
		Crude oil/petroleum: Grimmer et al., 1983a
		Coal tar/pitch: Borwitzky et al., 1977; Borwitzky and Schomburg, 1979; Burchill et al., 1982a; Nishioka et al., 1985a, 1986b
		Coal/coal products: Lee et al., 1977; White and Lee, 1980; Later et al., 1981; Lee et al., 1980; Burchill et al., 1982b; Chiu et al., 1983; Walsh et al., 1983; Nakamura, 1983; Burchill et al., 1983; Kong et al., 1982, 1984; Willey et al., 1981b; Nishioka et al., 1986b; White and Lee, 1980; Lee et al., 1980
		Shale oil: Chiu et al., 1983; Willey et al., 1981a,b; Kong et al., 1984
		Sediment/soil: West et al., 1986
		Air: Howard and Mills, 1983; Grimmer et al., 1985; Tong and Karasek, 1984; Chiu et al., 1983
		Water: Kveseth et al., 1982; Vassilaros et al., 1982a; West et al., 1985
		Fish/marine organisms: Vassilaros et al., 1982b; Kveseth

Compound	Mass	Sources and references
Phenaleno[1,9-bc]thiophene (**84**)	208	Crude oil/petroleum: Nishioka et al., 1985a
Anthra[1,2-b]thiophene (**69**)	234	Coal tar/pitch: Nishioka et al., 1985a Coal tar: Nishioka et al., 1985a Coal/coal products: Nakamura, 1983; Wise et al., 1983
Anthra[2,1-b]thiophene (**70**)	234	Coal products: Wise et al., 1983
Anthra[2,3-b]thiophene (**71**)	234	Coal products: Wise et al., 1983 Shale oil: Kong et al., 1984
Phenanthro[1,2-b]thiophene (**72**)	234	Coal tar: Nishioka et al., 1985a Coal products: Nakamura, 1983; Castle et al., 1983 Fish: Vassilaros et al., 1982a
Phenanthro[2,1-b]thiophene (**73**)	234	Crude oil: Payzant et al., 1983 Coal products: Nakamura, 1983; Wise et al., 1983
Phenanthro[2,3-b]thiophene (**74**)	234	Coal tar: Nishioka et al., 1986b Coal products: Nakamura, 1983; Wise et al., 1983
Phenanthro[3,2-b]thiophene (**75**)	234	Coal tar: Nishioka et al., 1986b Coal products: Nakamura, 1983; Wise et al., 1983
Phenanthro[3,4-b]thiophene (**76**)	234	Coal tar: Nishioka et al., 1985a Coal products: Nakamura, 1983; Wise et al., 1983
Phenanthro[4,3-b]thiophene (**77**)	234	Coal tar: Nishioka et al., 1985a Coal products: Nakamura, 1983; Wise et al., 1983
Phenanthro[9,10-b]thiophene (**78**)	234	Coal tar: Nishioka et al., 1985a Coal products: Nakamura, 1983; Wise et al., 1983 Fish: Vassilaros et al., 1982b
Benzo[b]naphtho[1,2-b]thiophene (**85**)	234	Crude oil/petroleum: Oshima et al., 1966; Carruthers and Stewart, 1967; Grimmer et al., 1983a; et al., 1982; Lee et al., 1982; Baumann et al., 1982; West et al., 1985 Foodstuffs: Kveseth et al., 1982; Vassilaros et al., 1982a Sewage: Kveseth et al., 1982 Carbon black: Lee and Hites, 1976; Fitch et al., 1978; Locati et al., 1979; Alsberg et al., 1982; Colmsjö and Östman, 1982

Table 11 cont.

Compound	Mole weight	Occurrence
		Coal tar/pitch: Schultz et al., 1965; Nishioka et al., 1985a, 1986b; Burchill et al., 1982a
		Coal/coal products: Kong et al., 1984; Nielsen, 1984; Wise et al., 1983; Kong et al., 1982; Nishioka et al., 1986b; Lucke et al., 1985; Willey et al., 1981b
		Shale oil: Kong et al., 1984; Willey et al., 1981b
		Sediments/soil: Lee et al., 1982; West et al., 1985
		Air: Nielsen, 1984; Hites et al., 1981; Lee et al., 1982; Grimmer et al., 1983b, 1985; Howard and Mills, 1983
		Water: Grimmer et al., 1981c; Vassilaros et al., 1982a
		Fish/marine organisms: Vassilaros et al., 1982a,b; Lee et al., 1982
		Technical products: Grimmer et al., 1981a
		Carbon black: Silva et al., 1982
Benzo[b]naphtho[2,1-d]thiophene (86)	234	Crude oil/petroleum: Grimmer et al., 1983a; DGMK, 1983; Ho et al., 1975
		Coal tar/pitch: Lee et al., 1980; Wilson et al., 1984; Kong et al., 1982, 1984; Nakamura, 1983; Wise et al., 1983; Nishioka et al., 1985a, 1986b; Kruber and Grigoleit, 1954; Burchill et al., 1982a
		Coal/coal products: Nishioka et al., 1986b; Lucke et al., 1985; Kong et al., 1982, 1984; Lee et al., 1980; Willey et al., 1981b
		Shale oil: Chiu et al., 1983; Kong et al., 1984; Willey et al., 1981b
		Sediment/soil: Vassilaros et al., 1982b; Lee et al., 1982; Wise et al., 1986; West et al., 1985, 1986

Air: Grimmer et al., 1983b; Lee et al., 1982; Bhide et al., 1984; Tong and Karasek, 1984; Kaschani, 1983; Grimmer et al., 1980b, 1985; Yu and Hites, 1981; Ratajzak et al., 1982; Chiu et al., 1983

Water: Grimmer and Naujack, 1979

Fish/marine organisms: Vassilaros et al., 1982a,b; Lee et al., 1982

Sewage: Grimmer et al., 1978a, 1980a

Carbon black: Lee and Hites, 1976a

Technical products: Grimmer et al., 1981b; Eyres, 1981; Kaishev et al., 1961; Grimmer and Böhnke, 1976; Grimmer and Glaser, 1975; Karcher et al., 1981

Crude oil/petroleum: Mel'nikova et al., 1981; Grimmer et al., 1978b; Melikadse and Gverdtsiteli, 1975; Brodskii et al., 1977; Lyapina et al., 1980a,b; Teplitskaya et al., 1981; Smith et al., 1983; Katti et al., 1984

Coal tar/pitch: Mlochowski and Skrzywan, 1969; Kruber and Rappen, 1940; Lang and Eigen, 1967; Nishioka et al., 1985a, 1986b; Burchill et al., 1982a

Coal/coal products: Kong et al., 1982, 1984; Nakamura, 1983; Wise et al., 1983; Burchill et al., 1978; Nishioka et al., 1986b; Lucke et al., 1985; Willey et al., 1981b

Shale oil: Kong et al., 1984; Willey et al., 1981b

Sediments/soil: West et al., 1985

Air: Grimmer et al., 1983b, 1985

Water: Vassilaros et al., 1982a

Fish/marine organisms: Vassilaros et al., 1982a,b

Sewage: Kveseth et al., 1982

Technical products: Karcher et al., 1981

Benzo[b]naphtho[2,3-d]thiophene (87)

234

Table 11 *cont.*

Compound	Mole weight	Occurrence
[1]Benzothieno[2,3-*b*][1]benzothiophene (*88*)	240	Crude oil/petroleum; Hunt and Shabanowitz, 1982; Drushel and Sommers, 1966
		Coal products: Kong et al., 1982
[1]Benzothieno[3,2-*b*][1]benzothiophene (*89*)	240	Crude oil/petroleum: Drushel and Sommers, 1966
Benzo[1,2]phenaleno[4,3-*bc*]thiophene (*144*)	258	Coal products: Nakamura, 1983
Benzo[1,2]phenaleno[3,4-*bc*]thiophene (*145*)	258	Coal products: Nakamura, 1983
Benzo[2,3]phenanthro[4,5-*bcd*]thiophene (*154*)	258	Coal tar/pitch: Burchill et al., 1982a; Nishioka et al., 1986b
		Coal/coal products: Nakamura, 1983; Kong et al., 1982, 1984; Wise et al., 1983; Nishioka et al., 1986b
		Sediments/soil: West et al., 1986
		Carbon black: Silva et al., 1982; Colmsjö et al., 1982; Colmsjö and Östman, 1982
		Technical products: Karcher et al., 1979, 1981; Depaus, 1979
Chryseno[4,5-*bcd*]thiophene (*155*)	258	Coal tar/pitch: Nishioka et al., 1986b
		Coal/coal products: Nakamura, 1983; Kong et al., 1982, 1984; Karcher et al., 1981; Wise et al., 1983; Nishioka et al., 1986b; Lee et al., 1980
		Shale oil: Kong et al., 1984
		Carbon black: Sugiura et al., 1983; Colmsjö and Östman, 1982
		Technical products: Depaus, 1979; Karcher et al., 1979
Pyreno[1,2-*b*]thiophene (*162*)	258	Coal products: Nakamura, 1983
Pyreno[2,1-*b*]thiophene (*163*)	258	Coal products: Nakamura, 1983
		Shale oil: Kong et al., 1984
Pyreno[4,5-*b*]thiophene (*164*)	258	Coal products: Nakamura, 1983
Acenaphtho[3,4-*b*]benzo[*d*]thiophene (*123*)	260	Crude oil/petroleum: Lyapina et al., 1980a,b

Compound	Mass	References
Benzo[10,11]chryseno[4,5-*bcd*]thiophene (*196*)	282	Sediments/soil: Colmsjö *et al.*, 1982 Carbon black: Colmsjö and Östman, 1982
Benzo[4,5]triphenyleno[1,12-*bcd*]thiophene (*197*)	282	Sediments/soil: Colmsjö *et al.*, 1982 Carbon black: Colmsjö and Östman, 1982
Perylo[1,12-*bcd*]thiophene (*198*)	282	Coal tar/pitch: Borwitzky *et al.*, 1977; Nishioka *et al.*, 1986*b*; Burchill *et al.*, 1982*a* Coal products: Nishioka *et al.*, 1986*b* Carbon black: Colmsjö *et al.*, 1982; Colmsjö and Östman, 1982; Lee and Hites, 1976 Technical products: Karcher *et al.*, 1979
Anthra[1,2-*b*]benzo[*d*]thiophene (*139*)	284	Coal products: Nakamura, 1983; Wise *et al.*, 1983
Anthra[2,3-*b*]benzo[*d*]thiophene (*141*)	284	Crude oil/petroleum: Teplitskaya *et al.*, 1981; Akhobadze *et al.*, 1977
Benzo[*b*]phenanthro[1,2-*d*]thiophene (*146*)	284	Air: Murayama and Moriyama, 1982
Benzo[*b*]phenanthro[2,1-*d*]thiophene (*147*)	284	Coal/coal products: Nakamura, 1983; Wise *et al.*, 1983; Kong *et al.*, 1984
Benzo[*b*]phenanthro[2,3-*d*]thiophene (*148*)	284	Sediments/soil: Wise *et al.*, 1986
Benzo[*b*]phenanthro[3,2-*d*]thiophene (*149*)	284	Coal products: Nakamura, 1983
Benzo[*b*]phenanthro[3,4-*d*]thiophene (*150*)	284	Coal products: Nakamura, 1983
Benzo[*b*]phenanthro[9,10-*d*]thiophene (*152*)	284	Coal products: Nakamura, 1983
Dinaphtho[1,2-*b*:1',2'-*d*]thiophene (*156*)	284	Coal products: Nakamura, 1983 Coal tar/pitch: Borwitzky and Schomburg, 1979; Shultz *et al.*, 1965
Dinaphtho[1,2-*b*:2',1'-*d*]thiophene (*157*)	284	Air: Kumanova and Vasileva, 1983
Dinaphtho[1,2-*b*:2',3'-*d*]thiophene (*158*)	284	Coal products: Nakamura, 1983 Coal tar/pitch: Nishioka *et al.*, 1986*b*
Dinaphtho[2,1-*b*:1',2'-*d*]thiophene (*159*)	284	Coal products: Nakamura, 1983; Nishioka *et al.*, 1986*b* Sediments/soil: Wise *et al.*, 1986; West *et al.*, 1986
Dinaphtho[2,3-*b*:2',3'-*d*]thiophene (*161*)	284	Coal/coal products: Gundermann and Fuhrmann, 1978 Technical products: Karcher *et al.*, 1979, 1981 Coal/coal products: Nakamura, 1983 Technical products: Karcher *et al.*, 1979

Table 11 cont.

Compound	Mole weight	Occurrence
Triphenyleno[2,1-b]thiophene (*168*)	284	Coal/coal products: Nakamura, 1983; Kong et al., 1984; Willey et al., 1981b
Triphenyleno[1,12-bcd]thiophene (*170*)	284	Crude oil/petroleum: Grimmer et al., 1983a Coal tar/pitch: Karcher et al., 1981; Nishioka et al., 1986b Coal/coal products: Kong et al., 1982; Nishioka et al., 1986b Sediments/soil: Colmsjö and Östman, 1982 Air: Grimmer et al., 1985 Carbon black: Fitch et al., 1978; Fitch and Smith, 1979; Colmsjö and Östman, 1982 Technical products: Grimmer et al., 1981a
Benzo[6,7]perylo[1,12-bcd]thiophene (*223*)	306	Carbon black: Alsberg et al., 1982; Stenberg and Alsberg, 1981; Lee and Hites, 1976; Colmsjö and Östman, 1982
Napthofluorenothiophenes	322	Sediments/soil: Wise et al., 1986
Diacenaphtho[1,2-b:1',2'-d]thiophene (*219*)	332	Air: Greinke and Lewis, 1979a
Naphtho[2',3':9,10]phenanthro[4,5-bcd]thiophene (*202*)	334	Coal/coal products: Kong et al., 1984
Dibenzo[4,5:6,7]perylo[1,12-bcd]thiophene (*232*)	356	Carbon black: Peaden et al., 1980
Coroneno[3,2,1-bcd][1]benzothiophene (*235*)	380	Carbon black: Peaden et al., 1980
Phenanthro[5',4',3',2':4,5,6,7]perylo[1,12-bcd]thiophene (*236*)	380	Carbon black: Peaden et al., 1980

* Under the terms used in the column 'occurrence' the following matrices have been summarized: crude oil/petroleum = crudes, petroleum fractions, gasoline; coal tar/pitch = tars, pitches, anthracene oil, bitumen; coal/coal products = coal, coke, coal oil, coal liquids, hard-coal and brown-coal combustion effluents; sediments/soil = river and lake sediments, soils, minerals; air = includes also industrial areas (coke plants, aluminium plants etc); fish/marine organisms = fish, mussels, plankton, algae; foodstuffs = smoked and dried meat, vegetables etc.; technical products = hydrocarbons, motor oils (fresh and used).

According to their formation during fossilation of biomass, thiaarenes are found in coal and crude oil as well as in products related to these fossil fuels such as petroleum fractions, motor oil, shale oil, coal liquids, coal tars and pitches, and other coal-derived technical products. From these materials they may be transferred directly, by technical processes (coke plants etc.), by tanker-damage induced oil-spills, or by combustion processes into the environment. Accordingly, they are also detectable in sediments and in water, in marine organisms such as fish, mussels, algae etc. as well as in the matrix air, from where they may pollute vegetables and soil surfaces so that finally they are also found in various foodstuffs. Thiaarenes have been found in sewage, in carbon blacks, in tobacco smoke and in many other matrices. Table 11 lists references for the predominant sources of thiaarenes in the environment. Further details may be found in Chapter 2 under the various compounds.

1.6   Synthesis of thiaarenes

In this chapter some generally applicable methods for the synthesis of thiaarenes are discussed. There are, however, many other and more specific routes which have been applied to the preparation of various thiaarenes. Some of them are presented in Chapter 2 in which the various thiaarenes are treated. An excellent review on this subject has been published by Klemm (1982).

In view of its formal simplicity, sulfur insertion into aromatic ring systems seems to be the most tempting method in thiaarene synthesis. However, in most cases, this method leads to mixtures of isomers. For instance, sulfur insertion (or sulfur bridging) into *p*-terphenyl results in the formation of two isomers – benzo[2,1-*b*:3,4-*b'*]bis[l]benzothiophene and benzo[1,2-*b*:5,4-*b'*]bis[l]benzothiophene; and in case of *m*-terphenyl even to three isomers – benzo[1,2-*b*:3,4-*b'*]bis[l]benzothiophene, benzo[1,2-*b*:5,4-*b'*]bis[l]benzothiophene and benzo[1,2-*b*:4,5-*b'*]bis[1]benzothiophene. In most of the experiments in which this route has been used poor yields have been obtained.

Table 12 summarizes some results of attempts to synthesize thiaarenes by sulfur insertion into aromatic compounds by heating them in mixture with sulfur and aluminium chloride.

Better results sometimes are achieved by the method used by Klemm in which aromatic compounds react with hydrogen sulfide in the presence of an oxide catalyst such as $Al_2O_3/MoO_3/CoO$ or $MgO/Cr_2O_3/Al_2O_3$ at elevated temperatures (Klemm *et al.*, 1979*a*). However, sulfur insertion and extrusion (hydrodesulfuration) are reversible processes which often favour the unwanted sulfur extrusion. Some experiments on sulfur

Table 12. *Examples of sulfur insertion into aromatic compounds by treatment with sulfur/$AlCl_3$ at elevated temperatures*

Starting material	Product	Yield (%)	Reference
Biphenyl	Dibenzothiophene(**29**)	60–80	Gilman and Jacoby, 1938 Chapiro and Gach, 1933 Tschunkur and Himmer, 1934 Voronkov and Faitel'son, 1967
2-Phenylnaphthalene	Benzo[*b*]naphtho[2,1-*d*]thiophene (**86**)	1	Klemm *et al.*, 1978 Kruber and Rappen, 1940
p-Terphenyl	Benzo[1,2-*b*:4,5-*b'*]bis[1]benzothiophene (**180**) Benzo[2,1-*b*:3,4-*b'*]bis[1]benzothiophene (**184**)	2 3	Rao and Tilak, 1958
m-Terphenyl	Benzo[1,2-*b*:3,4-*b'*]bis[1]benzothiophene (**176**) Benzo[1,2-*b*:4,5-*b'*]bis[1]benzothiophene (**180**) Benzo[1,2-*b*:5,4-*b'*]bis[1]benzothiophene (**181**)	2 1 3	Pandya *et al.*, 1959*b*
3-Phenylbenzo[*b*]thiophene	[1]Benzothieno[3,2-*b*][1]benzothiophene (**89**)	5	Murthy *et al.*, 1961
2,2'-bis-Benzo[*b*]thiophene	Thieno[3,2-*b*:4,5-*b'*]bis[1]benzothiophene*	16	Pandya *et al.*, 1959*b*

* Also formed by sulfur insertion into 2,3'- and in 3,3'-bis-benzo[*b*]thiophene (Murthy *et al.*, 1961).

insertion by oxide-catalyzed H_2S-treatment of polycyclic aromatic hydrocarbons are summarized in Table 13.

Plain heating of polycyclic aromatic hydrocarbons with sulfur at 190–320°C has also been applied to achieve sulfur bridging (see Table 14 for a summary). The formation of thiaarenes from partially hydrogenated bay-region containing polycyclic aromatic hydrocarbons by heating in a sealed glass ampoule with sulfur has been described by Colmsjö *et al.* (1985). In some cases two sulfur atoms are inserted under these conditions. The authors found that the yield could not be enhanced by adding catalysts like $AlCl_3$, $SnCl_4$, or $FeCl_3$ (Table 14).

In most of the thiaarene syntheses aromatic systems are enlarged by ring annulation. When thiophene ring(s) are already present in the precursor and the additionally formed ring is carbocyclic this route is called homoannulation. When the thiophene ring is newly formed, the term thiannulation is used.

A very common and successfully applied method has been introduced by Tilak and his working group (Tilak thiannulation). In this route mainly arene thiols are condensed with α-haloketones resulting in α-(arylthio)ketones which then may be cyclized by treatment with polyphosphoric acid. Dehydrogenation with selenium or palladium/charcoal aromatized the product to the corresponding thiaarene system. The synthesis of naphtho[1,2-*b*:5,6-*b'*]bis[1]benzothiophene carried out by Desai and Tilak (1961) may be taken as an example:

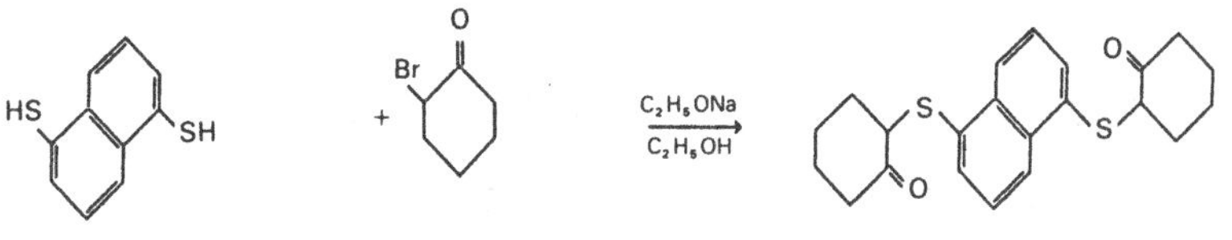

naphthalene-   2-bromocyclohexanone   1,5-bis[2-oxocyclohexylthio]
1,5-dithiol   naphthalene

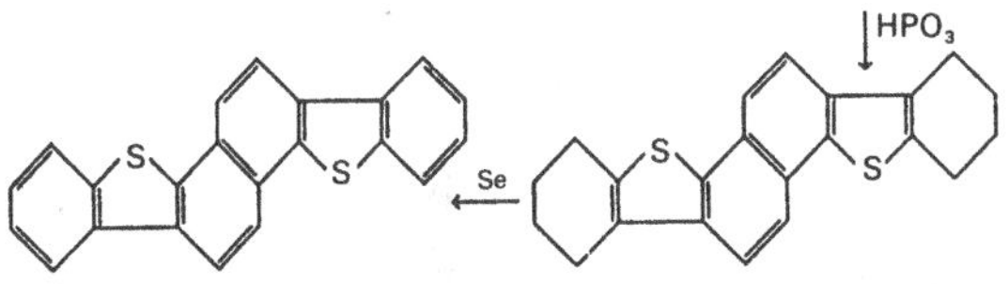

naphtho[1,2-*b*:5,6-*b'*]   1,2,3,4,8,9,10,11-octahydronaphtho
bis[1]benzothiophene   [1,2-*b*:5,6-*b'*]bis[1]benzothiophene

The Tilak-thiannulation has been widely used and many thiaarene systems have been obtained through this reaction sequence (Table 15).

Table 13. *Examples of sulfur insertion into aromatic compounds by treatment with hydrogen sulfide and heterogenous oxide catalyst at elevated temperatures*

Starting material	Product	Conditions	Yield (%)	Reference
Biphenyl	Dibenzothiophene (29)	FeS, 85% purity; 630°C	0	Klemm et al., 1970
		Al_2O_3(13%)/SiO_2(87%); 630°C	31	
		Al_2O_3(Houdry HA 100), 630°C	33	
		Al_2O_3(Harshaw Al-0104T); 630°C	35	
		Al_2O_3(90%)/ThO_2(10%); 630°C	54	
		Al_2O_3(95%)/Cr_2O_3(5%); 630°C	56	
		Al_2O_3(81%)/Cr_2O_3(19%); 630°C	57	
		Al_2O_3(86%)/Cr_2O_3(12%)/MgO(2%); 630°C	59	
Styrene	Benzo[b]thiophene (3)	Al_2O_3/FeS; 600°C	63	Klemm et al., 1979a
Phenanthrene	Phenanthro[4,5-bcd]-thiophene (80)	CoO/MoO_3/Al_2O_3; 430–600°C	29	Klemm et al., 1978
		Al_2O_3(86%)/Cr_2O_3(12%)/MgO(2%); 630°C	39	Klemm et al., 1970
Triphenylene	Triphenyleno[1,12-bcd]-thiophene (170)	CoO(3%)/MoO_3(12%)/Al_2O_3(85%); 500°C	18	Klemm and Lawrence, 1979
2-Phenylnaphthalene	Benzo[b]naphtho[2,1-d]-thiophene (86)	CoO/MoO_3/Al_2O_3; 430–600°C	24	Klemm et al., 1978
	Benzo[b]naphtho[2,3-d]-thiophene (87)		1	

Table 14. *Examples of sulfur insertion into aromatic compounds by treatment with sulfur at elevated temperatures*

Starting material	Product	Yield (%)	Reference
Biphenyl	—	0	Klemm et al., 1970
3-Phenylbenzo[b]thiophene	[1]Benzothieno[2,3-b][1]benzothiophene (88)	20	Murthy et al., 1961
3,3'-bis-Benzo[b]thiophene	Thiopyrano[2,3-b:4,5,6-c'd']thiophene	51	Murthy et al., 1961
3-Phenylthieno[2,3-b][1]benzothiophene	Thieno[2,3-b:5,4-b']bis[1]benzothiophene	20	Murthy et al., 1961
2,2-bis-Benzo[b]thiophene	Thieno[3,2-b:4,5-b']bis[1]benzothiophene	51	Dayagi et al., 1970
1,1'-Diphenylethene	[1]Benzothieno[2,3-b][1]benzothiophene (88)	54	Dayagi et al., 1970
1-Ethylacenaphthylene	Acenaphtho[1,2-b]thiophene (50)	15	Morel and Mollier, 1965
1-Propylacenaphthylene	8-Methyl-acenaphtho[1,2-b]thiophene	15	Morel and Mollier, 1965
1-Isopropyl-acenaphthylene	9-Methyl-acenaphtho[1,2-b]thiophene	15	Morel and Mollier, 1965
Dodecahydrotriphenylene	Triphenyleno[1,12-bcd]thiophene + triphenyleno-[1,12-bcd:4,5-b'c'd']dithiophene (170)	18 + 2	Colmsjö et al., 1985
4,5,10,11-Tetrahydrochrysene (?)	Chryseno[4,5-bcd]thiophene + chryseno-[4,5-bcd:10,11-b'c'd']dithiophene (155)	6 + 1.8	Colmsjö et al., 1985
1,2,3,10,11,12-Hexahydroperylene	Perylo[1,12-bcd]thiophene (198)	13	Colmsjö et al., 1985
1,2,3,6,7,8,10,11,12-Decahydrobenzo[e]pyrene	Benzo[4,5]triphenyleno[1,12-bcd]thiophene (197)	—	Colmsjö et al., 1985

Table 15. *Some thiaarene systems synthesized by thiannulation*

Starting material	Product	Yield (%)	Reference
2-Bromocyclohexanone + naphthalene-1-thiol	Benzo[b]naphtho[2,1-d]thiophene (86)	55	Rabindran and Tilak, 1953b
2-Bromocyclohexanone + naphthalene-2-thiol	Benzo[b]naphtho[1,2-d]thiophene (85)	—	Campaigne and Osborn, 1968; Rabindran and Tilak, 1953b
2-Bromocyclohexanone + benzo[b]thiophene-2-thiol	[1]Benzothieno[2,3-b][l]benzothiophene (88)	41	Mitra et al., 1957
2-Bromocyclohexanone + benzene-1,3-dithiol	Benzo[1,2-b:3,4-b']bis[1]benzothiophene (176)	14	Rao and Tilak, 1954
2-Bromocyclohexanone + benzene-1,3-dithiol	Benzo[1,2-b:4,5-b']bis[1]benzothiophene (180) + benzo[1,2-b:4,3-b']bis[1]benzothiophene (178)	11 + 15	Rao and Tilak, 1958
2-Bromocyclohexanone + 2,5-dimethylbenzene-1,3-dithiol	6,12-Dimethylbenzo[1,2-b:5,4-b']bis[1]benzothiophene	69	Pillai et al., 1963
2-Bromocyclohexanone + 1-chloro-benzene-2,4-dithiol	Benzo[1,2-b:3,4-b']bis[1]benzothiophene (176)	—	Rao and Tilak, 1954
2-Chlorocyclohexanone + phenanthrene-9-thiol	Benzo[b]phenanthro[9,10-d]thiophene (152)	26	Wilputte and Martin, 1956

2-Chlorocyclohexanone + 2-methyl-naphthalene-1-thiol	6-Methyl-8,9,10,11-tetrahydrobenzo[k]thioxanthene	—	Muller and Cagniant, 1968
2-Chlorocyclohexanone + acenaphthene-3-thiol	Acenaphtho[3,4-b]benzo[d]thiophene (123)	—	Faller and Cagniant, 1968
2-Bromotetralone + benzenethiol	Benzo[b]naphtho[1,2-d]thiophene (85)	25	Campaigne and Osborn, 1968
2-Bromotetralone + naphthalene-1-thiol	Dinaphtho[1,2-b:1′,2′-d]thiophene (156)	—	Rabindran and Tilak, 1953c
2-Bromotetralone + naphthalene-2-thiol	Dinaphtho[2,1-b:1′,2′-d]thiophene (159)	—	Rabindran and Tilak, 1953c
3-Chloro-2-decalone + naphthalene-1-thiol	Dinaphtho[1,2-b:2′,3′-d]thiophene (158)	—	Wilputte and Martin, 1956
3-Chloro-2-decalone + naphthalene-2-thiol	Dinaphtho[2,1-b:2′,3′-d]thiophene (160)	—	Wilputte and Martin, 1956
3-Chloro-2-decalone + phenanthrene-9-thiol	Naphtho[2,3-b]phenanthro[9,10-d]thiophene (201)	—	Wilputte and Martin, 1956
α-Chloroacetone + naphthalene-1,5-dithiol	1,6-Dimethyl-naphtho[1,2-b:5,6-b′]dithiophene	14	Desai and Tilak, 1961
α-Chloroacetone + naphthalene-1,3-dithiol	3,6-Dimethyl-naphtho[1,2-b:3,4-b′]dithiophene	18	Desai and Tilak, 1961
Bromoacetaldehydedimethylacetale + naphthalene-2,7-dithiol	Naphtho[2,1-b:7,8-b′]dithiophene (102)	—	Desai and Tilak, 1961
α-Bromoacetophenone + naphthalene-2-thiol	Benzo[1,2]phenaleno[4,3-bc]thiophene (144)	4	Pratap et al., 1982a

Special forms of thiannulation are the base-catalyzed Hinsberg reaction in which 1,2-diketones are condensed with thiodiglycolic esters to thiaarenes (Hinsberg, 1910), and intramolecular thiannulation. Following the first route, phenanthro[9,10-*c*]thiophene has been obtained from phenanthrene-9,10-quinone (Kochkanyan *et al.*, 1974; Hauptmann *et al.*, 1969) and the acenaphtho[1,2-*c*]thiophene system has been prepared with acenaphtho-1,2-quinone as starting material (Birch and Crombie, 1971; Koshelev and Plakidin, 1973). Elegant syntheses of dinaphtho[1,2-*b*:2′,1′-*d*]thiophene (Wilputte and Martin, 1956) and dinaphtho[2,1-*b*:1′,2′-*d*]thiophene (Gogte *et al.*, 1960) have been achieved by intramolecular thiannulation of 1,1′-dinaphthylsulfoxide and 2,2′-dinaphthylsulfone, respectively. Examples for other intramolecular thiannulations are presented under benzo[1,2-*b*:5,4-*b*′]bis[1]benzothiophene (Grandolino, 1961) and anthra[1,9-*bc*:5,10-*b*′*c*′]dithiophene (Wudl *et al.*, 1979) in Chapter 2.

For homoannulations three methods are of outstanding importance: (a) the Elbs pyrolysis (Elbs cyclodehydration), (b) the Photocyclization, (c) the acid-catalyzed cyclization. In the first method aroylthiophenes with a methyl substituent in the *ortho*-position to the carbonyl group are heated for 1–3 h to 350–450°C during which time ring closure takes place. In most cases poor yields are observed and rearrangements may also occur (Croisy *et al.*, 1984). Moreover, yields very much depend on the temperature and sometimes several isomers are formed which are difficult to separate (see Table 16). The method was introduced to thiaarene synthesis by Buu–Hoi and Hoan (1948) and by Werner (1949). It has been applied to synthesize benzo[*b*]naphtho[2,1-*d*]thiophene from 3-(2-methylbenzoyl)-benzo[*b*]thiophene (Badger and Christie, 1958). More recently the Elbs pyrolysis procedure has been used by Croisy *et al.* (1984) to synthesize benzo[*b*]naphtho[2,1-*d*]thiophene and its [2,3-*d*]-isomer as well as a number of benzo[*b*]phenanthrothiophenes from ortho-methylated aroylbenzo[*b*]thiophenes. Some selected examples for the application of the Elbs pyrolysis in thiaarene synthesis are summarized in Table 16.

A large number of thiaarenes has been prepared by photocyclization (mercury lamp) of 1-aryl-2-thiaarenyl-substituted ethenes and propenes. The reaction is carried out in an inert solvent such as cyclohexane or benzene in the presence of iodine. First experiments were carried out by Carruthers and Stewart (1965*a*) who synthesized various monomethyl-substituted benzo[*b*]naphtho[2,1-*d*]thiophenes by this procedure. In a series of publications the synthesis of 3–6 rings-containing thiaarenes by photocyclization has been described. In most cases the 1,2-disubstituted ethenes serving as starting materials were prepared by Wadsworth–Emmons reaction between diethyl-, thenyl- benzyl-, benzo[*b*]thenyl-, or naphthyl methylphosphonates and various aryl- or thiaarylaldehydes. Following this route, naphthothiophenes, phenanthrothiophenes, benzo[*b*]naphtho[1,2-*d*]- and -[2,1-*d*]thiophenes as well as their methyl derivatives, triphenylenothiophenes, benzophenalenothiophenes, benzophenanthrothiophenes, anthrabenzothiophenes, dinaphthothiophenes, thienodibenzothiophenes, benzobisbenzothiophenes, benzothienodibenzothiophenes, and naphthobisbenzothiophenes have been prepared. The application of the photocyclization to thiaarene synthesis has been thoroughly reviewed by Castle *et al.* (1984). Some examples for it are summarized in Table 17.

The synthesis of dinaphtho[1,2-*b*:1',2'-*d*]thiophene from 2-styrylnaphtho[1,2-*b*]thiophene which may be obtained by Wadsworth-Emmons condensation of naphtho[1,2-*b*]thiophene-2-aldehyde and diethyl benzylphosphonate may illustrate the synthesis of thiaarenes by photocyclization:

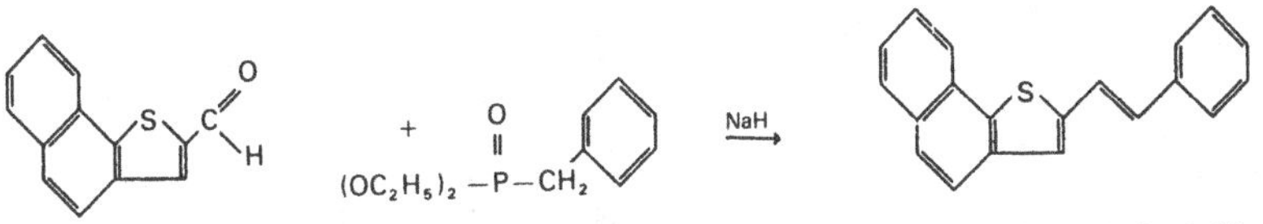

naphtho[1,2-*b*]thio   diethyl benzylphosphonate   2-styrylnaphtho[1,2-*b*]
phene-2-aldehyde   thiophene

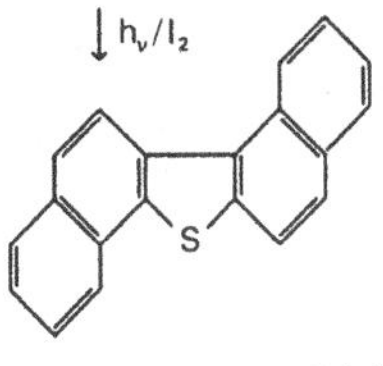

dinaphtho[1,2-*b*:1',2'-*d*]thiophene

The formation of dibenzothiophenes from diphenylsulfides by photocyclization has been described by Zeller and Petersen (1975), and Bluemer *et al.* (1977) reported on the formation of dinaphthothiophenes from 1,2'- and from 2,2'-dinaphthylsulfide.

A common reaction in the synthesis of polycyclic aromatic hydrocarbons, the Haworth homoannulation procedure, which makes use of the proton- or Lewis acid-catalyzed ring closure of aryl-butyric acid to aromatic tetrahydroketo acids, has also been applied to thiaarene synthesis. Campaigne and Osborn (1968) described the synthesis of benzo[*b*]naphtho[2,3-*d*]thiophene from 4-(2-dibenzothienyl)-1-butyric acid via 7,8,9,10-tetrahydrobenzo[*b*]naphtho[2,3-*d*]thiophene. Ring closure with polyphosphoric acid or sulfuric acid resulted in yields of some

Table 16. *Some applications of the Elbs pyrolysis to the synthesis of thiaarenes*

Starting material	Product	Yield (%)	Reference
2-Benzoyl-3-methylbenzo[b]thiophene	Benzo[b]naphtho[2,3-d]thiophene (87)	5–8	Werner, 1949
		1*	Croisy et al., 1984
		3**	Croisy et al., 1984
		9***	Croisy et al., 1984
3-(2-Methylbenzoyl)benzo[b]thiophene	Benzo[b]naphtho[2,1-d]thiophene (86)	—	Buu-Hoï et al., 1969
		20	Badger and Christie, 1958
		2.5*	Croisy et al., 1984
		3.5**	Croisy et al., 1984
		64.5***	Croisy et al., 1984
2-(2-Methylbenzoyl)benzo[b]thiophene	Benzo[b]naphtho[2,1-d]thiophene (86)	3*	Croisy et al., 1984
		2**	Croisy et al., 1984
		2.5***	Croisy et al., 1984
	Benzo[b]naphtho[2,3-d]thiophene (87)	2*	Croisy et al., 1984
		4.5**	Croisy et al., 1984
		30***	Croisy et al., 1984
3-Benzoyl-2-methylbenzo[b]thiophene	Benzo[b]naphtho[2,1-d]thiophene (86)	0.75*	Croisy et al., 1984
		1**	Croisy et al., 1984
		4***	Croisy et al., 1984
	Benzo[b]naphtho[2,3-d]thiophene (87)	1.5*	Croisy et al., 1984
		2**	Croisy et al., 1984
		6***	Croisy et al., 1984

3-(2-Methylnaphthoyl)benzo[b]thiophene	Benzo[b]phenanthro[3,2-d]thiophene (*149*)	2.5	Croisy et al., 1984
	Benzo[b]phenanthro[2,3-d]thiophene (*148*)	1	Croisy et al., 1984
	Benzo[b]phenanthro[3,4-d]thiophene (*150*)	35	Croisy et al., 1984
	Benzo[b]phenanthro[3,2-d]thiophene (*149*)	54	Badger and Christie, 1956a, 1958
2-(2-Methylnaphthoyl)benzo[b]thiophene	Benzo[b]phenanthro[3,2-d]thiophene (*149*)	4	Croisy et al., 1984
	Benzo[b]phenanthro[2,3-d]thiophene (*148*)	10	Croisy et al., 1984
	Benzo[b]phenanthro[2,1-d]thiophene (*147*)	3	Croisy et al., 1984
3-(1-Naphthoyl)-2-methylbenzo[b]thiophene	Benzo[b]phenanthro[3,2-d]thiophene (*149*)	25	Croisy et al., 1984
	Benzo[b]phenanthro[2,3-d]thiophene (*148*)	6	Croisy et al., 1984
	Benzo[b]phenanthro[3,4-d]thiophene (*150*)	6	Croisy et al., 1984
2-(1-Naphthoyl)-3-methylbenzo[b]thiophene	Benzo[b]phenanthro[2,3-d]thiophene (*148*)	20.5	Croisy et al., 1984
3-(2-Methylnaphthoyl)dibenzothiophene	Anthra[2,3-b]benzo[d]thiophene (*141*)	—	Cherry et al., 1967
5-(2-Methylbenzoyl)benzo[b]thiophene	Anthra[2,3-b]thiophene (*71*)	10	Faller, 1968
	Anthra[2,1-b]thiophene (*70*)	25	Faller, 1968
7-(2-Methylbenzoyl)benzo[b]thiophene	Anthra[1,2-b]thiophene (*69*)	20	Faller, 1968
3-(4-Indanoyl)benzo[b]thiophene	Acenaphtho[3,4-b]benzo[d]thiophene (*123*)	—	Faller, 1967
2-(4-Indanoyl)benzo[b]thiophene	Acenaphtho[4,3-b]benzo[d]thiophene (*124*)	33	Faller, 1967
5-(4-Indanoyl)benzo[b]thiophene	Aceanthreno[9,10-b]thiophene (*128*)	15	Faller, 1966b

* At cyclization temperatures of 360°C, ** 390°C, and *** 420°C.

Table 17. *Examples for the photocyclization of 1,2-substituted ethenes in thiaarene synthesis*

Starting material	Product	Yield (%)	Reference
1-(3-Thienyl)-2-(1-naphthyl)ethene	Phenanthro[1,2-*b*]thiophene (**72**)	32	Carruthers and Stewart, 1965*a*
1-(2-Thienyl)2-(1-naphthyl)ethane	Phenanthro[2,1-*b*]thiophene (**73**)	88	Carruthers and Stewart, 1965*a*
1-(3-Thienyl)-2-(2-naphthyl)ethene	Phenanthro[4,3-*b*]thiophene (**77**)	75	Carruthers and Stewart, 1965*a*
1-(2-Thienyl)-2-(2-naphthyl)ethene	Phenanthro[3,4-*b*]thiophene (**76**)	17	Carruthers and Stewart, 1965*a*
3-Styrylbenzo[*b*]thiophene	Benzo[*b*]naphtho[2,1-*d*]thiophene (**86**)	72	Davies *et al.*, 1957; Campaigne and Osborn, 1968
2-Styrylbenzo[*b*]thiophene	Benzo[*b*]naphtho[1,2-*d*]thiophene (**85**)	51	Campaigne and Osborn, 1968; Rabindran and Tilak, 1953*a*
1-(2-Thienyl)-2-(1-naphthyl)propene	10-Methylphenanthro[2,1-*b*]thiophene	19	Pratap *et al.*, 1981*b*
5-Methyl-2-styrylthiophene	1-Methylnaphtho[2,1-*b*]thiophene	41	Tominaga *et al.*, 1981*b*
2-(3-Benzo[*b*]thienyl)-1-phenylpropene	6-Methylbenzo[*b*]naphtho[2,1-*d*]thiophene	73	Thompson *et al.*, 1981
2-(9-Phenanthrylethenyl)thiophene	Triphenyleno[1,2-*b*]thiophene (**167**)	20	Pratap *et al.*, 1981*a*
2-(9-Phenanthrylethenyl)thiophene	Triphenyleno[2,1-*b*]thiophene (**168**)	70	Pratap *et al.*, 1981*a*
1-Phenylnaphtho[2,1-*b*]thiophene	Benzo[1,2]phenaleno[4,3-*bc*]thiophene (**144**)	5	Tominaga *et al.*, 1982*a*
1-(4-Methyl-2-thienyl)-2-(1-naphthyl)ethene	3-Methylphenanthro[2,1-*b*]thiophene	84	Tominaga *et al.*, 1982*a*
o-Methylstyryl-2-benzo[*b*]thiophene	4-Methylbenzo[*b*]naphtho[1,2-*d*]thiophene	42	Tominaga *et al.*, 1982*a*
p-Methylstyryl-2-benzo[*b*]thiophene	2-Methylbenzo[*b*]naphtho[1,2-*d*]thiophene	45	Tominaga *et al.*, 1982*a*
m-Methylstyryl-2-benzo[*b*]thiophene	1- + 3-methylbenzo[*b*]naphtho[1,2-*d*]thiophene	10 + 22	Tominaga *et al.*, 1982*a*
5-Methyl-2-styrylbenzo[*b*]thiophene	10-Methylbenzo[*b*]naphtho[1,2-*d*]thiophene	45	Tominaga *et al.*, 1982*a*
6-Methyl-2-styrylbenzo[*b*]thiophene	9-Methylbenzo[*b*]naphtho[1,2-*d*]thiophene	45	Tominaga *et al.*, 1982*a*
7-Methyl-2-styrylbenzo[*b*]thiophene	8-Methylbenzo[*b*]naphtho[1,2-*d*]thiophene	40	Tominaga *et al.*, 1982*a*

3-Chloro-4-methyl-2-styrylbenzo[b]thiophene	11-Methylbenzo[b]naphtho[1,2-d]thiophene	34	Tominaga et al., 1982a
1-(2-Benzo[b]thienyl)-2-phenylpropene	5-Methylbenzo[b]naphtho[1,2-d]thiophene	52	Tominaga et al., 1982a
o-Methylstyryl-3-benzo[b]thiophene	4-Methylbenzo[b]naphtho[2,1-d]thiophene	80	Tominaga et al., 1982b
p-Methylstyryl-3-benzo[b]thiophene	2-Methylbenzo[b]naphtho[2,1-d]thiophene	60	Tominaga et al., 1982b
m-Methylstyryl-3-benzo[b]thiophene	1- + 3-Methylbenzo[b]naphtho[2,1-d]thiophene	17 + 24	Tominaga et al., 1982b
1-(3-Benzo[b]thienyl)-2-phenylpropene	5-Methylbenzo[b]naphtho[2,1-d]thiophene	50	Tominaga et al., 1982b
2-(3-Benzo[b]thienyl)-1-phenylpropene	6-Methylbenzo[b]naphtho[2,1-d]thiophene	60	Tominaga et al., 1982b
2-(7-Methyl-3-benzo[b]thienyl)-3-phenyl-2-propenoic acid	10-Methylbenzo[b]naphtho[2,1-d]thiophene	60	Tominaga et al., 1982b
2-(5-Methyl-3-benzo[b]thienyl)-3-phenyl-2-propenoic acid	8-Methylbenzo[b]naphtho[2,1-d]thiophene	52	Tominaga et al., 1982b
2-(4-Methyl-3-benzo[b]thienyl)-3-phenyl-2-propenoic acid	7-Methylbenzo[b]naphtho[2,1-d]thiophene	36	Tominaga et al., 1982b
2-(6-Methyl-3-benzo[b]thienyl)-3-phenyl-2-propenoic acid	9-Methylbenzo[b]naphtho[2,1-d]thiophene	48	Tominaga et al., 1982b
2-(1-Naphthylethenyl)benzo[b]thiophene	Benzo[b]phenanthro[1,2-b]thiophene (*146*)	41	Davies and Porter, 1957a
2-(2-Naphthylethenyl)benzo[b]thiophene	Benzo[b]phenanthro[4,3-d]thiophene (*151*)	25	Davies and Porter, 1957a
3-(1-Naphthylethenyl)benzo[b]thiophene	Benzo[b]phenanthro[2,1-d]thiophene (*147*)	10	Croisy et al., 1975
3-(2-Naphthylethenyl)benzo[b]thiophene	Anthra[1,2-b]benzo[d]thiophene + benzo[b]phenanthro[3,4-d]thiophene (*139*) + (*150*)	—	Croisy et al., 1975
2-Styryldibenzothiophene	Benzo[b]phenanthro[4,3-b]thiophene + benzo[b]phenanthro[2,3-d]thiophene (*151*) + (*148*)	50 + 37	Pillai et al., 1963
4-Styryldibenzothiophene	Benzo[b]phenanthro[2,1-d]thiophene (*147*)	83	Croisy et al., 1975
2-Styrylthiophene	Naphtho[2,1-b]thiophene (*32*)	75	Tedjamulia et al., 1983b
2-Styrylnaphtho[1,2-b]thiophene	Dinaphtho[1,2-b:1',2'-d]thiophene (*156*)	72	Rabindran and Tilak, 1953c
2-Styrylnaphtho[2,1-b]thiophene	Dinaphtho[2,1-b:1',2'-d]thiophene (*159*)	45	Rabindran and Tilak, 1953c
3-Styrylnaphtho[1,2-b]thiophene	Dinaphtho[1,2-b:2',1'-d]thiophene (*157*)	76	Clarke et al., 1973
5-Methyl-2-styrylthiophene	2-Methylnaphtho[2,1-b]thiophene	30	Tominaga et al., 1983
4-Methyl-2-styrylthiophene	1-Methylnaphtho[2,1-b]thiophene	61	Tominaga et al., 1983

Table 17 cont.

Starting material	Product	Yield (%)	Reference
1-Thienyl-2-phenylpropene	5-Methylnaphtho[2,1-b]thiophene	56	Tominaga et al., 1983
1-Phenyl-2-thienylpropene	4-Methylnaphtho[2,1-b]thiophene	38	Tominaga et al., 1983
2-(2-Thienylethenyl)benzo[b]thiophene	Thieno[3,2-a]dibenzothiophene	88	Kudo et al., 1984
2-(3-Thienylethenyl)benzo[b]thiophene	Thieno[2,3-a]dibenzothiophene	83	Kudo et al., 1984
3-(2-Thienylethenyl)benzo[b]thiophene	Thieno[2,3-c]dibenzothiophene	80	Kudo et al., 1984
3-(3-Thienylethenyl)benzo[b]thiophene	Thieno[3,2-c]dibenzothiophene	21	Kudo et al., 1984
1,2-bis(2-Benzo[b]thienyl)ethene	Benzo[1,2-b:4,3-b′]bisbenzo[b]thiophene (178)	85	Kudo et al., 1984
1-(2′-benzo[b]thienyl)-2-(3′-benzo[b]thienyl)-ethene	Benzo[1,2-b:3,4-b′]bisbenzo[b]thiophene (176)	84	Kudo et al., 1984
1,2-bis(3,3′-Benzo[b]thienyl)ethene	Benzo[2,1-b:3,4-b′]bisbenzo[b]thiophene (184)	28	Kudo et al., 1984
1-(4-Dibenzothienyl)-2-(2-thienyl)ethene	Benzo[b]thieno[4,5-c]dibenzothiophene	75	Kudo et al., 1984
1-(4-Dibenzothienyl)-2-(3-thienyl)ethene	Benzo[b]thieno[7,6-c]dibenzothiophene	62	Kudo et al., 1984
2-(2-Thienylethenyl)dibenzothiophene	Benzo[b]thieno[4,5-a]dibenzothiophene + benzo[b]thieno[5,4-d]dibenzothiophene	65 + 20	Kudo et al., 1984
2-(3-Thienylethenyl)dibenzothiophene	Benzo[b]thieno[7,6-a]dibenzothiophene + benzo[b]thieno[6,7-b]dibenzothiophene	57 + 19	Kudo et al., 1984
1-(2-Benzo[b]thienyl)-2-(2-dibenzothienyl)ethene	Naphtho[2,1-b:7,6-b′]bisbenzo[b]thiophene (215) + naphtho[2,1-b:7,8-b′]bisbenzo[b]thiophene (216)	16 + 42	Tedjamulia et al., 1984
1-(3-Benzo[b]thienyl)-2-(2-dibenzothienyl)ethene	Naphtho[1,2-b:7,6-b′]bisbenzo[b]thiophene (212) + naphtho[1,2-b:7,8-b′]bisbenzo[b]thiophene (213)	23 + 42	Tedjamulia et al., 1984
1-(2-Benzo[b]thienyl)-2-(1-dibenzothienyl)ethene	Naphtho[1,2-b:6,5-b′]bisbenzo[b]thiophene (211)	82	Tedjamulia et al., 1984
1-(2-Benzo[b]thienyl)-2-(1-dibenzothienyl)ethene	Naphtho[2,1-b:6,5-b′]bisbenzo[b]thiophene (214)	12	Tedjamulia et al., 1984
1-(2-Benzo[b]thienyl)-2-(4-dibenzothienyl)ethene	Naphtho[1,2-b:6,5-b′]bisbenzo[b]thiophene (211)	79	Tedjamulia et al., 1984

30% (Campaigne and Osborn, 1968; Gilman and Jacoby, 1938) and the use of $PCl_5/SnCl_4$ in benzene was even more efficient (Bachman and Wilds, 1940). Wolff–Kishner reduction and subsequent dehydrogenation of the tetrahydro derivative with palladium/charcoal or selenium gives the parent thiaarene:

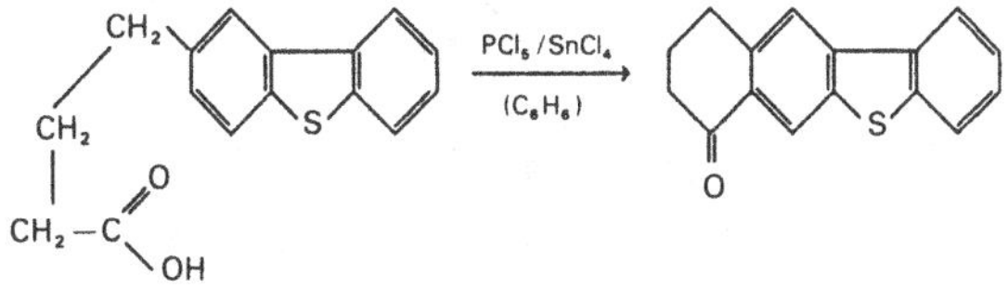

4-[2-dibenzothienyl]butyric acid

7-oxo-7,8,9,10-tetrahydrobenzo[*b*]-naphtho[2,3-*d*]thiophene

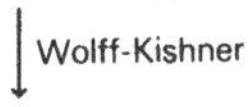

| Wolff-Kishner

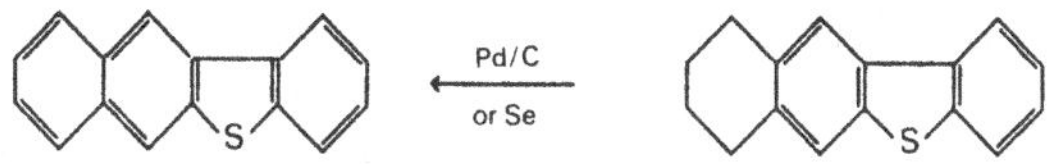

benzo[*b*]naphtho[2,3-*d*]thiophene

7,8,9,10-tetrahydrobenzo[*b*]naphtho-[2,3-*d*]thiophene

The method has also been used by Schroeder and Weinmayer (1952) to prepare variously substituted naphtho[2,3-*b*]thiophene-4,9-quinones from thenoyl-benzoic acids:

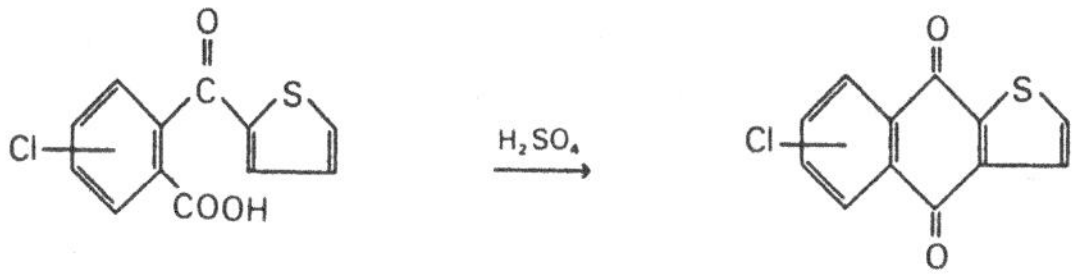

Cyclization may also be successful when γ-thiaarylbutyric acids are heated with P_2O_5 *in vacuo* (Ricci *et al.*, 1971).

Condensation with phthalic anhydride or naphthalene-2,3-dicarboxylic anhydride may be used instead of succinic anhydride for adding two or three rings to a thiaarene system. These ortho-carboxyaroylation procedures require Friedel-Crafts conditions and lead to thiaarenoyl-arenecarboxylic acids and sometimes already to cyclized quinones. As an example, naphtho[1,2-*b*]thiophene yields dinaphtho[1,2-*b*:2',3'-*d*]thiophene upon condensation with phthalic anhydride, ring closure with polyphosphoric acid and subsequent reduction (Armarego, 1960):

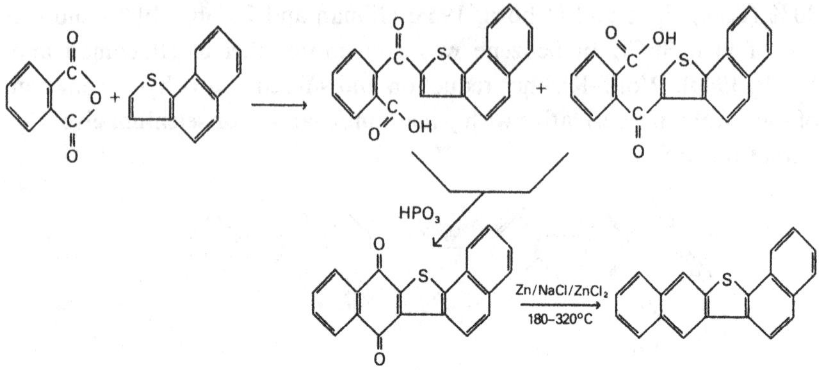

As may be seen from this example, the reaction is expected to lead to mixtures of isomers when a substituted anhydride is used for the condensation.

A related procedure is known under the term 'Bradsher reaction' during which dithiarylmethanes are treated with 1,1-dichlorodimethylether (Ahmed *et al.*, 1970, 1973):

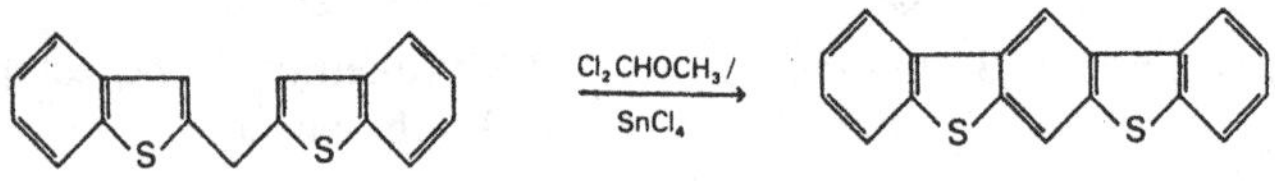

There are many more reactions which have been applied for the synthesis of thiaarenes in special cases. Examples are given in Chapter 2, such as Diels–Alder reaction between quinones and vinylthiophenes (Faller, 1968), condensation of thiaarenealdehydes with thiaaryl- or aryl-5,5-dimethyl-2-oxazoline (Iwao *et al.*, 1980), the application of the Pschorr reaction (Wilputte and Martin, 1956), the use of sulfones self-condensation (Davies *et al.*, 1952*ab*; Bordwell *et al.*, 1951; Taylor and Wallace, 1968) or condensation with vinylarenes (Davies and Porter 1957*a*), condensation of diazomethylarylthiophenes (Munro and Sharp, 1984), sulfuration of haloarylalkynes with subsequent cyclization etc. In this chapter only those routes have been regarded which have been applied to a great number of thiaarene systems.

1.7   Biological activity

1.7.1   *Balance of biological effects in environmental matrices*

Although it is well documented that polycyclic aromatic hydro-carbons contribute considerably, and in some cases almost exclusively, to the carcinogenic potency of environmental matter such as automotive exhaust (Grimmer *et al.*, 1983*c*, 1984), hard coal combustion exhaust

(Grimmer *et al.*, 1986), and used motor oil (Grimmer *et al.*, 1982; Grimmer, 1982) in different animal test systems, little is known about the carcinogenic potential of thiaarenes which are also present in these matrices. Effluents from coal combustion especially contain larger amounts of thiaarenes (Grimmer *et al.*, 1985, 1986; Schmidt *et al.*, 1986, 1987) and it may be expected that part of the carcinogenic effect can be attributed to this class of compounds. The same holds for the mutagenic potential of the above matrices (Dehnen *et al.*, 1977; Talcott and Wei, 1977; Pitts *et al.*, 1977; Tokiwa *et al.*, 1977; Teranishi *et al.*, 1978; Commoner, 1977). Tables 18 and 19 exhibit the balances of the carcinogenic and mutagenic effects as measured in the original matrix and in various fractions thereof. Unfortunately, also in case of the mutagenicity studies no attempt to calculate the contribution of thiaarenes to the total effect has been undertaken.

1.7.2 *Mutagenicity*

Since many of the thiaarenes became available in pure form during the past ten years, especially by the synthetic efforts of Iwao *et al.* (1980), Tominaga *et al.* (1981*a,b*, 1982*a,b,c*); Kudo *et al.* (1984, 1985); Pratap *et al.* (1981*a,b*, 1982*a,b*); Thompson *et al.* (1981); Tedjamulia *et al.* (1983*a,b,c*, 1984), their mutagenic activities in the Ames' *Salmonella typhimurium* assay could be measured. Pelroy *et al.* (1983) tested various 3- and 4-rings-containing thiaarenes in strain TA 98 and TA 100 with and without S9-mix activation and McFall *et al.* (1984) have investigated the methyl-substituted derivatives of these compounds in strain TA 98 with S9-mix activation. Karcher *et al.* (1981) also presented data on the mutagenic potential of some 3–5 rings-containing thiaarenes (dibenzothiophene, phenanthro[4,5-*bcd*]thiophene, benzo[2,3]phenanthro[4,5-*bcd*]thiophene, triphenyleno[1,12-*bcd*]thiophene and dinaphtho[2,1-*b*:1′,2′-*d*]thiophene) in the strains TA 98, TA 100 and in *Escherichia coli* strain PKM 101. The data of these tests are tabulated in Tables 20 and 21.

Among the 3-rings-containing thiaarenes only naphtho[1,2-*b*]thiophene proved to be mutagenic. Methyl-substitution in the inactive dibenzothiophene did not alter the mutagenic activity since no effect was found in any of the four methyldibenzothiophenes.

Among the 4-rings-containing thiaarenes various active compounds were found, the most mutagenic one of which was phenanthro[3,4-*b*]thiophene. The isomeric phenanthro[4,3-*b*]thiophene exhibits only a low activity in TA 100 indicating that the position of the sulfur plays a key role in the biological effect. Moreover, such findings obviously cannot be

Table 18. *Portions of carcinogenicity of various fractions obtained by chemical separation of environmental materials (related to the original matrix)*

Matrix (Ref.)	Bioassay used	Fraction	Weight (% of the fraction)	Portion of carcinogenicity (%)
Vehicle exhaust condensate (Grimmer et al., 1983c)	Mice, topical application onto the skin	Original material	100	100
		PAC-free fraction	83.5	8.6
		2–3 rings-containing PAC	13.0	3.4
		more than 3 rings-cont. PAC	3.5	105.6
Vehicle exhaust condensate (Grimmer et al., 1984)	Rats, implantation into the lung	Original material	100	100
		PAC-free fraction	87.3	8.3
		2–3 rings-containing PAC	9.9	16.2
		more than 3 rings-cont. PAC	2.8	81.0
Used motor oil (Grimmer et al., 1982)	Mice, topical application onto the skin	Original material	100	100
		PAC-free fraction	91.6	2.9
		2–3 rings-containing PAC	7.3	14.6
		more than 3 rings-cont. PAC	1.1	82.5
Hard coal combustion emission (Grimmer et al., 1986)	Mice, topical application onto the skin	Original material	100	100
		PAC-free fraction	52.9	3.5
		2–3 rings-containing PAC	24.4	3.5
		more than 3 rings-cont. PAC	22.7	93.0

PAC = polycyclic aromatic compounds.

Table 19 *Distribution of mutagenic activity in aromatic fractions obtained from a synfuel by Sephadex LH 20 partition chromatography (Guerin et al., 1978)*

Subfraction	Weight (% of fraction)	Revertants per mg of fraction*	
		−S9	+S9
Original material (aromatic fraction)	100	60	160
High molecular weight compounds	5.7	0	0
Aliphatic + 1 ring-containing PAC	47.0	0	0
2 rings-containing PAC	33.7	0	0
3 rings-containing PAC	8.0	0	1000
4 rings-containing PAC	2.7	1600	4000
5 rings-containing PAC	0.6	2600	3800
more than 5 rings-containing PAC	0.5	600	1500
Total	98.2	62	214

* Number of revertants from *Salmonella typhimurium* strain TA 98 by use of plate assay with 2×10^8 bacteria per plate. +S9 and −S9 indicate that tests were carried out with or without metabolic activation by a S9-fraction of a liver homogenate obtained from Aroclor 1254-pretreated rats.

Table 20. *Mutagenicity of 3- and 4-rings-containing thiaarenes in* Salmonella typhimurium *strains TA 98 and TA 100 with and without S9-mix (Standard Ames plate test. S9-mix was obtained from Aroclor-induced Sprague-Dawley rats)* (*Pelroy* et al.,*1983; McFall* et al., *1984*)

Compound	µg/plate	TA 98		TA 100	
		+S9	−S9	+S9	−S9
Dibenzothiophene	0	101 ± 17	85 ± 8	221 ± 20	221 ± 20
	164	126 ± 14	80 ± 10	284 ± 21*	304 ± 21*
	328	88 ± 4	83 ± 3	294 ± 34*	294 ± 34*
1-Methyldibenzothiophene***	0	38 ± 1	—	—	—
	10	40 ± 17	—	—	—
	100	42 ± 5	—	—	—
2-Methyldibenzothiophene***	0	30–2	—	—	—
	10	30 ± 1	—	—	—
	100	24 ± 2	—	—	—
3-Methyldibenzothiophene***	0	30 ± 2	—	—	—
	10	16 ± 2	—	—	—
	100	22 ± 4	—	—	—
4-Methyldibenzothiophene***	0	40 ± 5	—	—	—
	10	40 ± 5	—	—	—
	100	45 ± 6	—	—	—
Naphtho[2,3-*b*]thiophene	0	62 ± 6	85 ± 8	223 ± 16	221 ± 29
	100	18 ± 2	—	165 ± 21	—
	200	66 ± 8	76 ± 10*	222 ± 32	228 ± 18*
Naphtho[2,1-*b*]thiophene	0	62 ± 6	32 ± 6	223 ± 16	221 ± 20
	100	49 ± 14	23 ± 1*	157 ± 3	167 ± 11*
	200	41 ± 4	21 ± 0**	173 ± 23	152 ± 12**
Naphtho[1,2-*b*]thiophene	0	34 ± 4	32 ± 0	217 ± 19	221 ± 20
	100	186 ± 50	—	1185 ± 11	174 ± 10*
Benzo[*b*]naphtho[2,3-*d*]-thiophene	0	31 ± 2	38 ± 2	193 ± 13	221 ± 0
	100	34 ± 2	42 ± 1*	220 ± 3	231 ± 15*
	200	36 ± 9	27 ± 4	170 ± 1	218 ± 12
1-Methylbenzo[*b*]naphtho-[2,3-*b*]thiophene***	0	40 ± 8	—	—	—
	10	38 ± 4	—	—	—
	100	60 ± 15	—	—	—
2-Methylbenzo[*b*]naphtho-[2,3-*b*]thiophene***	0	40 ± 8	—	—	—
	10	35 ± 6	—	—	—
	100	40 ± 12	—	—	—
3-Methylbenzo[*b*]naphtho-[2,3-*b*]thiophene***	0	40 ± 8	—	—	—
	10	46 ± 0	—	—	—
	100	32 ± 8	—	—	—
4-Methylbenzo[*b*]naphtho-[2,3-*b*]thiophene***	0	42 ± 5	—	—	—
	10	54 ± 1	—	—	—
	100	106 ± 20	—	—	—
6-Methylbenzo[*b*]naphtho-[2,3-*b*]thiophene***	0	42 ± 5	—	—	—
	10	37 ± 6	—	—	—
	100	45 ± 4	—	—	—
7-Methylbenzo[*b*]naphtho-[2,3-*b*]thiophene***	0	42 ± 5	—	—	—
	10	42 ± 1	—	—	—
	100	34 ± 8	—	—	—

Table 20 (*cont.*)

Compound	µg/plate	TA 98 +S9	TA 98 −S9	TA 100 +S9	TA 100 −S9
8-Methylbenzo[b]naphtho-[2,3-b]thiophene***	0	39 ± 7	—	—	—
	10	28 ± 3	—	—	—
	100	46 ± 5	—	—	—
9-Methylbenzo[b]naphtho-[2,3-b]thiophene***	0	39 ± 7	—	—	—
	10	44 ± 5	—	—	—
	100	33 ± 4	—	—	—
10-Methylbenzo[b]naphtho-[2,3-b]thiophene***	0	39 ± 7	—	—	—
	10	39 ± 3	—	—	—
	100	43 ± 7	—	—	—
11-Methylbenzo[b]naphtho-[2,3-b]thiophene***	0	27 ± 1	—	—	—
	10	46 ± 7	—	—	—
	100	32 ± 8	—	—	—
Anthra[1,2-b]thiophene	0	34 ± 2	38 ± 2	193 ± 13	221 ± 20
	100	77 ± 19	31 ± 5*	415 ± 23	231 ± 15*
	200	104 ± 4	36 ± 4**	416 ± 10	218 ± 11**
Anthra[2,1-b]thiophene	0	34 ± 2	38 ± 2	193 ± 13	221 ± 20
	100	54 ± 5	23 ± 4*	639 ± 6	276 ± 6
	200	110 ± 3	34 ± 5**	584 ± 28	235 ± 36*
Anthra[2,3-b]thiophene	0	39 ± 9	32 ± 7	185 ± 14	180 ± 20
	100	115 ± 23	52 ± 7	409 ± 104	212 ± 20
	200	125 ± 10	40 ± 2	611 ± 3	195 ± 0
Benzo[b]naphtho[1,2-d]-thiophene	0	36 ± 1	32 ± 0	217 ± 19	221 ± 20
	100	26 ± 2	27 ± 4*	186 ± 4	259 ± 11*
	200	24 ± 7	35 ± 13**	164 ± 21	247 ± 10**
1-Methylbenzo[b]naphtho-[1,2-d]thiophene***	0	38 ± 1	—	—	—
	10	42 ± 1	—	—	—
	100	108 ± 7	—	—	—
2-Methylbenzo[b]naphtho-[1,2-d]thiophene***	0	40 ± 1	—	—	—
	10	26 ± 13	—	—	—
	100	24 ± 11	—	—	—
3-Methylbenzo[b]naphtho-[1,2-d]thiophene***	0	38 ± 1	—	—	—
	10	54 ± 2	—	—	—
	100	151 ± 1	—	—	—
4-Methylbenzo[b]naphtho-[1,2-d]thiophene***	0	34 ± 0	—	—	—
	10	67 ± 10	—	—	—
	100	34 ± 10	—	—	—
5-Methylbenzo[b]naphtho-[1,2-d]thiophene***	0	34 ± 0	—	—	—
	10	28 ± 3	—	—	—
	100	33 ± 1	—	—	—
6-Methylbenzo[b]naphtho-[1,2-d]thiophene***	0	36 ± 2	—	—	—
	10	42 ± 5	—	—	—
	100	42 ± 13	—	—	—
8-Methylbenzo[b]naphtho-[1,2-d]thiophene***	0	36 ± 2	—	—	—
	10	47 ± 16	—	—	—
	100	28 ± 2	—	—	—
9-Methylbenzo[b]naphtho-[1,2-d]thiophene***	0	36 ± 2	—	—	—
	10	50 ± 19	—	—	—
	100	30 ± 5	—	—	—

Table 20 (cont.)

Compound	μg/plate	TA 98		TA 100	
		+S9	−S9	+S9	−S9
10-Methylbenzo[b]naphtho-[1,2-d]thiophene***	0	27 ± 1	—	—	—
	10	22 ± 1	—	—	—
	100	25 ± 3	—	—	—
11-Methylbenzo[b]naphtho-[1,2-d]thiophene***	0	27 ± 1	—	—	—
	10	36 ± 11	—	—	—
	100	28 ± 4	—	—	—
Benzo[b]naphtho[2,1-d]thiophene	0	36 ± 1	32 ± 0	217 ± 19	221 ± 20
	100	31 ± 6	27 ± 3*	305 ± 6	260 ± 7*
	200	49 ± 2	32 ± 1**	312 ± 4	215 ± 18**
1-Methylbenzo[b]naphtho-[2,1-d]thiophene***	0	34 ± 9	—	—	—
	10	36 ± 1	—	—	—
	100	86 ± 6	—	—	—
2-Methylbenzo[b]naphtho-[2,1-d]thiophene***	0	34 ± 9	—	—	—
	10	44 ± 8	—	—	—
	100	52 ± 9	—	—	—
3-Methylbenzo[b]naphtho-[2,1-d]thiophene***	0	26 ± 3	—	—	—
	10	24 ± 3	—	—	—
	100	22 ± 9	—	—	—
4-Methylbenzo[b]naphtho-[2,1-d]thiophene***	0	26 ± 3	—	—	—
	10	26 ± 2	—	—	—
	100	32 ± 2	—	—	—
5-Methylbenzo[b]naphtho-[2,1-d]thiophene***	0	22 ± 4	—	—	—
	10	32 ± 9	—	—	—
	100	42 ± 4	—	—	—
6-Methylbenzo[b]naphtho-[2,1-d]thiophene***	0	22 ± 4	—	—	—
	10	32 ± 6	—	—	—
	100	241 ± 38	—	—	—
7-Methylbenzo[b]naphtho-[2,1-d]thiophene***	0	36 ± 2	—	—	—
	10	40 ± 1	—	—	—
	100	36 ± 4	—	—	—
8-Methylbenzo[b]naphtho-[2,1-d]thiophene***	0	40 ± 8	—	—	—
	10	50 ± 5	—	—	—
	100	62 ± 1	—	—	—
9-Methylbenzo[b]naphtho-[2,1-d]thiophene***	0	34 ± 0	—	—	—
	10	30 ± 1	—	—	—
	100	55 ± 3	—	—	—
10-Methylbenzo[b]naphtho-[2,1-d]thiophene***	0	40 ± 8	—	—	—
	10	41 ± 10	—	—	—
	100	35 ± 6	—	—	—
Phenanthro[2,3-b]thiophene	0	62 ± 6	32 ± 0	217 ± 19	221 ± 20
	100	59 ± 5	27 ± 3*	244 ± 4	207 ± 7*
	200	50 ± 5	32 ± 1**	244 ± 3	166 ± 8**
Phenanthro[3,2-b]thiophene	0	62 ± 6	32 ± 0	223 ± 16	221 ± 20
	100	76 ± 12	32 ± 3*	271 ± 11	232 ± 26*
	200	67 ± 9	27 ± 2**	269 ± 4	221 ± 2**
Phenanthro[1,2-b]thiophene	0	62 ± 6	32 ± 0	223 ± 16	221 ± 20
	100	49 ± 1	34 ± 2*	197 ± 5	238 ± 4*
	200	60 ± 1	32 ± 7**	224 ± 6	227 ± 12**

Table 20 (*cont.*)

Compound	μg/plate	TA 98 + S9	TA 98 − S9	TA 100 + S9	TA 100 − S9
Phenanthro[2,1-*b*]thiophene	0	62 ± 2	32 ± 0	223 ± 16	221 ± 20
	100	61 ± 5	30 ± 4*	278 ± 26	280 ± 12*
	200	50 ± 10	27 ± 0**	285 ± 9	26 ± 1**
Phenanthro[3,4-*b*]thiophene	0	99 ± 10	85 ± 8	223 ± 16	221 ± 20
	2	—	—	386 ± 92	—
	4	—	—	907 ± 397	—
	8	—	—	1585 ± 25	—
	10	—	—	1277 ± 243	—
	11	412 ± 15	70 ± 5	—	—
	20	—	—	1158 ± 19	—
	22	741 ± 22	75 ± 2	—	—
	25	—	—	—	215 ± 10
	50	—	—	681 ± 50	201 ± 5
Phenanthro[4,3-*b*]thiophene	0	62 ± 6	85 ± 8	223 ± 16	221 ± 20
	100	14 ± 1	81 ± 10*	256 ± 8	127 ± 12*
	200	30 ± 3	95 ± 5**	219 ± 44	112 ± 0**
Phenanthro[9,10-*b*]thiophene	0	62 ± 6	85 ± 8	223 ± 16	221 ± 20
	100	62 ± 3	71 ± 9*	224 ± 3	232 ± 45*
	200	55 ± 3	77 ± 7**	216 ± 34	228 ± 7**

* 250μg/plate; ** 500 μg/plate; *** all with 20% S9 mix; — = no data available.

extrapolated to polycyclic aromatic hydrocarbons since both of the aforementioned thiaarenes are isosteric to benzo[*c*]phenanthrene which is a moderate mutagen (Croisey-Delcey *et al.*, 1979). Among those compounds being isosteric to the weakly mutagenic benz[*a*]anthracene (anthra[1,2-*b*]thiophene, anthra[2,1-*b*]thiophene, benzo[*b*]naphtho[2,3-*d*]thiophene, phenanthro[2,3-*b*]thiophene, phenanthro[3,2-*b*]thiophene) as well as among those being isosteric to the weak mutagen chrysene (benzo[*b*]naphtho[2,1-*d*]thiophene, phenanthro[1,2-*b*]thiophene, phenanthro[2,1-*b*]thiophene) great variations of mutagenicity are found. Several of the various methyl derivatives of benzo[*b*]naphtho[1,2-*d*]-, -[2,1-*d*]- and -[2,3-*d*]thiophene were found to be mutagenic. The most potent of this group was 6-methyl-benzo[*b*]naphtho[2,1-*d*]thiophene; others were 1-methyl- and 3-methyl-benzo[*b*]naphtho[1,2-*d*]thiophene, 1-methyl-benzo[*b*]naphtho[2,1-*d*]thiophene and 4-methyl-benzo[*b*]naphtho[2,3-*d*]thiophene. It is noteworthy that 6-methyl-benzo[*b*]naphtho[2,1-*d*]thiophene is isosteric to the potent mutagen and carcinogen 5-methylchrysene. Out of all methylchrysenes this compound also exhibits the most pronounced biological activity. On the other hand, no correspondence can be observed in case of benzo[*b*]naphtho[2,3-*d*]thiophene

Table 21. *Mutagenicity of some 3-, 4-, and 5-rings-containing thiaarenes in microbial test systems (Karcher et al., 1981)*

Compound	μg/plate	TA 98*	TA 100*	PKM 101*
Control	—	36(21)	85(72)	35(47)
Dibenzothiophene	1	27(17)	67(45)	56(28)
	5	27(17)	69(46)	61(29)
	10	30(17)	72(48)	61(29)
	20	30(15)	78(45)	63(30)
Phenanthro[4,5-*bcd*]thiophene	0.5	73(27)	86(74)	93(70)
	1	85(22)	92(84)	84(68)
	2	81(23)	83(67)	78(65)
	5	51(17)	78(64)	75(65)
Benzo[*b*]naphtho[2,1-*d*]-	1	37(11)	63(46)	23(12)
thiophene	5	40(13)	72(47)	25(12)
	10	44(12)	79(46)	24(13)
	20	48(14)	82(48)	26(11)
Benzo[2,3]phenanthro[4,5-*bcd*]-	0.5	122(14)	150(63)	95(47)
thiophene	1	206(13)	241(55)	176(57)
	2	220(11)	248(56)	190(50)
	5	141(10)	247(51)	121(52)
Triphenyleno[1,12-*bcd*]-	1	38(22)	64(44)	35(18)
thiophene	5	41(24)	69(46)	43(16)
	10	42(23)	71(46)	45(18)
	20	44(24)	73(46)	50(16)
Dinaphtho[2,1-*b*:1,2'-*d*]-	1	32(21)	49(41)	30(17)
thiophene	5	35(19)	58(42)	38(16)
	10	36(22)	63(43)	40(15)
	20	37(22)	78(48)	43(17)
Benzo[*a*]pyrene	0.5	78	93	65
(positive control)	1	117	134	96
	2	277	407	138
Aflatoxin B$_1$	1	850	902	440

All data given are averages of 3–5 determinations. Values in parentheses refer to revertents observed in the absence of NADP.
* TA 98 and TA 100 = *S. typhimurium*; PKM 101 = *E.coli.*

and its isoster benz[*a*]anthracene. The most active compounds are 7- and 12-methyl-benz[*a*]anthracene being isosteric to 6- and 11-methylbenzo[*b*]naphtho[2,3-*d*]thiophene for both of which no mutagenic effect could be found. If there be *any* correlation between the chemical structure of polycyclic aromatic hydrocarbons and thiaarenes and their mutagenic potentials it is most complex and not yet understood.

Benzo[2,3]phenanthro[4,5-*bcd*]thiophene exhibits an outstanding mutagenic activity exceeding even that of benzo[*a*]pyrene to which it is the homocyclic isoster (Karcher *et al.*, 1981). Grünbauer and Wegener (1983) carried out Hückel molecular orbital calculations (HMO) for benzo[*a*]pyrene and some thiaarene isosters trying to explain the comparatively high mutagenic potential of benzo[2,3]phenanthro[4,5-*bcd*]thiophene. They also predicted a mutagenic potency of benzo[4,5]phenaleno[1,9-*bc*]thiophene on the base of similar metabolic pathways for thiaarenes and polycyclic aromatic hydrocarbons. However, as is shown in Section 1.8 the metabolism of both classes of compounds does not follow the same routes since the predominant primary metabolites of thiaarenes in rat liver are sulfones, not phenols and dihydrodiols as are found with hydrocarbons.

Table 22 presents data on the mutagenicity of some sulfoxides, sulfones, and of a quinone which have been identified as metabolites of the corresponding thiaarenes (dibenzothiophene, benzo[*b*]naphtho[1,2-*d*]thiophene, benzo[*b*]naphtho[2,1-*d*]thiophene, benzo[*b*]naphtho[2,3-*d*]thiophene, and triphenyleno[1,12-*bcd*]thiophene) (Jacob *et al.*, 1987*a*).

No mutagenicity was observed in case of dibenzothiophene, triphenyleno[1,12-*bcd*]thiophene, the three isomeric benzonaphthothiophenes, benzo[*b*]naphtho[2,3-*d*]thiophene-6,11-quinone, and the sulfones of benzo[*b*]naphtho[1,2-*d*]- and -[2,3-*d*]thiophene. Weakly mutagenic were all five sulfoxides tested and dibenzothiophenesulfone, whereas benzo[*b*]naphtho[2,1-*d*]thiophene sulfone was found to be a potent mutagen (Jacob *et al.*, 1987*a*).

Recently also some azadibenzothiophenes (1-, 2-, 3-, and 4-azadibenzothiophene) have been tested for mutagenicity in *S. typhimurium* strain TA 98 and were found to be inactive (Nishioka *et al.*, 1986*c*) in contrast to aminodibenzothiophenes which were active in the same strain (Nishioka *et al.*, 1985*c*).

1.7.3 Carcinogenicity

The carcinogenicity of thiaarenes has not yet been studied systematically. It has been observed, however, that the carcinogenic potency of crude oil fractions may depend on their sulfur content. Desulfuration of such fractions decreased their biological activity and resulfuration could partially or completely restore it (Horton *et al.*, 1963, 1965; Bingham and Horton, 1966). Tilak (1960) reported on the carcinogenic potencies of various 4- and 5-rings-containing thiaarenes, and since then no fundamental and comparative investigation of this subject has been published. Tilak compared the carcinogenic potential of a number of thiaarenes which are isosteric to 7,12-dimethylbenz[*a*]anthracene, dibenz[*a,h*]anthracene, 7,14-dimethyldibenz[*a,h*]anthracene, dibenz[*a,j*]anthracene, 7,14-dimethyldibenz[*a,j*]anthracene, benzo[*c*]phe-

Table 22. *Mutagenicity of some thiaarene metabolites* (*sulfoxides, sulfones, quinones*) *in* S. typhimurium *strains TA 98 and TA 100 with and without S9-mix* (*Jacob* et al., *1987*a)

Compound	Dose (μg/plate)	Revertants/plate			
		TA 98		TA 100	
		+S9	−S9	+S9	−S9
Dibenzothiophene	0	25±2	19±2	127±3	96±6
	1	20±2	20±1	111±10	95±5
	5	21±1	16±2	116±6	106±3
	25	21±3	15±2	126±6	107±7
	125	21±1	14±1	123±3	102±5
Dibenzothiophene-5-oxide	0	29±2	21±2	139±2	106±4
	1	36±3	22±1	144±1	127±4
	5	34±1	24±1	152±3	122±2
	25	30±3	20±1	155±2	127±4
	125	28±1	21±2	156±3	120±1
Dibenzothiophene-5,5-dioxide	0	32±3	16±2	117±4	97±1
	1	39±1	20±1	115±2	129±2
	5	34±3	17±1	126±1	136±3
	25	28±1	14±1	133±1	150±1
	125	19±1	11±1	146±1	168±2
Benzo[*b*]naphtho[1,2-*d*]-thiophene	0	37±1	24±2	147±4	107±3
	1	58±3	30±3	164±3	142±4
	5	41±3	29±2	155±3	131±6
	25	36±1	26±3	150±7	119±1
	125	34±1	22±1	143±9	114±4
Benzo[*b*]naphtho[1,2-*d*]-thiophene-7-oxide	0	42±1	33±2	148±2	104±2
	1	49±3	32±1	152±1	95±2
	5	42±3	31±3	173±2	73±1
	25	34±1	27±1	194±3	40±3
	125	30±1	25±1	227±7	15±1
Benzo[*b*]naphtho[1,2-*d*]-thiophene-7,7-dioxide	0	36±4	27±3	142±5	105±5
	1	31±2	36±1	123±2	112±1
	5	34±3	26±2	106±2	129±3
	25	50±2	27±1	119±3	123±6
	125	46±1	29±3	110±10	134±4
Benzo[*b*]naphtho[2,1-*d*]-thiophene	0	37±1	24±2	147±4	107±3
	1	47±1	30±2	149±5	165±6
	5	41±2	29±3	137±5	106±5
	25	38±2	24±1	177±5	117±5
	125	37±3	21±2	197±6	122±2
Benzo[*b*]naphtho[2,1-*d*]-thiophene-11-oxide	0	42±2	33±2	148±2	104±2
	1	54±2	36±2	143±2	146±3
	5	45±3	34±3	143±2	164±3
	25	45±1	32±2	183±3	176±2
	125	33±3	31±1	224±5	180±2
Benzo[*b*]naphtho[2.1-*d*]-thiophene-11,11-dioxide	0	36±4	27±3	142±5	105±5
	1	34±5	103±2	137±5	138±3
	5	35±2	105±3	131±3	127±3

Table 22 (*cont.*)

Compound	Dose (µg/plate)	TA 98 +S9	TA 98 −S9	TA 100 +S9	TA 100 −S9
	25	43 ± 1	109 ± 7	120 ± 4	131 ± 2
	125	39 ± 2	90 ± 7	125 ± 3	131 ± 4
Benzo[*b*]naphtho[2,3-*d*]-thiophene	0	37 ± 1	24 ± 2	147 ± 4	107 ± 3
	1	55 ± 2	37 ± 1	169 ± 1	126 ± 5
	5	40 ± 0	27 ± 2	158 ± 5	113 ± 5
	25	40 ± 1	29 ± 1	144 ± 7	104 ± 5
	125	24 ± 2	21 ± 3	134 ± 5	98 ± 6
Benzo[*b*]naphtho[2,3-*d*]-thiophene-5-oxide	0	42 ± 2	33 ± 2	148 ± 2	104 ± 2
	1	61 ± 2	55 ± 1	143 ± 5	137 ± 4
	5	47 ± 2	43 ± 3	149 ± 4	152 ± 4
	25	43 ± 4	33 ± 4	156 ± 3	153 ± 2
	125	38 ± 2	33 ± 1	175 ± 5	166 ± 2
Benzo[*b*]naphtho[2,3-*d*]-thiophene-5,5-dioxide	0	36 ± 4	27 ± 3	142 ± 5	105 ± 5
	1	56 ± 3	30 ± 4	138 ± 2	127 ± 6
	5	48 ± 6	30 ± 3	136 ± 1	154 ± 3
	25	45 ± 3	31 ± 3	129 ± 1	122 ± 5
	125	46 ± 4	25 ± 3	110 ± 3	122 ± 6
Benzo[*b*]naphtho[2,3-*d*]-thiophene-6,11-quinone	0	33 ± 3	19 ± 1	127 ± 4	94 ± 5
	1	31 ± 2	19 ± 1	168 ± 2	122 ± 3
	5	36 ± 1	23 ± 3	146 ± 9	117 ± 4
	25	37 ± 3	26 ± 2	124 ± 6	113 ± 3
	125	40 ± 1	36 ± 1	124 ± 6	111 ± 3
Triphenylene[1,12-*bcd*]-thiophene	0	34 ± 3	23 ± 3	112 ± 5	101 ± 6
	1	40 ± 1	24 ± 2	110 ± 3	118 ± 5
	5	30 ± 1	28 ± 0	118 ± 1	131 ± 4
	25	29 ± 1	21 ± 2	118 ± 2	109 ± 1
	125	27 ± 2	20 ± 1	104 ± 3	105 ± 4
Triphenylene[1,12-*bcd*]-thiophene-4-oxide	0	34 ± 1	19 ± 1	142 ± 3	116 ± 3
	1	50 ± 1	38 ± 1	122 ± 4	105 ± 4
	5	52 ± 1	38 ± 2	146 ± 2	127 ± 2
	25	46 ± 1	35 ± 1	155 ± 2	144 ± 3
	125	54 ± 1	37 ± 2	179 ± 3	152 ± 3

nanthrene, chrysene, and benzo[*c*]chrysene. For instance, 7,11-dimethyl-phenanthro[2,3-*b*]thiophene, and 6,11-dimethylanthra[1,2-*b*]thiophene were found to be potent carcinogens, whereas 6,11-dimethylbenzo[*b*]naphtho[2,3-*d*]thiophene proved to be only slightly active in the mouse skin painting assay and inactive by subcutaneous injection (Hartwell, 1951). Two isosters of the very potent carcinogen dibenz[*a,h*]anthracene, namely benzo[*b*]phenanthro[2,3-*d*]thiophene and benzo[1,2-*b*:4,5-*b*′]bis[1]benzothiophene, were found to be inactive (Waravdekar and Ranadive, 1957).

However, isosters of 7,14-dimethyldibenz[*a,h*]anthracene, namely 7,13-dimethylbenzo[*b*]phenanthro[2,3-*d*]thiophene and 6,12-dimethylbenzo-[1,2-*b*:4,5-*b'*]bis[1]benzothiophene exhibited strong carcinogenic activities (Tilak, 1951*a,b*; Waravdekar and Ranadive, 1957; Ranadive and Mashelkar, 1972). Dinaphtho[2,1-*b*:1',2'-*d*]thiophene, an isoster of the the moderately active carcinogen dibenz[*a,j*]anthracene, was found to be inactive (Rabindran and Tilak, 1953*c*), and two isosters of 7,14-dimethyldibenz[*a,j*]anthracene were found to be strong carcinogens, namely 7,13-dimethylbenzo[*b*]phenanthro[3,2-*d*]thiophene and 6,12-benzo[1,2-*b*:5,4-*b'*]bis[1]benzothiophene (Tilak, 1951*a,b*; Waravdekar and Ranadive, 1957). Naphtho[2,1-*b*:7,8-*b'*]dithiophene, [1]benzothieno[2,3-*b*][1]benzothiophene and benzo[*b*]naphtho[1,2-*d*]thiophene, all of which are isosteric to the moderately carcinogenic benzo[*c*]phenanthrene, were found to be inactive (Waravdekar and Ranadive, 1957; Ranadive *et al.*, 1963; Dannenberg, 1960; Hartwell, 1951). Two isosters of the weak carcinogen chrysene were also inactive as carcinogens, [1]benzothieno[3,2-*b*][1]benzothiophene (Waravdekar and Ranadive, 1957) and naphtho[2,1-*b*:6,5-*b'*]dithiophene, whereas there are contradictory results on a third isoster, benzo[*b*]naphtho[2,1-*d*]thiophene for which negative (Hartwell, 1951; Waravdekar and Ranadive, 1957) and positive responses (Croisy *et al.*, 1984) in animal test systems have been reported. In a recent study a carcinogenic potential of this thiaarene comparable to that of chrysene has been found, when applied by injection into the lung of rats (Brune and Deutsch-Wenzel, 1986).

After subcutaneous injection dinaphtho[1,2-*b*:1',2'-*d*]thiophene, being isosteric to benzo[*c*]chrysene, was found to be active (Tilak, 1960). Zajdela and coworkers (referred to in Croisy *et al.*, 1984) have tested some thiaarenes for carcinogenicity by subcutaneous injection into mice. They found that benzo[*b*]naphtho[2,1-*d*]thiophene (isosteric to chrysene), benzo[*b*]phenanthro[3,4-*d*]thiophene (isosteric to benzo[*c*]chrysene), benzo[*b*]phenanthro[3,2-*d*]thiophene (isosteric to dibenz[*a,h*]anthracene), and benzo[*b*]phenanthro[2,3-*d*]thiophene (isosteric to dibenz[*a,h*]anthracene) were more potent carcinogens than their carbocyclic isosters. The structures of the thiaarenes tested and those of their carbocyclic isosters are given in Fig. 10.

As emphasized for the mutagenic effect, no simple correlation between the carcinogenic potential of carbocyclic systems and of their isosteric thiaarenes exists. Further systematic investigations on the biological testing and on the metabolism of thiaarenes are required before comparative conclusions on the structure-dependence of carcinogenicity can be

Fig. 10. Thiaarenes and their carbocyclic isosters which have been tested for carcinogenicity.

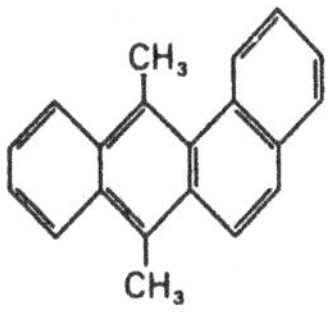

(+++)*

7,12-Dimethylbenz[a]anthracene

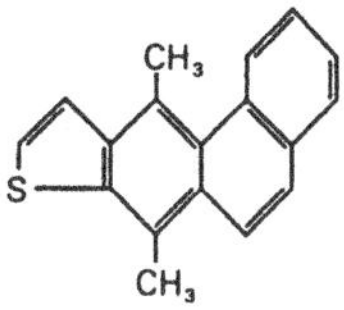

(++)

7,11-Dimethylphenanthro[2, 3-b]thiophene

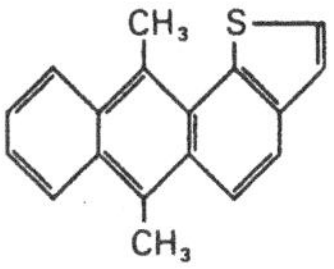

(++)

6,11-Dimethylanthra[1,2-b]thiophene

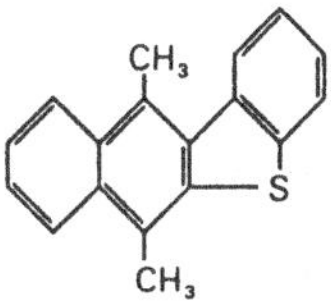

(+)

6,11-Dimethylbenzo[b]naphtho[2,3-d]thiophene

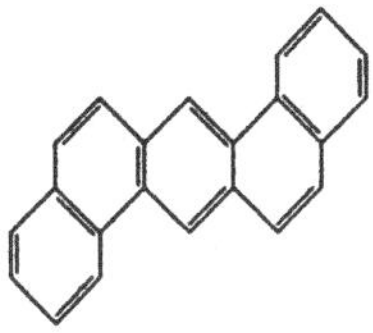

(+++)

Dibenz[a, h]anthracene

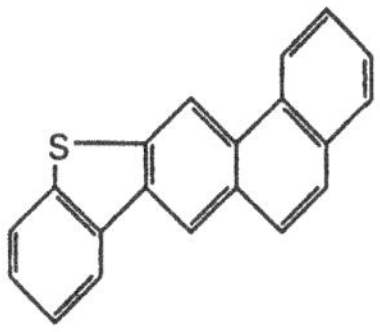

(-)

Benzo[b]phenanthro[2,3-d]thiophene

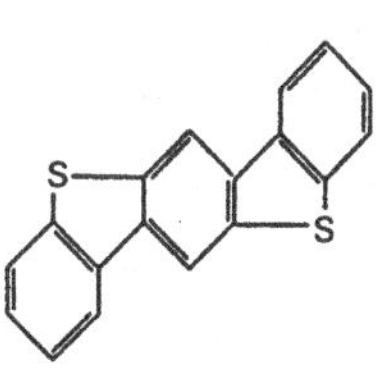

(-)

Benzo[1,2-b : 4,5-b']bis[1]benzothiophene

(*continued*)

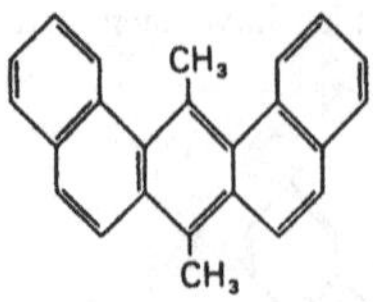

(+)

7,14-Dimethyldibenz[*a, h*]anthracene

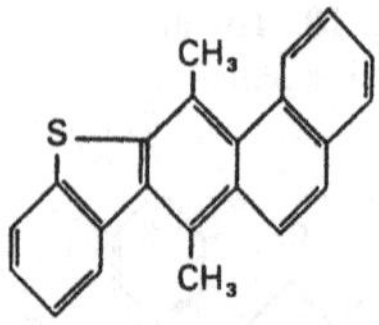

(+)

7,13-Dimethylbenzo[*b*]phenanthro
[2, 3-*d*]thiophene

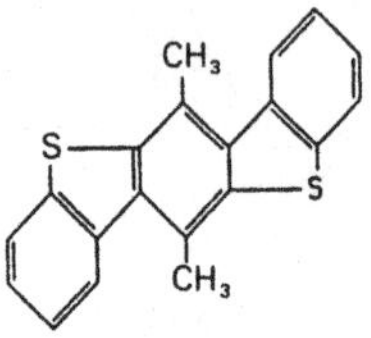

(+ +)

6,12-Dimethylbenzo[1,2-*b* : 4, 5-*b′*]
bis[1]benzothiophene

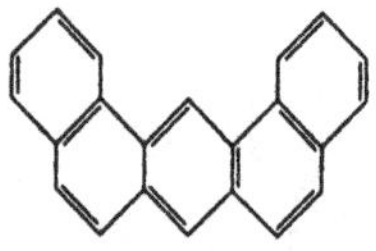

(+ +)

Dibenz[*a, j*]anthracene

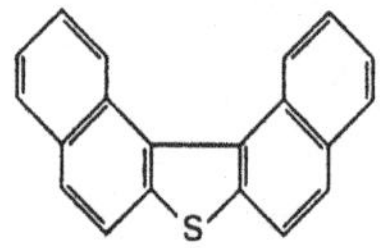

(−)

Dinaphtho[2,1-*b* : 1′,2′-*d*]thiophene

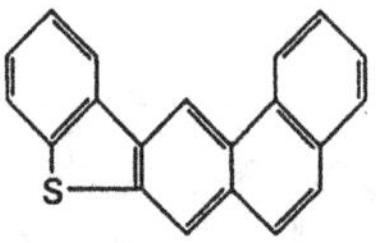

(?)

Benzo[*b*]phenanthro[3,2-*d*]thiophene

(+)

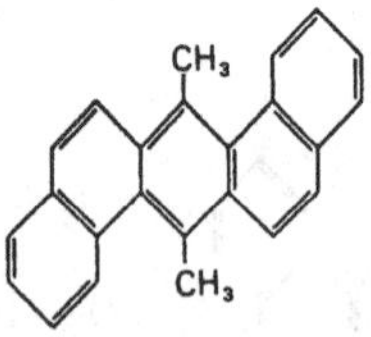

7,14-Dimethyldibenz[*a, j*]anthracene

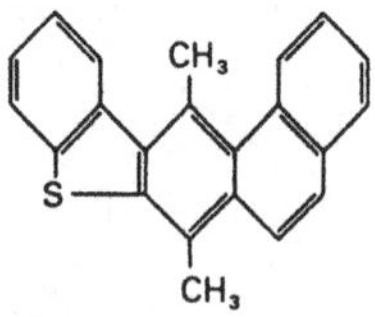

(++)

7,13-Dimethylbenzo[*b*]phenanthro
[3,2-*d*]thiophene

(*continued*)

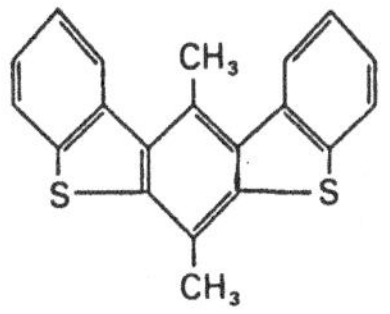

6,12-Dimethylbenzo[*1, 2-b* : 5, 4-*b'*]
bis[1]benzothiophene

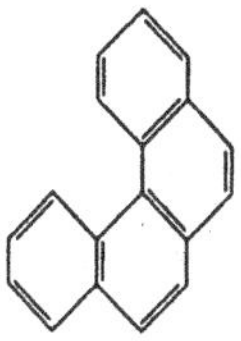

(++)

(+/++)

Benzo[*c*]phenanthrene

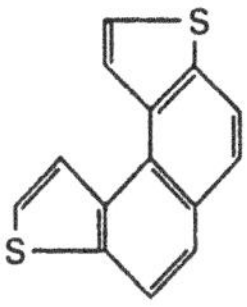

(-)

Naphtho[2, 1-*b* : 7, 8-*b'*]dithiophene

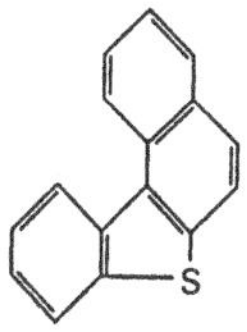

(-)

Benzo[*b*]naphtho[1, 2-*d*]thiophene

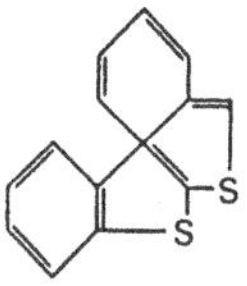

(-)

[1]Benzothieno[2,3-*b*][1]benzothiophene

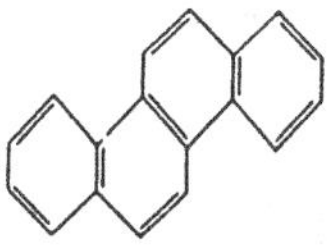

(+)

Chyrsene

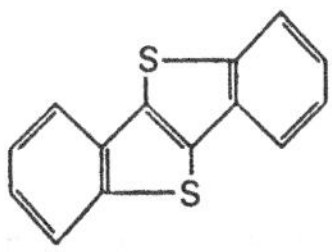

(-)

[1]Benzothieno[3, 2-*b*][1]benzothiophene

(continued)

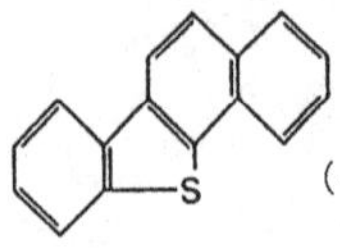

(-/+)

Benzo[*b*]naphtho[2,1-*d*]thiophene

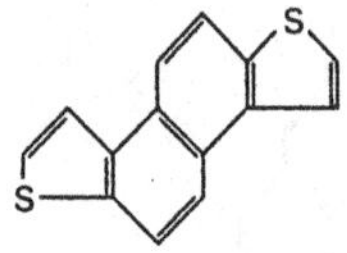

(-)

Naphtho [2, 1-*b*: 6, 5-*b'*]dithiophene

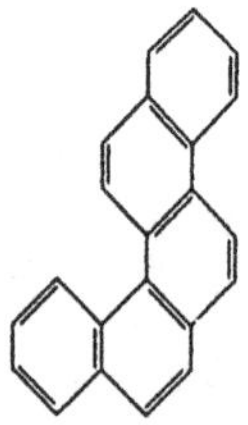

(++)

Benzo[*c*]chrysene

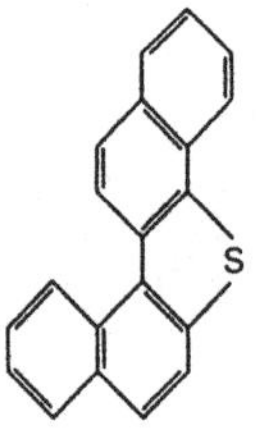

(+)

Dinaphtho[1, 2-*b*: 1',2' -*d*]thiophene

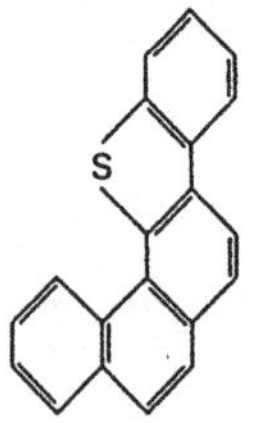

(++)

Benzo[*b*]phenanthro[3,4-*d*]thiophene

* + + + = very potent carcinogen; + + = potent carcinogen; + = weak or moderate carcinogen;
— = inactive. Where two designations are given contradictory data exist in the literature.

drawn. Many thiaarene systems have been prepared during the last decade, providing an excellent potential for future biological experiments.

1.7.4 Other biological effects

It has been reported that dibenzothiophene may influence the hatchability of *Artemia* eggs (Kuwabara *et al.*, 1980) and that it inhibits the mitochondrial phosphorylation in goldfish liver (Ogata and Hasegawa, 1982). Wofford and Neff (1978) provided data on the median lethal concentration (LC_{50}) in 96 h to grass shrimp (*Palaemonetes pugio*) and sheep's-head minnow (*Cyprinodon variegatus*) to be 0.28 and 3.18 ppm, respectively.

1.8 Metabolism of thiaarenes
1.8.1 Metabolic pathways

There are only a few investigations which have dealt with the metabolism of thiaarenes so this subject remains a domain for future scientific activities. Although the physico-chemical properties of thiaarenes very much resemble those of the corresponding carbocyclic isosters, their metabolic behaviour is dictated by the sensitivity of the sulfur atom to oxidation. Hence, enzymic oxidation by cytochrome P450-dependent mixed-function oxidases results predominantly in the formation of sulfoxides and sulfones rather than in the formation of ring-oxidation products such as epoxides, phenols and dihydrodiols which are observed with isosteric carbocyclic substrates.

Lu *et al.* (1978) investigated sulfoxidation in a marine model ecosystem. Vignier *et al.* (1985) and Berthou and Vignier (1986) studied the metabolism of dibenzothiophene with liver microsomes of Wistar rats pretreated with Aroclor 1254 (single dose of 500 mg/kg body weight), 3-methylcholanthrene (40 mg/day/kg b.w., 3 days), dibenzothiophene (40 mg/day/kg b.w., 3 days) and phenobarbital (80 mg/day/kg b.w., 4 days) and after HPLC separation identified dibenzothiophene-5-oxide and dibenzothiophene-5,5-dioxide by mass spectrometry. They found quantitatively high and qualitatively similar inducing rates for the monooxygenase system by three of these inducers (Aroclor 25 times, 3-methylcholanthrene 24 times, phenobarbital 26 times), whereas the induction rate by the substrate (dibenzothiophene) was found to be not significant ($f = 1.2$). More recently, Jacob *et al.* (1986*b*) studied the metabolism of 4–5 rings-containing thiaarenes (benzo[*b*]naphtho[1,2-*d*]-, -[2,1-*d*]- and -[2,3-*d*]thiophene as well as triphenyleno[1,12-*bcd*]thiophene) with liver microsomes of untreated and variously pretreated Wistar rats by means of GC/MS. They presented evidence for S-oxidation as a predominant pathway of the oxidative metabolism. Main metabolites were sulfones followed by the corresponding sulfoxides. Apart from S-oxidation also ring-oxidation was observed in the three benzonaphtho-thiophenes investigated yielding sulfone phenols. A non-κ-region dihy-drodiol was detected as a metabolite of benzo[b]naphtho[1,2-d]thiophene, and a 6,11-quinone has been identified as a metabolite of benzo[b]naphtho[2,3-d]thiophene. Induction rates after treatment with DDT (200 mg/day/kg b.w., single dose, orally) or benzo[k]fluoranthene (40 mg/day/kg b.w., for three days, intraperitoneally) were found to be 1.2–2.4 and 2.6, respectively (Table 23 and Fig. 11). No resemblance was observed between the metabolite patterns of the thiaarenes investigated and their carbocyclic isosters (benzo[c]phenanthrene, chrysene, benz[a]anthracene and benzo[e]pyrene).

In a study of the stereochemistry of sulfoxide formation during the enzymic oxidation of a number of diaryl-, alkyl- and dialkyl sulfides with liver microsomes of phenobarbital-induced rats Takata *et al.* (1983) found that the oxidation takes place at the less-hindered side of the sulfide to optically active sulfoxides, e.g. enzymic oxidation of *trans*-thiadecalines and 4-(*p*-chlorophenyl)thiane resulted in equatorial sulfoxides. They also studied the cytochrome P450-dependent oxidation of 2-methyl-2,3-dihydrobenzo[b]thiophene to four stereoisomeric sulfoxides. Fukushima *et al.* (1978), Takahasi *et al.* (1978), and Watanabe *et al.* (1981a) studied the S-oxidation and S-dealkylation of sulfides as model compounds by a reconstituted cytochrome P450 system and later Watanabe *et al.* (1981b) investigated the oxidation of thioanisole derivatives by a reconstituted system of purified cytochrome P450 from rabbit liver catalyzing S-oxidation of this substrate. Their results suggested that the S-oxidation of sulfides is initiated by one-electron transfer to the active species of the enzyme which they formulated as:

$$\text{Aryl}-\overset{\cdot\cdot}{\text{S}}-\text{CH}_3 \longrightarrow \text{Aryl}-\overset{+}{\text{S}}-\text{CH}_3 + (\text{FeO})^{2+} \longrightarrow \text{Aryl}-\overset{\text{O}}{\underset{\uparrow}{\text{S}}}-\text{CH}_3 + \text{Fe}^{3+}$$

$$e^- \searrow$$

$$\text{Cyt P450(Fe O)}^{3+}$$

At least for acyclic sulfoxide substrates, Tatsumi *et al.* (1983) provided evidence that liver aldehyde oxidase (EC 1.2.3.1) from rabbits and guinea pigs catalyzes the reduction of sulfoxides to sulfides. It is not yet proven, however, whether this holds also for thiaarene sulfoxides.

In a series of papers Jacob *et al.* (1983, 1986a, 1987b), Norpoth *et al.* (1984), and Kemena *et al.* (1987) demonstrated that benzo[b]naphtho[1,2-d]- and [2,1-d]thiophene are weak to moderate inducers of the mon-

Table 23. *Metabolites of benzo[b]naphtho[1,2-d]- [2,1-d]-, -[2,3-d] thiophene and triphenyleno[1,12-bcd]thiophene formed by liver microsomes of untreated and variously pretreated Wistar rats (Jacob et al., 1986b)*

Substrate	Pretreatment	Metabolites formed (nmol/mg microsomal protein)		
		Sulfone/sulfoxide	Sulfonephenol	Other
Benzo[b]naphtho[1,2-d]thiophene	none	9.43	2.07	—
	DDT	15.57	12.03	—
	BkF*	30.03	—	0.44**
Benzo[b]naphtho[2,1-d]thiophene	none	8.00	—	—
	DDT	7.39	4.15	—
Benzo[b]naphtho[2,3-d]thiophene	none	7.17	—	—
	DDT	6.43	—	10.49***
Triphenyleno[1,12-bcd]thiophene	none	5.16	—	—
	DDT	6.25	—	—

* BkF = benzo[k]fluoranthene; ** non-K-region dihydrodiol; *** 6,11-quinone.

Fig. 11. Structures of metabolites formed from various 4–5 rings-containing thiaarenes with rat liver microsomes (Jacob *et al.*, 1986*b*).

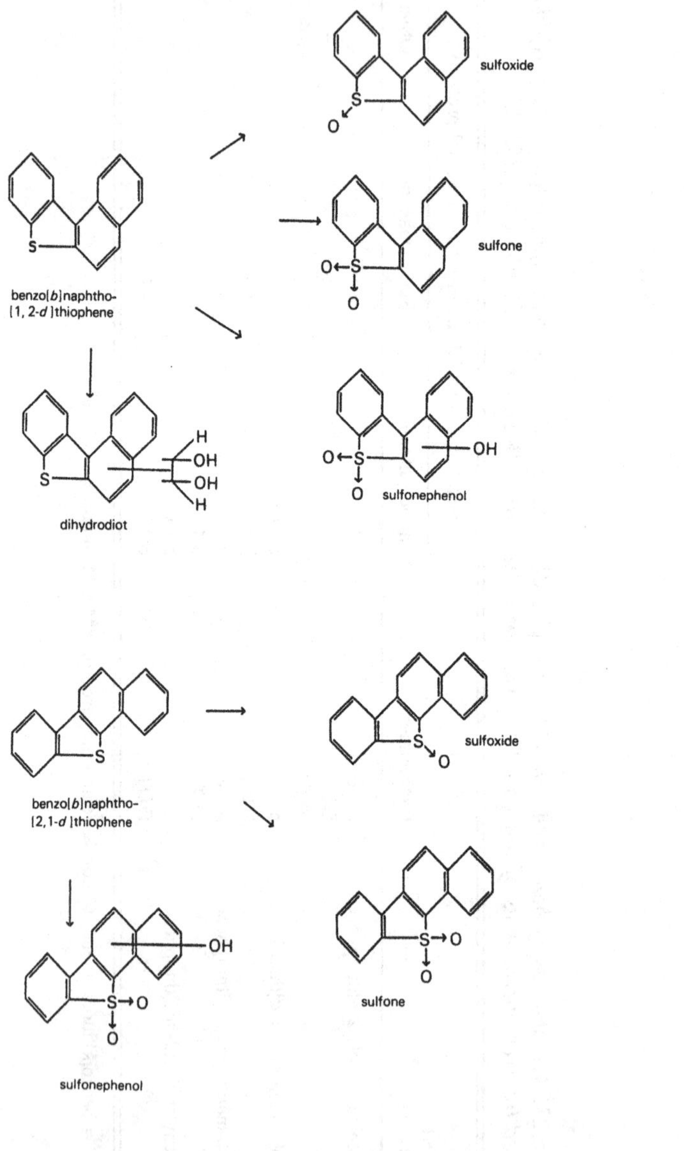

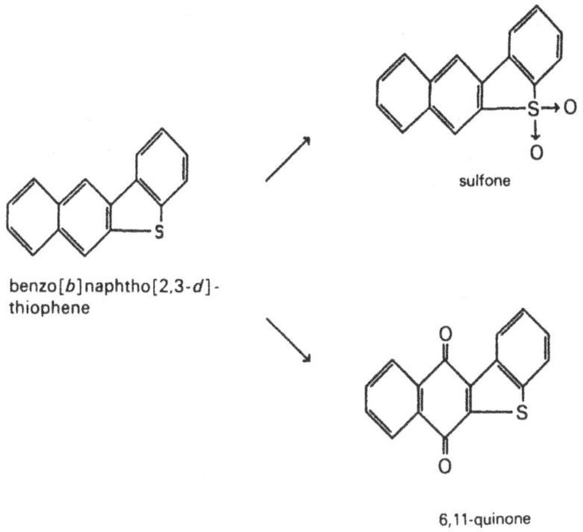

benzo[*b*]naphtho[2,3-*d*]-
thiophene

sulfone

6,11-quinone

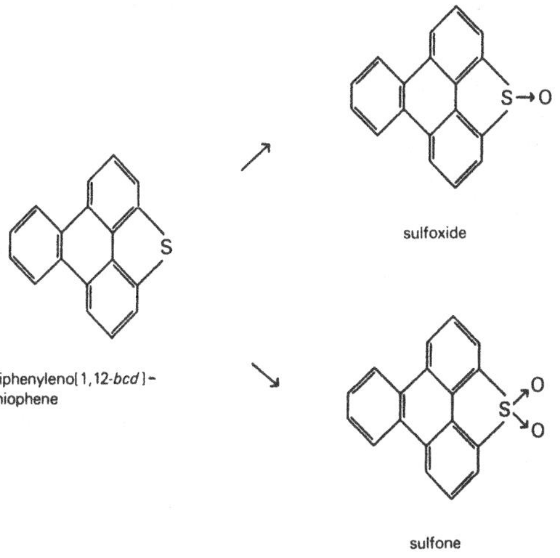

triphenyleno[1,12-*bcd*]-
thiophene

sulfoxide

sulfone

Table 24. *Induction factors for the specific oxidation of benz[a]anthracene and chrysene by liver mircosomes of thiaarene-pretreated in comparison to untreated Wistar rats (Jacob* et al., *1983, 1986, 1987*b)

Substrate	Induction with	
	Benzo[*b*]naphtho-[1,2-*d*]thiophene	Benzo[*b*]naphtho-[2,1-*d*]thiophene
Benz[a]*anthracene*		
Total turnover	1.0	1.7
5,6-Oxidation	2.5	3.8
8,8-Oxidation	1.9	3.2
10,11-Oxidation	0.4	0.5
IF(5,6/8,9)*	1.3	1.2
Chrysene		
Total turnover	5.5	3.1
1,2-Oxidation	4.7	4.8
3,4-Oxidation	4.8	2.6
IF(1,2/3,4)*	1.0	1.8

* IF(5,6/8,9) and IF(1,2/3,4) = ratio of the induction factors for the 5,6- and 8,9-oxidation of benz[*a*]anthracene and the 1,2- and 3,4-oxidation of chrysene (for structure see Fig. 12).

Fig. 12. Positions which are predominantly oxidized in chrysene and benz[*a*]anthracene with liver microsomes of Wistar rats pretreated with benzo[*b*]naphtho[1,2-*d*]- or -[2,1-*d*]thiophene.

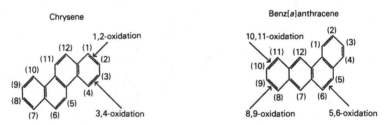

oxygenases which catalyze PAH-oxidation. They reported on the specific alterations of the metabolism of benz[*a*]anthracene and chrysene with liver microsomal preparations obtained from thiaarene-pretreated Wistar rats. In Table 24 the induction effects on the various regiospecific oxidation rates (Fig. 12) of the above PAH substrates are summarized.

The above results, although obtained with rat liver microsomes, correspond to the mutagenic response to benz[*a*]anthracene in the Ames test with *S. typhimurium* strain TA 100 using activation by S9-fractions from mice which were pretreated with benzo[*b*]naphtho-[1,2-*d*]-, -[2,1-*d*]-, or -[2,3-*d*]-thiophene. Inducing potencies measured as increase of revertant numbers were found to be 1.6 for the [1,2-*d*]-isomer and 2.8 for the [2,1-*d*]-isomer, whereas the [2,3-*d*]-isomer was found to be inactive (Norpoth *et al.*, 1984).

1.8.2 Bioaccumulation and elimination

Thiaarenes have been investigated with regard to bioaccumulation and toxicity in marine organisms (Lu *et al.*, 1978; Giddings, 1979; Nakamura and Kashimoto, 1979*b*; Neff, 1979; Ogata *et al.*, 1980*a,b*; Fink and Smith, 1936; Adlard, 1972; Vassilaros *et al.*, 1982*a*; Grahl-Nielsen *et al.*, 1978; Dillon *et al.*, 1978; VanderMeulen, 1981; Clement *et al.*, 1980; Mironov and Shchekaturina, 1981; Ogata and Miyake, 1981; Ogata and Fujisawa, 1980; Eastmond *et al.*, 1984). The transfer of benzo[*b*]thiophene and its alkylated homologues to marine organisms (Ogata *et al.*, 1980*b*, 1981*a*; Ogata and Miyake, 1978, 1979) and their enrichment by a factor of 10^3 in the mussel *Mytilus edulis* has been reported by Ogata *et al.* (1981*b*). Eastmond *et al.* (1984) showed that for benzo[*b*]thiophene bioconcentration is more pronounced than for naphthalene in the water flea *Daphnia magna*. The same holds for the isosteric pair benzo[*b*]naphtho[2,1-*d*]thiophene and chrysene (Eastmond *et al.*, 1984), whereas comparable rates of bioaccumulation in *Daphnia* were observed for the isosters phenanthrene and dibenzothiophene, both being also similar to anthracene (Eastmond *et al.*, 1984; Herbes and Risi, 1978), although their water solubilities differ almost by a factor of 10^2 (phenanthrene 1002 μg/L and anthracene 44.6 μg/L at 25–27°C) (May *et al.*, 1978). Generally speaking, it seems that thiaarenes are more bioaccumulated than their carbocyclic isosters.

Eastmond *et al.* (1984) also studied the elimination of polycyclic aromatic hydrocarbons and thiaarenes in *Daphnia*, but did not find a clear trend. Naphthalene was more rapidly eliminated than benzo[*b*]thiophene, but similar elimination rates were found for the pairs dibenzothiophene/phenanthrene and benzo[*b*]naphtho[2,1-*d*]thiophene/chrysene. The accumulation and a retarded release of dibenzothiophene and its methyl derivatives in oysters (*Crassostrea virginica*) and in mummichogs (*Fundulus heteroclitus*) have been studied by Bieri and Stamoudis (1977) and by Bieri *et al.* (1977).

Although monoxygenase activities have been extensively measured in many tissues of various organisms and the metabolism of polycyclic aromatic hydrocarbons (especially benzo[*a*]pyrene) studied, no such systematic investigation on thiaarenes have been undertaken.

The microbial degradation of dibenzothiophene by various soil and marine micro-organisms has been described (Fedorak and Westlake, 1983*b*, 1984; Foght *et al.*, 1983; Finnerty *et al.*, 1983; Kargi and Robinson, 1984). The metabolic pathways of dibenzothiophene in *Pseudomonas* species have been studied in detail (Kodama *et al.*, 1970, 1973; Koehler *et al.*, 1978; Yamada *et al.*, 1968) (see Section 2.2 under dibenzothiophene).

2

Compounds

Following the Chemical Abstract parent compounds handbook the structures are listed according to increasing ring sizes i.e. thiapyrans appear after thiophenes. Partial structures are abbreviated as C_4S standing for a thiophene, C_5S for a thiopyran, C_5 for a cyclopenta- and C_6 for a benzene ring.

2.1 Bicyclic compounds
C_4S–C_5

$$C_7H_6S \text{ (m.w.: 122)}$$

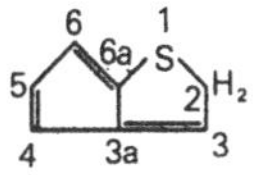

2H-cyclopenta[b]thiophene

(1)

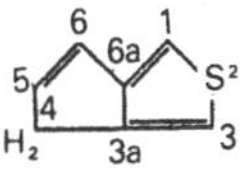

4H-cyclopenta[c]thiophene

(2)

Apart from a number of substituted thiophenes and thiacyclopentanes, some bicyclic thiophenes of the above type were detected in petroleum fractions (Birch, 1953). The [b]-isomer was found to be less stable than the [c]-isomer which has been synthesized from 1,3-dichloro-5,6-dihydro-4H-cyclopenta[c]thiophene-6-ol by treatment with p-toluenesulfonic acid (p-TSA) and subsequent dechlorination with copper powder (Skramstad, 1969):

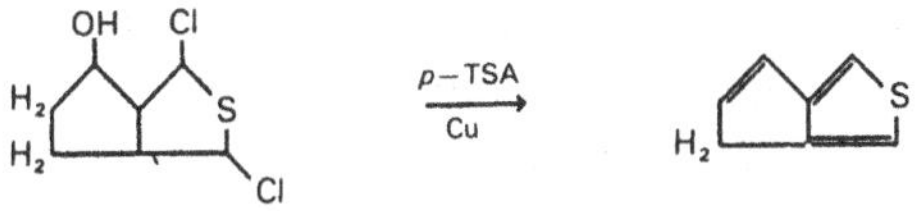

(2)

$C_4S–C_6$

Benzo[b]thiophene (syn.: 1-thiaindene; thianaphthene; thionaphthene; 1-benzothiophene; benzothiofuran)

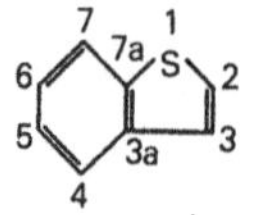

m.w.: 134 (C_8H_6S)
m.p.: 31.3°C
b.p.: 219.9°C (760 mm)

(3)

The chemistry of benzo[b]thiophene and its derivatives has been thoroughly reviewed by Hartough and Meisel (1954), Iddon and Scrowston (1970) and by Scrowston (1981). Benzo[b]thiophene or derivatives may be obtained by catalytic dehydrocyclization of 2-ethylbenzenethiols (Hansch et al., 1956) or by cyclization of arylthioacetaldehyde diethylacetales (Rabindran and Tilak, 1951b).

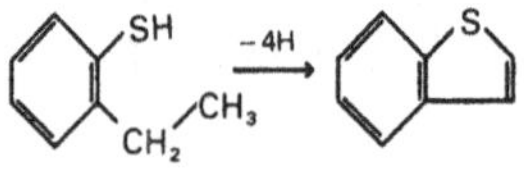

(3)

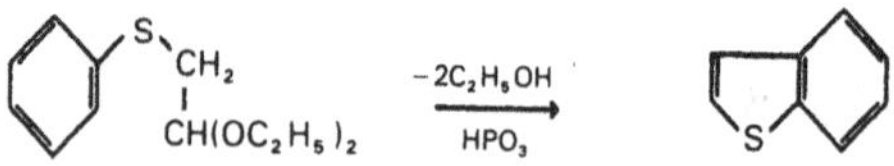

(3)

It is also formed by Al_2O_3/FeS-catalyzed reaction of styrene with H_2S in up to 63% yield (Moore and Greensfelder, 1947; Klemm et al., 1979a) and in low yield during the pyrolysis of thiophene (Fields and Meyerson, 1966).

UV spectra of benzo[b]thiophene and various of its derivatives have been published (Iddon and Scrowston, 1970; Friedel and Orchin, 1951). However, differences in the spectra from variously substituted benzo[b]thiophenes generally do not allow a definite identification of isomers in mixtures. Fluorescence- (Kharitonova, 1963), phosphorescence- (Heckman, 1959), IR- (Derkosch and Specht, 1962), mass- (Porter, 1967), ^{1}H–NMR- (Caddy et al., 1968; Chapman et al., 1968) as well as ^{13}C–NMR-spectra also have been recorded. Qualitative analysis of benzo[b]thiophenes in complex mixtures has been carried out by quasilinear luminescence spectroscopy (Akhobadze et al., 1976, 1977).

Benzo[b]thiophene tends to polymerize and therefore should be stored in the dark in a freezer. In most chemical reactions, benzo[*b*]thiophene is attacked at the C-3- (and C-2-) position. Halogenation and Friedel–Crafts acylation result in 2- and/or 3-substitution (Van Zyl *et al.*, 1966; Royer *et al.*, 1962). The 2-position is preferred in derivatives already substituted at the 3-position (Gaertner, 1952). Sulphonation results also in 3-substitution (Boswell *et al.*, 1968; Pailer and Romberger, 1961). Nitration forms a series of mononitro compounds among which 3-nitrobenzo[*b*]thiophene predominates (56%) followed by almost equal amounts of 4- (13%), 2- (12%), 7- (11%) and 6-nitrobenzo[*b*]thiophene (10%) (Gronowitz and Dahlgren, 1977), whereas no nitration at C-5 was observed (Armstrong *et al.*, 1969). Cautious reduction of benzo[*b*]thiophene with Na/C_2H_5OH gives 2,3-dihydrobenzo[*b*]thiophene. More rigid hydrogenation catalyzed by CoO(or NiO)-MoO_3-Al_2O_3 eliminates sulphur from benzo[*b*]thiophenes (hydrodesulfuration). This plays a role in removing these compounds from petroleum fractions (hydrofining) (Watkins and DeRossett, 1957). Oxidation of benzo[*b*]thiophene with tert.-butylhypochlorite in methanol or butanol or with *p*-nitroperbenzoic acid forms the sulfoxide (Geneste *et al.*, 1975, 1977a,b,c) whereas treatment with peracetic acid leads to the sulfone, which, however, readily reacts by self-condensation.

Benzo[*b*]thiophenes occur in crude oil and accordingly in petroleum distillates (Kuras *et al.*, 1982; Nesterenko *et al.*, 1983; Poirier and Smiley, 1984; Johansen, 1977; Parfenova *et al.*, 1977; Mel'nikova *et al.*, 1979, 1980, 1981; Vol'tsov and Lyapina, 1980; Numanov, 1977; Drushel and Sommers, 1967; Nishioka *et al.*, 1985a; Potolovskii *et al.*, 1977; Brodskii *et al.*, Lyapina *et al.*, 1980a,b; Mostecky, 1982; for earlier published data see Iddon and Scrowston, 1970) and several approaches for their separation were carried out e.g. by complexing with $TiCl_4$ (Nesterenko *et al.*, 1983). They have been detected in coal tar (Lang and Eigen, 1967; Taits *et al.*, 1984; Lee *et al.*, 1980; Burchill *et al.*, 1982a,b; White and Lee, 1980; Vassilaros *et al.*, 1982c), in coal tar pitch (Van Grass *et al.*, 1981; Nishioka *et al.*, 1985a; Weissgerber and Kruber, 1920; Weissgerber and Moehrle, 1921; Willey *et al.*, 1981b), anthracene oil (Burchill *et al.*, 1982b), in coal liquification products (Nishioka *et al.*, 1985a; Kong *et al.*, 1984; White and Lee, 1980; Lee *et al.*, 1980), in shale and shale oils (van Grass *et al.*, 1981; Willey *et al.*, 1981a,b; Kong *et al.*, 1984) and as by-product in crude and commercial naphthalene (Navivach *et al.*, 1982; McKague and Meier, 1984; Kazarova *et al.*, 1979) from which benzo[*b*]thiophene has been removed by fractional crystallization (Jakubczyk and Rabczuk, 1979). Benzo[*b*]thiophenes were found in used crankcase oil (Peake and Parker, 1980), in sediments (Bates and Carpenter, 1979b), in tobacco smoke (Schmid *et al.*, 1985), in air and absorbed to airborne matter (Dimitriev *et al.*, 1984; Hanson *et al.*, 1980; Chiu *et al.*, 1983) as well as in water (Warner, 1975; Winters and Parker, 1977) in which the parent compound exhibits a comparatively high solubility (113 ppm) (Vassilaros *et al.*, 1982*a*) and from which it is together with alkylated homologues transferred to marine organisms (Ogata *et al.*, 1981*a,b*; Ogata and Miyake, 1978, 1979) and enriched up to thousand-fold e.g. in the mussel *Mytilus edulis* (Ogata *et al.*, 1981*b*). Microbial degradation of benzo[*b*]thiophene has been observed (Fedorak and Westlake, 1983*a,b*, 1984; Bohonos *et al.*, 1977). The occurrence of benzo[*b*]thiophene in foodstuffs and in rat liver has been reported (Ogata and Miyake, 1980; Ogata and Fujisawa, 1983), and it has been detected in some unusual sources such as the volatiles of off-flavoured unblanched green peas (*Pisum sativum*) (Murray *et al.*, 1976) and in the volatile flavour components of white bread crust (Folkes and Gramshaw, 1981).

In most of the above matrices also alkyl-substituted benzo[*b*]thiophenes were found, and hydroxybenzo[*b*]thiophenes (4- and 6-OH-benzo[*b*]thiophene) were found in coal tar (Lang and Eigen, 1967) and coal liquid (Nishioka *et al.*, 1985*a*).

Benzo[c]thiophene (synonyms: 2-thiaindene, isothianaphthene, isothionaphthene, isobenzothiophene).

m.w.: 134 (C_8H_6S)
m.p.: 53–55°C

(4)

The chemistry of benzo[*c*]thiophene has been reviewed by Iddon (1972). It can be synthesized by catalytic dehydrogenation of 1,3-dihydrobenzo[*c*]thiophene under nitrogen at 330°C and 20 Torr (Mayer *et al.*, 1962, 1963) or by heating 1,3-dibenzo[*c*]thiophene-2-oxide with neutral alumina to 120–130°C (Cava *et al.*, 1971). Due to the high reactivity of the 1- and 3-positions, benzo[*c*]thiophene is an unstable compound. The 1,3-dihydro derivative (2-thiaindane; m.p. 23°C) is also oxygen sensitive. It can be readily separated by reaction with Hg-(II)-acetate forming a water-soluble adduct from which it can be recovered by acidification. Due to the low stability of benzo[*c*]thiophene and its derivatives, these compounds have not been found in environmental matter. A derivative of the 4,5,6,7-tetrahydrobenzo[*c*]thiophene, 1,4,4-trimethyl-4,5,6,7-tetrahydrobenzo[*c*]thiophene (*5*), has been detected in refinery products of Middle East crude oil (Birch *et al.*, 1959).

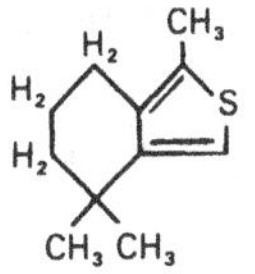

m.w.: 180 ($C_{11}H_{16}S$)

1,4,4-trimethyl-4,5,6,7-tetrahydrobenzo[c]thiophene
(5)

C_5S–C_6

None of the isomeric benzothiopyrans have been detected in natural sources or in environmental matter. However, the occurrence of the perhydro-1-benzothiopyran (6) in crude petroleum distillates (190–360°C) was reported (Lyapina *et al.*, 1982).

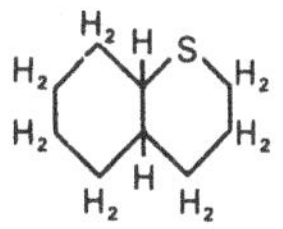

m.w.: 156 ($C_9H_{16}S$)

perhydro-1-benzothiopyran
(6)

2.2 Tricyclic compounds
C_4S–C_5–C_5

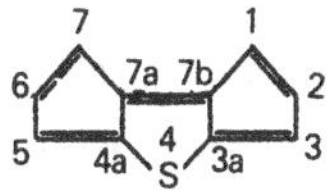

m.w.: 158 ($C_{10}H_6S$)

dicyclopenta[b,d]thiophene
(7)

The compound was found as a minor constituent of Usinskaya heavy petroleum (Mel'nikova *et al.*, 1981).

C_4S–C_5–C_6
8H-*indeno[2,1-*b]*thiophene*

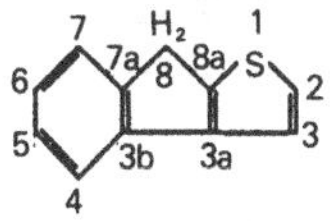

m.w.: 172 ($C_{11}H_8S$)

(8)

Dimethyl-8*H*-indeno[2,1-*b*]thiophene (m.w.: 200) was indentified in a distillation fraction of a sulfur-rich shale oil (Pailer and Berner-

Fenz (1973) and synthesized from 3-phenyl-2,5-thiophenedicarboxylic acid via the diacylchloride which, after cyclization to 8-oxo-8*H*-indeno-[2,1-*b*]thiophene-2-carboxylic acid and decarboxylation, gives the corresponding ketone which yields the thiophene by Wolff–Kishner reduction (MacDowell and Patrick, 1967*a*):

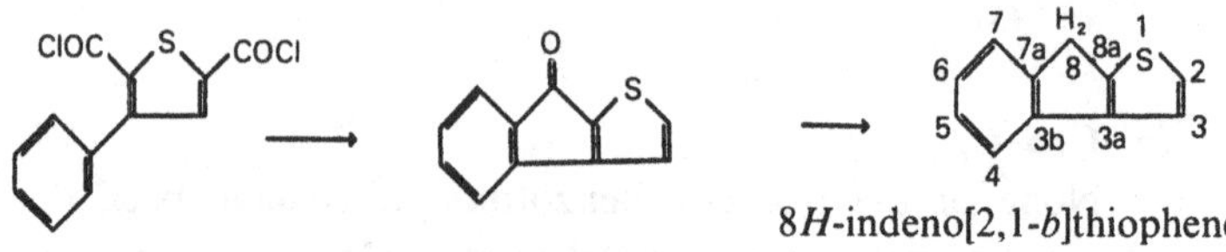

8*H*-indeno[2,1-*b*]thiophene

5H-*indeno[5,6-b]thiophene*

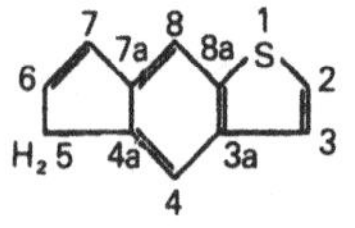

m.w.: 172 ($C_{11}H_8S$)

(9)

5*H*-indeno[5,6-*b*]thiophene (*9*) has been detected in various crude oils (Lyapina *et al.*, 1980*b*, 1982; Mel'nikova *et al.*, 1981); the synthesis of its 6,7-dihydro-product has been published by Pailer and coworkers (Pailer and Gruenhaus, 1974; Gruenhaus *et al.*, 1976).

The syntheses of various other indenothiophenes have been described. The 4*H*-indeno[1,2-*b*]thiophene (*10*) system can be obtained in 92% yield by decomposing 3-diazoethyl-2-phenylthiophene in boiling dimethylformamide (Munro and Sharp, 1984):

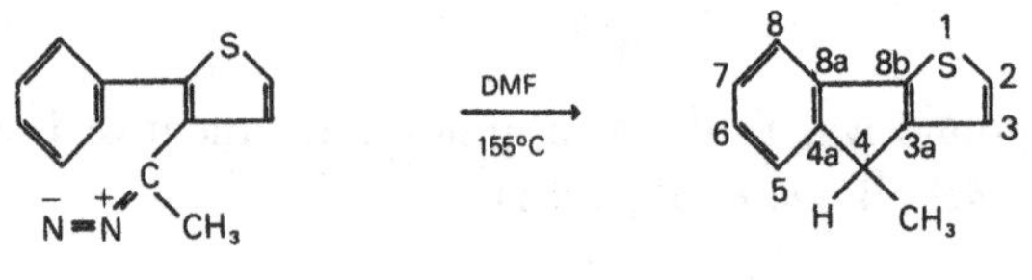

4*H*-indeno[1,2-*b*]- and 8*H*-indeno[1,2-*c*]thiophene (*11*) (MacDowell and Jeffries, 1970) as well as indeno[4,5-*b*]-, indeno[5,4-*b*]- and indeno[5,6-*b*]thiophene with a hydrogenated cyclopenta ring were synthesized by Pailer *et al.* (1976), Pailer and Gruenhaus (1974), and Gruenhaus *et al.* (1976).

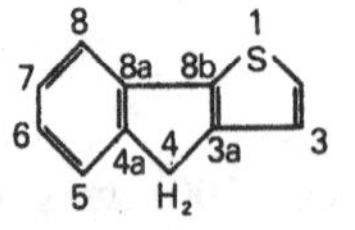

4*H*-indeno[1,2-*b*]thiophene
m.w.: 172 ($C_{11}H_8S$)

(10)

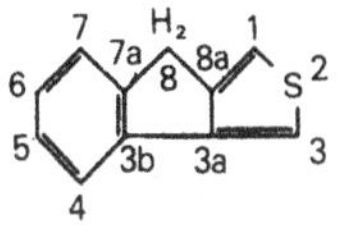

8*H*-indeno[1,2-*c*]thiophene
m.w.: 172 (C$_{11}$H$_8$S)

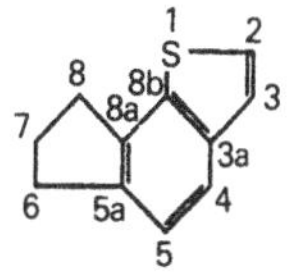

(*11*)

7,8-dihydro-6*H*-indeno[4,5-*b*]thiophene
m.w.: 174 (C$_{11}$H$_{10}$S)

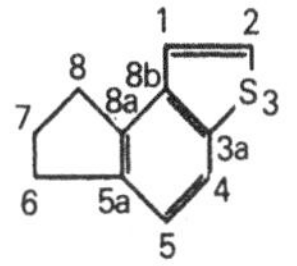

(*12*)

7,8-dihydro-6*H*-indeno[5,4-*b*]thiophene
m.w.: 174 (C$_{11}$H$_{10}$S)

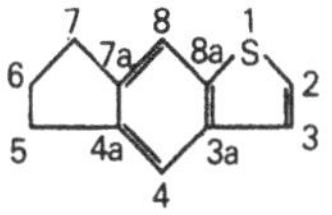

(*13*)

6,7-dihydro-5*H*-indeno[5,6-*b*]thiophene
m.w.: 174 (C$_{11}$H$_{10}$S)

(*14*)

C$_4$S–C$_4$S–C$_6$

There are only a few indications for the presence of benzodithiophenes in fossil fuels (Drushel and Sommers, 1966; Pailer and Berner-Fenz, 1973), 1-methylbenzo[1,2-*b*:4,3-*b'*]dithiophene (*15*) was found in shale oil (98).

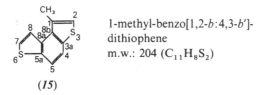

1-methyl-benzo[1,2-*b*:4,3-*b'*]-
dithiophene
m.w.: 204 (C$_{11}$H$_8$S$_2$)

(*15*)

Gronowitz and Dahlgren (1977) have synthesized the following benzodithiophenes by Wittig reaction of *o*-bromoformylthiophenes with *o*-bromothenyltriphenylphosphoranes, subsequent halogen–metal exchange with butyllithium and reaction with copper(II)chloride:

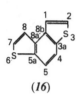

(16)

benzo[1,2-*b*:4,3-*b'*]dithiophene
m.w.: 190 ($C_{10}H_6S_2$)
(see also under: Rao and Tilak, 1957)

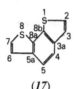

(17)

benzo[2,1-*b*:3,4-*b'*]dithiophene
m.w.: 190 ($C_{10}H_6S_2$)
(see also under: Rao and Tilak, 1958; Cagniant
and Kirsch, 1975; Wiersema and Gronowitz, 1970)

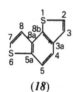

(18)

benzo[1,2-*b*:3,4-*b'*]dithiophene
m.w.: 190 ($C_{10}H_6S_2$)
(see also under: Rao and Tilak, 1954)

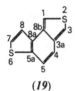

(19)

benzo[1,2-*b*:3,4-*c'*]dithiophene
m.w.: 190 ($C_{10}H_6S_2$)

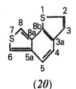

(20)

benzo[2,1-*b*:3,4-*c'*]dithiophene
m.w.: 190 ($C_{10}H_6S_2$)
(see also under: Ricci *et al.*, 1969)

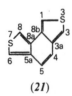

(21)

benzo[1,2-*c*:3,4-*c'*]dithiophene
m.w.: 190 ($C_{10}H_6S_2$)
(see also under: MacDowell and Maxwell, 1970)

The synthesis of the following isomers or their derivatives has also been
described (references in brackets):

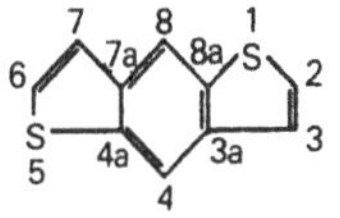

(22)

benzo[1,2-*b*:4,5-*b'*]dithiophene
m.w.: 190 ($C_{10}H_6S_2$)
(see also under: Ricci *et al.*, 1969; Aggarwal and MacDowell, 1979; Kossmehl *et al.*, 1983; Caullet *et al.*, 1967; MacDowell and Wisowaty, 1972; Buu-Hoi and Hoan, 1949; Rao and Tilak, 1957)

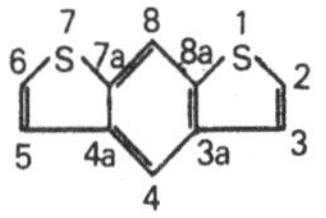

(23)

benzo[1,2-*b*:5,4-*b'*]dithiophene
m.w.: 190 ($C_{10}H_6S_2$)
(see also under: MacDowell and Wisowaty, 1972; Ahmed *et al.*, 1970)

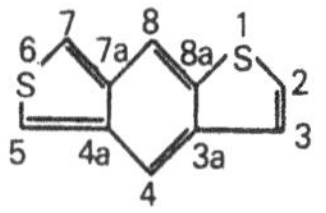

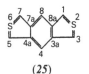

(24)

benzo[1,2-*b*:4,5-*c'*]dithiophene
m.w.: 190 ($C_{10}H_6S_2$)
(see also under: MacDowell and Wisowaty, 1972)

(25)

benzo[1,2-*c*:4,5-*c'*]dithiophene
m.w.: 190 ($C_{10}H_6S_2$)   m.p.: 112–113°C
(see also under: MacDowell and Wisowaty, 1972; Hart and Sasaoka, 1978)

It was observed that the [*b,c*]-fused systems tend to polymerize (Gronowitz and Dahlgreen, 1977).

NMR- (Blackburn *et al.*, 1972) and MCD-spectra of a number of benzodithiophenes have been recorded (Dahlgren *et al.*, 1979). For some isomers the π-electron structure has been calculated by DasGupta and Birss (1980) and by Güsten *et al.* (1969) indicating that the five-membered ring is the most reactive position of the molecule.

Compounds with two annelated thiophene rings (thienobenzothio-phenes) have been synthesized, e.g. thieno[2,3-*b*][1]benzothiophene (27) (Mitra *et al.*, 1957; Chapman *et al.*, 1970, 1971*a*; Sasaki *et al.*, 1982; Desai and Tilak, 1960) and thieno[3,2-*b*][1]benzothiophene (28) (Chapman *et al.*, 1970; Ricci *et al.*, 1971; Parham and Gadsby, 1960).

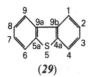
(27)

thieno[2,3-*b*][1]benzothiophene
m.w.: 190 ($C_{10}H_6S_2$)

(28)

thieno[3,2-*b*][1]benzothiophene
m.w.: 190 ($C_{10}H_6S_2$)

Substitution reactions such as halogenation, nitration, metalation, Friedel-Crafts acylation as well as Vilsmeier–Haack formylation preferentially take place at the C-2-position (Chapman *et al.*, 1971*b*) resulting in significant chemical shifts of the NMR-spectra (Ewing *et al.*, 1974).

$C_4S-C_6-C_6$

Various isomers of this formula are of environmental relevance and have been detected in various matrices.

Dibenzo[b,d]*thiophene* (29) (synonyms: biphenylene sulfide, diphenylene sulfide, 9-thiafluorene)

(29)

m.w.: 184 ($C_{12}H_8S$)
m.p.: 97°C
b.p.: 331.4°C

The chemistry of dibenzothiophene has been carefully reviewed by Ashby and Cook in 1974 who gave 525 references, and another 300 references can be found in *Chemical Abstracts* since then. Dibenzothiophene is widely distributed in the environment since it is a prominent component of crude oil (400 mg and more/kg) (Clugston *et al.*, 1972, 1974, 1976; Nuzzi and Casalini, 1978; Rebbert *et al.*, 1984; Nesterenko *et al.*, 1983; Grimmer and Böhnke, 1978; Grimmer *et al.*, 1983*a*; Drushel and Sommers, 1966); it has been detected in various petroleum fractions (Brodskii *et al.*, 1977; Mel'nikova *et al.*, 1979; Lohinska-Gasowska *et al.*, 1979; Baig *et al.*, 1982; Lyapina *et al.*, 1980*a*; Kuras *et al.*, 1982; Mostecky, 1982; Castex *et al.*, 1983; Poirier and Das, 1984; Poirier and Smiley, 1984), in motor oils (Arsic *et al.*, 1983; Peake and Parker, 1980; Grimmer *et al.*, 1981*a*; Kveseth *et al.*, 1982) in medical oils (Popl *et al.*, 1975), and in bitumen (Speight and Pancirov, 1983). It was also found in shale oils (Kong *et al.*, 1984; Willey *et al.*, 1981*a,b*), in coal (Ozdemir, 1971; Hayatsu *et al.*, 1975; White and Lee, 1980), coal-derived products (Lee *et al.*, 1980;

Kong *et al.*, 1982), coal oil, synfuels and coal liquification products (Nakamura, 1983; Willey *et al.*, 1981*b*; Wise *et al.*, 1983; Kong et al., 1984; Vo-dingh and Martinez, 1981; Fitch and Smith, 1979*a*; Later *et al.*, 1981; Holstein and Severin, 1982; Sharkey, 1976; White and Lee, 1980; Lee *et al.*, 1980; Kong *et al.*, 1982; Nishioka, 1986*b*), in coal tar (Borwitzky and Schomburg, 1978; Gerasimenko *et al.*, 1981; Burchill *et al.*, 1982*a*, 1983; Kruber, 1927; Kruber and Raeithel, 1954; Nishioka *et al.*, 1985*a*, 1986*b*), pitch (Burchill *et al.*, 1982*a*), in anthracene oil (Stadelhofer and Gerhards, 1981; Burchill, 1982*b*; Miki and Sugimoto, 1983), and in carbon black (Lee and Hites, 1976; Serth and Hughes, 1980). Accordingly, it is found in the combustion effluents of coal (2.8 mg/kg combusted coal) (Chiu *et al.*, 1983; Grimmer *et al.*, 1985), brown coal (0.1 mg/kg combusted material) (Grimmer *et al.*, 1983*b*), of gasoline (Howard and Mills, 1983) and of diesel (Choudhury and Bush, 1981; Yu and Hites, 1981; Howard and Mills, 1983). It has been detected in the working atmosphere of coke plants (Bjørseth *et al.*, 1978*a*,*b*; Murayama and Moriyama, 1982; Hung and Bernier, 1983), of aluminium reduction plants (Bjørseth *et al.*, 1978*b*, 1980, 1981) and also in emissions from incineration of combustible fractions of domestic wastes (Lunden *et al.*, 1982). It is a common aromatic pollutant of ambient air (Bjørseth and Lunde, 1977; Tong *et al.*, 1984; Moehnle *et al.*, 1984; York Research Group, 1979; Hanson *et al.*, 1977; Lee *et al.*, 1982) and it has been detected in tobacco smoke (Schmid *et al.*, 1985) and even in sauna air (Hasanen *et al.*, 1984). As a consequence of its presence in ambient air and its comparatively high solubility in water, it is found in vegetables (Beck and Stoebet, 1982) and in ground-, tap-, lake-, and sea-water (Hutchins and Ward, 1984; Gjessing *et al.*, 1984; Lygren *et al.*, 1984; Eganhouse and Kaplan, 1982; Kveseth *et al.*, 1982; Berglind, 1982; Mattox and Humenick, 1979; Hoffman *et al.*, 1984; Olufsen, 1980) into which it may enter from highway runoffs and pavement dusts but also from industrial discharges. Oil spills are the main source for the contamination of sea-water by dibenzothiophene (Berthou *et al.*, 1981; Calder and Boehm, 1979; Pearlman *et al.*, 1984). It is well known that dibenzothiophene can be transferred from petroleum spills to the aquatic environment, to fish and to other marine organisms in which it was found to be rather persistent (Oudot *et al.*, 1981). Hence, it is present in sediments (Teal *et al.*, 1978; Nakamura and Kashimoto, 1979*a*; Imanaka *et al.*, 1980; Bates and Carpenter, 1979*b*; Heit and Tan, 1979; Tan, 1979; Heit *et al.*, 1979; Lee *et al.*, 1982; Boehm *et al.*, 1982; Buchert *et al.*, 1982; Sporstol *et al.*, 1983), in mussels (Fukushima *et al.*, 1983; Kira *et al.*, 1983; Murray *et al.*, 1983; Mackie *et al.*, 1980) and many other marine products (Nakamura *et al.*, 1979; Nakamura and Kashimoto, 1977; Warner, 1975; Grahl-Nielsen *et al.*, 1978; Ogata and Miyake, 1978, 1980; Ogato *et al.*, 1979; Clarke and Law, 1981; Vassilaros *et al.*, 1982*a,b*; West *et al.*, 1985; Paasivirta *et al.*, 1981; Oudot *et al.*, 1981; Wise *et al.*, 1983; Galloway *et al.*, 1983; Herzschuh and Paasivirta, 1983; Ogata and Miyake, 1979; Warner, 1975; Ibe *et al.*, 1978; Lee *et al.*, 1982). Dibenzothiophene has also been found in sewage (Kveseth *et al.*, 1982), in avian tissues (Gay *et al.*, 1980), and in minerals (West *et al.*, 1985) and as a contaminant of reference compounds (Frycka, 1979; Kipot *et al.*, 1980).

The mono-, di- and higher-alkylated dibenzothiophenes are often found associated with the base compound in crudes (Carruthers, 1955; Carruthers and Douglas, 1957, 1964) and in coal tar (Lang and Eigen, 1967).

Dibenzothiophene may be synthesized by sulfur insertion into (Voronkov and Faitel'son, 1967; Obolentsev *et al.*, 1956; Klemm and Karchesy, 1978) or catalytic reaction of hydrogen sulfide with biphenyl (Patterson *et al.*, 1959) as well as by cyclization of 2,2'-dihydroxybiphenyl with phosphorous pentasulfide. An entrance to variously substituted dibenzothiophenes is provided by condensation of 2-chlorocyclohexanone with the corresponding benzenethiols, cyclization with P_2O_5 and subsequent dehydrogenation (Rabindran and Tilak, 1951*a*; McCall, 1953). Additional synthetic routes for the preparation of dibenzothiophenes were described such as photocyclization of dibenzosulfide (Zeller and Petersen, 1975), condensation of 2-allylbenzo[*b*]thiophene with dichloromethylbutylether/$SnCl_4$ (Ashby *et al.*, 1974), cyclization of 2,5-dipentenylthiophenes with $AlCl_3$ and subsequent dehydrogenation (Gourier and Canonne, 1970).

NMR-spectra (Bartle *et al.*, 1971*a*; Jones *et al.*, 1974), mass-, IR-, UV-, and, fluorescence-spectra (Nikitina *et al.*, 1972; Marty and Viallet, 1974), and quasilinear luminescence spectra (Teplitskaya *et al.*, 1981) have been published; most of them have been discussed and reviewed by Ashby and Cook (1974).

Oxidation of dibenzothiophene with peracids results in the 5-oxide or the 5,5-dioxide, the ratio of which depends on the reaction conditions and the excess of oxidation reagent (Sergienko *et al.*, 1960). The preparation of the sulfoxide by treatment of dibenzothiophene with N-bromo-caprolactam in the presence of water has been discussed by Sato *et al.* (1974). Reduction of dibenzothiophene with sodium in liquid ammonia gives 1,4-dihydrodibenzothiophene, whereas catalytic hydrogenation desulfurizes it to biphenyl. Electrophilic substitution of dibenzothiophene takes place at the 2-position, although the formation of small amounts of the 4-isomer has been observed. A nitro- or halo group in 2-position directs a second substituent into the 8-position, whereas the 3-nitro derivatives may be obtained after preceding sulfoxidation.

Evidence has been presented for an accumulation of dibenzothiophene and other polycyclic aromatic compounds from crude oils in various organisms, e.g. fish, crabs, clams, rotifers, water fleas, isopods etc. (Clement *et al.*, 1980; Ogato *et al.*, 1980*b*; Mironov and Shchekaturina, 1981; Ogata and Miyake, 1981; Ogata and Fujisawa, 1980; Eastmond *et al.*, 1984). Accumulation rate, persistence, and toxicity of dibenzothiophene seem to be greater than that of its PAH isoster phenanthrene (Eastmond *et al.*, 1984). Influence on the hatchability of *Artemia* dry eggs (Kuwabara *et al.*, 1980) and inhibition of goldfish liver mitochondrial phosphorylation (Ogata and Hasegawa, 1982) have been reported.

Dibenzothiophene is degraded by various soil and water microorganisms (Fedorak and Westlake, 1983*b*, 1984; Finnerty *et al.*, 1983; Foght *et al.*, 1983) and even by the thermophilic organism *Sulfolobus acidocaldarius* (Kargi and Robinson, 1984). Various *Pseudomonas* species; e.g. *Pseudomonas abikonensis* and *P. jianii*, can utilize dibenzothiophene as sole carbon source converting it to trans-4-(3-hydroxythiophene-2-yl)-2-oxo-3-butenoic acid and its hemiacetal and further to 3-hydroxy-2-formyl-benzo[*b*]thiophene and 3-methoxybenzo[*b*]thiophene-2-carboxylic acid (Kodama *et al.*, 1970, 1973; Koehler *et al.*, 1978; Yamada *et al.*, 1968). The microbial conversion of dibenzothiophene to the corresponding 5-oxide also has been observed (Kodama *et al.*, 1973; Koehler *et al.*, 1978).

Metabolites of dibenzothiophene formed by Pseudomonas species

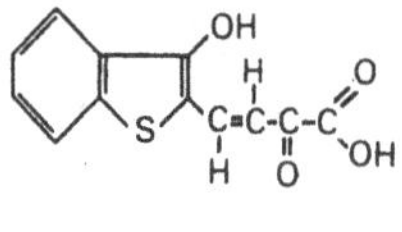

trans-4-(3-hydroxythiophen-2-yl)-2-oxo-3-butenoic acid

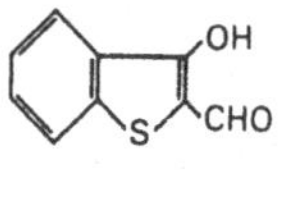

3-hydroxy-2-formyl-benzo[*b*]thiophene

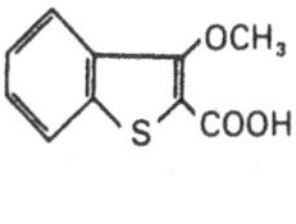

3-methoxybenzo[*b*]thiophene-2-carboxylic acid

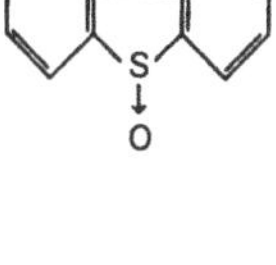

dibenzothiophene-5-oxide

Dibenzothiophene was found to be inactive as a mutagen in the Ames *S. typhimurium* test (Pelroy *et al.*, 1983; McFall *et al.*, 1984).

Naphtho[1,2-b]thiophene (synonym: 6,7-benzothianaphthene)

m.w.: 184 ($C_{12}H_8S$)
m.p.: 27–28°C

(*30*)

Naphtho[1,2-*b*]thiophene has been found in coal tar (Nishioka *et al.*, 1985*a*; Kruber and Raeithel, 1953; Borwitzky and Schomburg, 1979) and coal derived products (Nakamura, 1983; Lee *et al.*, 1980), e.g. in anthracene oil (Kruber and Raeithel, 1953; Proksch, 1966), and it has been tentatively identified in crude oil and shale oil (Nishioka *et al.*, 1985*a*). Its 3-ethyl-6,8-dimethyl derivative has been claimed to occur in high boiling petroleum distillates of Kuwait oil (Carruthers and Douglas, 1959). It has been synthesized by various routes such as decarboxylation of the 2-carboxyclic acid (Campaigne and Heaton, 1962), treatment of bis-(2-(β-naphthyl)ethyl)disulfide with iodine (Campaigne and Heaton, 1962), reduction of naphtho[1,2-*b*]thiophene-3-ol (Carruthers, 1953), treatment of the 2,3-dihydro derivative with chloranil (Banfield *et al.*, 1956*b*), or cyclization of (1-naphthothio)acetaldehyde diethylacetal with HPO_3 at 180°C/0.5 min (Banfield *et al.*, 1956*b*; Pandya and Tilak, 1959*a*), but other routes have also been described (Clarke *et al.*, 1973; Campaigne and Heaton, 1964; Tiecco *et al.*, 1970; Cagniant and Kirsch, 1975; Sidorenko *et al.*, 1983*a*; Anisimow *et al.*, 1983). 3-Methylnaphtho[1,2-*b*]thiophene can be obtained by cyclization of acetonyl-1-naphthylsulfide (Banfield *et al.*, 1956*a*), whereas the 2,3-dimethyl derivative has been synthesized by following the general route of condensation of benzene thiols with α-haloketones in the presence of 30% NaOH which yields arylketosulfides which can be cyclized in the presence of P_2O_5 or $ZnCl_2$ (Werner, 1949).

Bromination, formylation, Friedel-Crafts acetylation and lithiation occur at C-2; nitration gives 2- and 5-nitronaphtho[1,2-*b*]thiophene. Bromination and nitration of the 2-substituted compound takes place at C-5 (Clarke *et al.*, 1973). Cagniant *et al.* (1964*a*) reported on the substitution with higher alkylated naphtho[1,2-*b*]thiophenes. Oxidation of CrO_3 yields the 4,5-quinone (m.p. 218–219°C) (Kruber and Raeithel, 1953; Carruthers, 1953). Treatment with H_2O_2 in acetic acid gives the 1,1-dioxide (sulfone, m.p. 181–182°C) (Davies and Porter, 1956).

Naphtho[1,2-*b*]thiophene was found to be mutagenic in the Ames *S. typhimurium* test (Pelroy *et al.*, 1983).

Naphtho[1,2-c]thiophene (synonym: 4,5-benzoisothianaphthene)

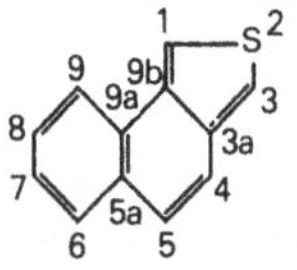

m.w.: 184 ($C_{12}H_8S$)

(*31*)

Because of its high diene reactivity and its low thermal stability this isomer has not been detected in environmental matter. It may be synthesized from 1-cyano-2-mercaptomethylnaphthalene by reduction with $NaBH_4/AlCl_3$ (3:1) giving 1,3-dihydronaphtho[1,2-*c*]thiophene (Stacy *et al.*, 1964), the S-oxide of which may be reduced and aromatized by heating with neutral alumina (Cava *et al.*, 1971) or with 30% aqueous NaOH (Horner *et al.*, 1976).

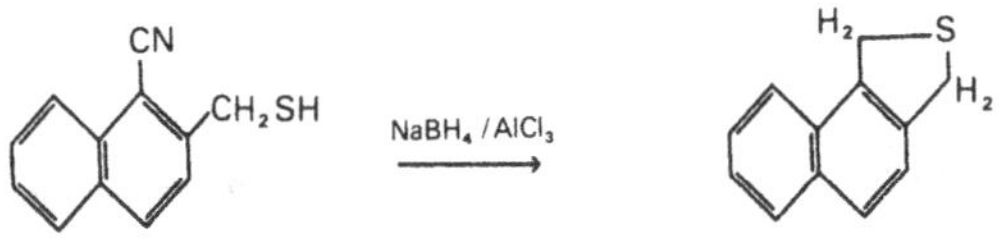

Naphtho[2,1-b]thiophene (synonym: 4,5-benzothianaphthene)

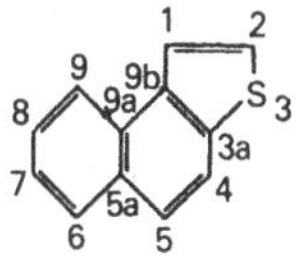

m.w.: 184 ($C_{12}H_8S$)
m.p.: 114–115°C

(*32*)

Naphtho[2,1-*b*]thiophene has been detected in coal-tar and anthracene oil (Kruber and Raeithel, 1953; Proksch, 1966; Nakamura, 1983; Nishioka *et al.*, 1985*a*), in synfuels (Kong *et al.*, 1984), and in shale oil (Willey *et al.*, 1981*b*). Various routes to obtain this thiaarene system have been reported, e.g. cyclization of 2-naphthyldimethoxyethylsulfide with P_2O_5/H_3PO_4 (Tilak, 1951*a*), reduction of 4.5-benzothioindoxyl (Carruthers, 1953), decarboxylation of naphtho[2,1-*b*]thiophene-2-carboxylic acid (Campaigne and Cline, 1956), acid-catalyzed cyclization of acetonylthionaphthol (Dann and Kokorudz, 1958), photocyclization of 2-styrylthiophene (Tominaga *et al.*, 1983; Carruthers and Stewart, 1965*a,b*), and cyclocondensation of naphthylacrylic acid with thionylchloride (Sidorenko *et al.*, 1983*a*). IR- (McDonald and Cook, 1967), UV- (Momicchioli and Rastelli, 1970), and NMR-spectral parameters (Ewing and Scrowston, 1971) as well as molecular orbital calculations (Trinajstic and Hinchliffe, 1968; Nair and Gogte, 1974) for naphtho[2,1-*b*]thiophene have been reported.

Nitration, formylation, acylation, bromination, mercuration, and lithiation of naphtho[2,1-*b*]thiophene occur at C-2; methyl-substitution at C-1 does not shift these reactions to other positions, whereas 1,2-dimethylnaphtho[2,1-*b*]thiophene is brominated at C-5 (Clarke *et al.*, 1969*a,b*). Naphtho[2,1-*b*]thiophene was found to be non-mutagenic in the Ames-Test (Pelroy *et al.*, 1983).

*Naphtho[2,3-*b]*thiophene* (synonym: 5,6-benzothianaphthene)

m.w.: 184 ($C_{12}H_8S$)
m.p.: 192–193°C

(33)

Naphtho[2,3-*b*]thiophene was found in anthracene oil (Proksch, 1966) and, as a consequence, also in commercial anthracene and phenanthrene standards (Frycka, 1979). It has been detected in coal tar (Nishioka *et al.*, 1985*a*, 1986*b*; Kruber and Raeithel, 1953), crude oil (Nishioka *et al.*, 1985*a*), in synfuels (Kong *et al.*, 1984), shale oil (Willey *et al.*, 1981*b*; Pailer and Berner-Fenz, 1973) and in sediments (Vassilaros *et al.*, 1982*c*; Lee *et al.*, 1982) from which it may be transferred to fish (Lee *et al.*, 1982; Vassilaros *et al.*, 1982*a,b*). Mass spectral data for this compound have been presented (Meyerson and Fields, 1968).

The compound can be synthesized from 3-amino-2-naphthoic acid by diazotization, subsequent treatment with Na_2S and reduction of the disulfide. The resulting 3-mercapto-2-naphthoic acid is condensed with bromoacetic acid, cyclized and reduced (Cagniant *et al.*, 1977). Carruthers *et al.* (1962) have synthesized naphtho[2,3-*b*]thiophene by cyclization of 4-(2,3-dihydro-5-benzo[*b*]thienyl)butyric acid and subsequent reduction and dehydrogenation of the resulting 2,3,5,6,7,8-hexahydro-8-oxonaphtho[2,3-*b*]thiophene. Diels-Alder reaction of 1,2-dimethylene-cyclohexane and thiophene-1,1-dioxide derivatives yields octahydro-naphtho[2,3-*b*]thiophene-1,1-dioxide and hence opens a door to tricyclic thiaarenes (Bailey and Cummings, 1954). Methods for the synthesis of aryl- and alkyl-substituted naphtho[2,3-*b*]thiophenes have been reported (Etienne, 1947). *p*-Quinones of naphtho[2,3-*b*]thiophene have also been synthesized (Schroeder and Weinmayer, 1952; MacDowell and Wisowaty, 1972).

Friedel-Crafts acetylation favours 3-substitution although in methylene chloride additional 4-acetylation is observed (Carruthers, 1963). Reduction of naphtho[2,3-*b*]thiophene with $Na/C_5H_{11}OH$ gives the 4,9- and 2,3-dihydro compounds. Naphtho[2,3-*b*]thiophene undergoes meso addition less readily than the isosteric anthracene (Carruthers, 1963).

No mutagenic activity could be found for this thiaarene (Pelroy *et al.*, 1983).

Naphtho[2,3-c]thiophene (synonym: 5,6-benzoisothianaphthene)

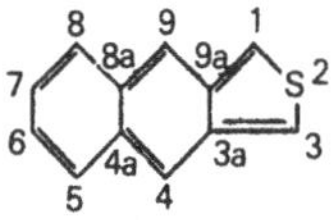

m.w.: 184 ($C_{12}H_8S$)

(*34*)

Due to its electronic configuration this compound is very unstable, although evidence has been presented for its formation from 1,3-dihydronaphtho[2,3-*c*]thiophene-2-oxide by pyrolytic dehydration on alumina (Cava *et al.*, 1971). 1,3-Dihydronaphtho[2,3-*c*]thiophene (m.p.: 169.5–170.5°C) has been synthesized by Cava and Muth (1960); its 4-phenyl derivative was obtained by reaction of 1-bromo-3-phenyl-propyne-2 with sodium sulfide and subsequent cyclization with potassium in butanol (Iwai and Ide, 1964):

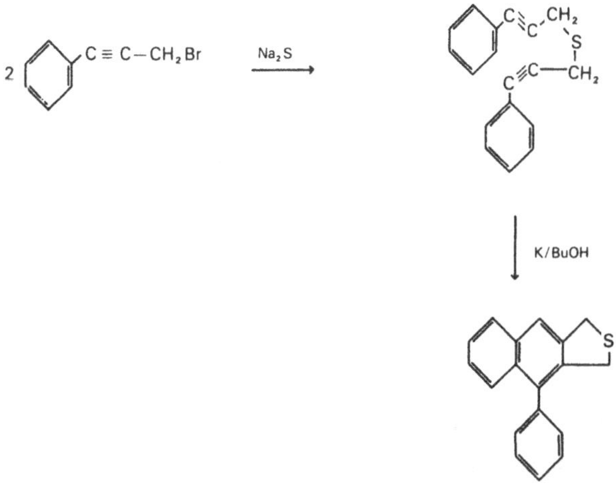

The stable 1,3-diphenylnaphtho[2,3-*c*]thiophene was prepared by S/O-exchange from 1,3-diphenylnaphtho[2,3-*c*]furan with P_2S_5 (Cava and VanMeter, 1962, 1969). The synthesis of 1,3,5,6,7,8-hexahydro-5,5,8,8-tetramethylnaphtho[2,3-*c*]thiophene has also been described by Folli *et al.* (1974).

2H-*Napththo[1,8-*bc]thiophene* (synonym: 1-thioacenaphthene; 1-thiacenaphthene)

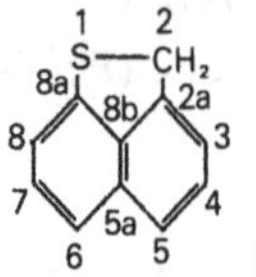

m.w.: 172 ($C_{11}H_8S$)

(*35*)

2*H*-Naphtho[1,8-*bc*]thiophene has been found in petroleum (Kuras *et al.*, 1982; Mostecky, 1982). Its 1-oxide has been synthesized from 8-mercapto-1-naphthoic acid via the thiolactone by reduction with $NaBH_4$ (Folli *et al.*, 1974). Other synthetic routes were also described (Hawthorne and Porter, 1966; Campaigne and Knapp, 1970; Neidlein and Humburg, 1979). The 2-methyl derivative can be obtained from (8-(methylthio)-1-naphthyl)diazomethane by thermolysis and photolysis (Bailey *et al.*, 1983) or by treatment of 2*H*-naphtho[1,8-*bc*]thiophene with butyllithium and iodomethane (Folli *et al.*, 1974).

In addition to the aforementioned tricyclic thiaarenes some petroleum-related systems such as methano- and ethano-bridged benzothiophenes have been synthesized, e.g. 4,7-methanobenzo[*b*]thiophene (*36*) (Birch *et al.*, 1956; Bimber *et al.*, 1964); 4,7-methanobenzo [*c*]thiophene (*37*) (Mark, 1962; Wilder and Feliu-Otero, 1965); 4,7-ethanobenzo[*c*]thiophene (*38*) (Birch *et al.*, 1956; Wynberg and Klunder, 1969; Wilder and Gratz, 1970).

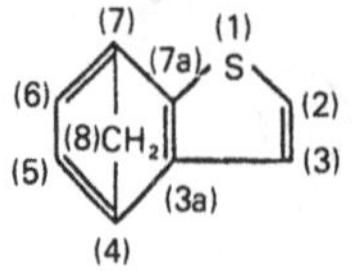

(*36*)

4,7-methanobenzo[*b*]thiophene

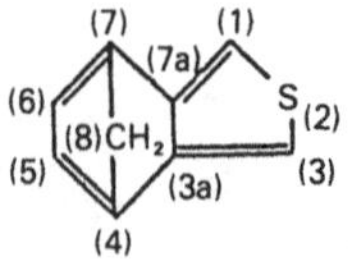

(*37*)

4,7-methanobenzo[*c*]thiophene

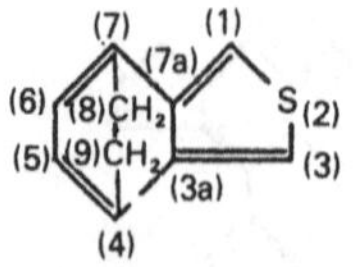

(*38*)

4,7-ethanobenzo[*c*]thiophene

$C_5S-C_6-C_6$

Compounds of this type (dibenzo- or naphthopyrans) are rarely found in environmental matter. However, great efforts have been made in synthesizing various isomers because of their importance as starting materials for the production of dyes and pharmaceuticals. For some of their derivatives also antimicrobial activity has been reported (Fedotova *et al.*, 1977).

Naphtho[1,8-bc]thiopyran (synonym: 1-thiaphenalene)

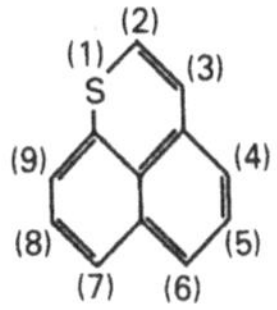

m.w.: 184 ($C_{12}H_8S$)

(*39*)

Various routes to obtain this system from which some industrial dyes are derived have been described (Pandya and Tilak, 1959a; O'Brien and Smith, 1963; Cook and Sutcliffe, 1968a: Chiang and Meinwald, 1981). Nitration of naphtho[1,8-*bc*]thiopyran gives 6- and 7-nitro-naphtho[1,8-*bc*]thiopyran in a ratio 10:1 (Cook and Sutcliffe, 1968b).

6H-*Dibenzo*[b,d]*thiopyran* (synonyms: 3,4-benzothiochromene; 9,10-dihydro-9-thiophenanthrene)

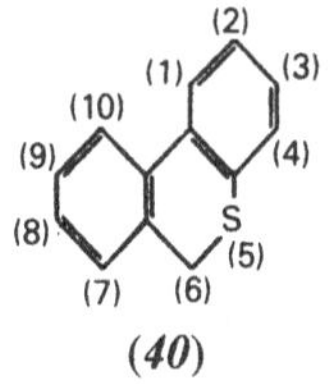

m.w.: 198 ($C_{13}H_{10}S$)

(*40*)

This compound can be obtained from ortho-phenyl-2-thiopheny-acetic acid by persulfate oxidation (Dewar *et al.*, 1972):

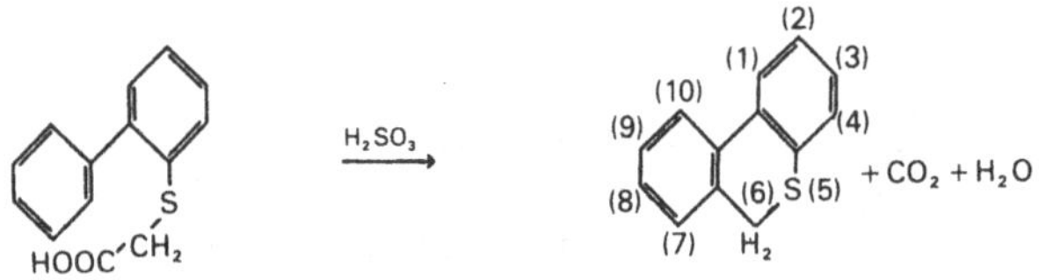

The formation of the fully aromatic system thiaphenanthrenium perchlorate has also been described (Lüttringhaus and Kolb, 1961; Jindal and Tilak, 1969):

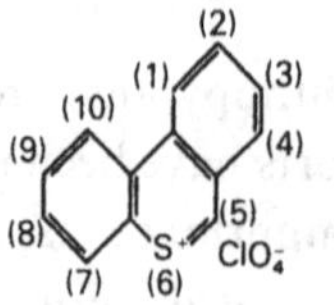

Syntheses of the following naphthothiopyran systems have been reported: 1*H*-naphtho[1,2-*c*]thiopyran (Cagniant *et al.*, 1966); 1*H*-naphtho[2,1-*b*]thiopyran (Cagniant and Cagniant, 1961); 1*H*-naphtho[2,3-*c*]thiopyran (Degani *et al.*, 1971); 4*H*-naphtho[1,2-*b*]thiopyran (Fedotova *et al.*, 1977); 2*H*-naphtho[1,2-*b*]thiopyran (Campaigne and Heaton, 1964; Ohmura *et al.*, 1982; Anisimow *et al.*, 1983); 2*H*-naphtho[2,1-*c*]thiopyran (Cagniant *et al.*, 1964*b*) and 2*H*-naphtho[2,3-*b*]thiopyran (Cagniant and Cagniant, 1961; Degani *et al.*, 1971):

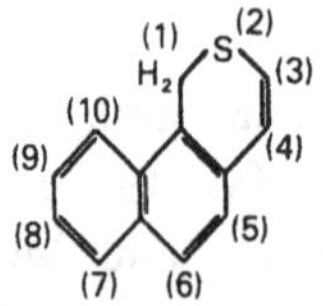

1*H*-naphtho[1,2-*c*]thiopyran
(synonyms: 7,8-benzoisotthiochromene;
3,4-dihydro-3-thiaphenanthrene
m.w.: 198 ($C_{13}H_{10}S$)

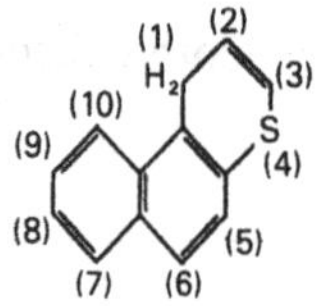

(41)

1*H*-naphtho[2,1-*b*]thiopyran
(synonyms: 5,6-benzothiochromene;
1,4-dihydro-1-thiaphenanthrene)
m.w.: 198 ($C_{13}H_{10}S$)

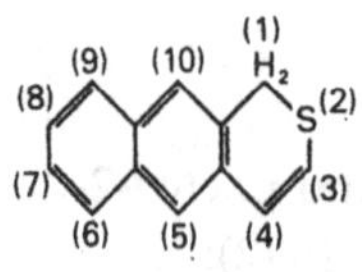

(42)

1*H*-naphtho[2,3-*c*]thiopyran
(synonyms: 6,7-benzoisothiochromene;
1,2-dihydro-2-thianthracene)
m.w.: 198 ($C_{13}H_{10}S$)

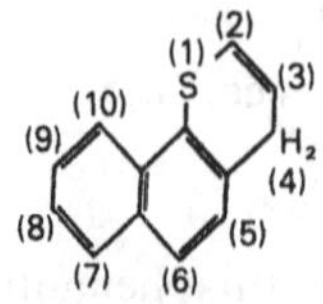

(43)

4*H*-naphtho[1,2-*b*]thiopyran
(synonyms: 7,8-benzo-4*H*-thiochromene;
1,4-dihydro-4-thiaphenanthrene)
m.w.: 198 ($C_{13}H_{10}S$)

(44)

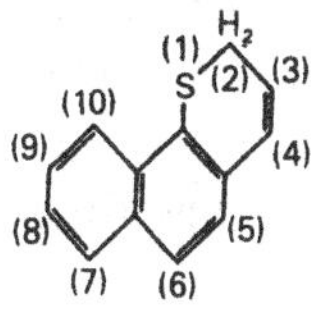

2*H*-naphtho[1,2-b]thiopyran
synonyms: 7,8-benzothiochromene;
3,4-dihydro-4-thiaphenanthrene
m.w.: 198 ($C_{13}H_{10}S$)

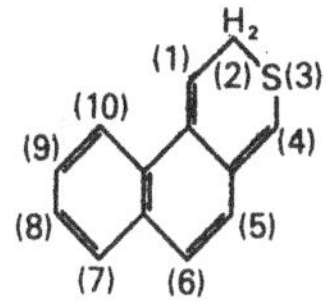

(45)

2*H*-naphtho[2,1-c]thiopyran
(synonyms: 5,6-benzo-3*H*-isothiochromene;
2,3-dihydro-2-thiaphenanthrene)
m.w.: 198 ($C_{13}H_{10}S$)

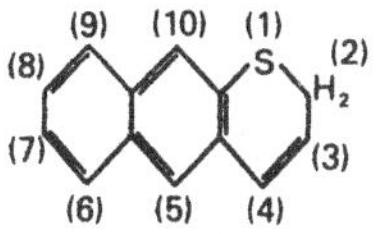

(46)

2*H*-naphtho[2,3-b]thiopyran
(synonyms: 6,7-benzothiochromene;
1,2-dihydro-1-thianthracene)
m.w. 198 ($C_{13}H_{10}S$)

(47)

Derivatives of 2*H*-naphtho[2,3-*b*]thiopyran such as perhydronaphtho[2,3-*b*]thiopyran have been found along with various completely and partially hydrogenated thiopyrans, benzothiopyrans and benzothiophenes in Western Surgut petroleum (Lyapina *et al.*, 1980*a,b*, 1982).

9H-*Thioxanthene* (synonyms: 2,3-benzo-4*H*-thiochromene; 9,10-dihydro-9-thianthracene)

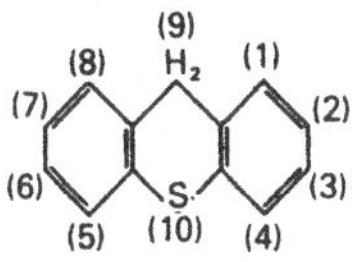

m.w.: 198 ($C_{13}H_{10}S$)

(48)

Several routes for the synthesis of this thiaarene have been described (Mayer, 1957; Bugakova and Rozantsev, 1964; Kharchenko and Krupina, 1967), e.g. condensation of benzenethiol and *o*-aminobenzoic acid in polyphosphoric acid yielding 70% thioxanthone which gives 9*H*-thioxanthene upon reduction (Mayer, 1957):

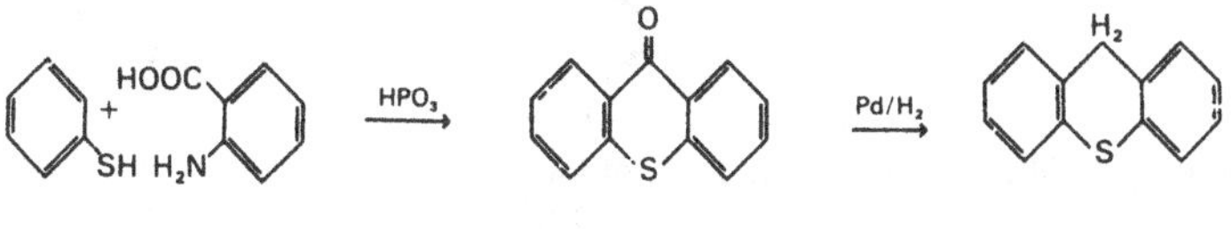

High-temperature reaction (450–650°C) between toluene and benzenethiol also results in the formation of 9*H*-thioxanthene (Voronkov *et al.*,
1977). A preventive and curative effect of thioxanthene and thioxanthone
against infections of tomatoes by *Fusarium oxysporum* has been reported
by Buchenauer (1971).

2.3   Tetracyclic compounds
$C_4S–C_5–C_5–C_6$

Only one compound of this structure, *as*-indaceno[4,5-*c*]thio-
phene (**49**) has so far been reported.

as-Indaceno[4,5-c]thiophene

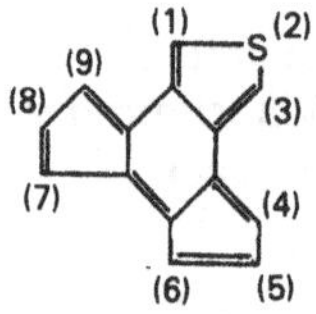

m.w.: 208 ($C_{14}H_8S$)

(**49**)

The 1,3,4,5,6,7,8,9-octahydro-*as*-indaceno[4,5-*c*]thiophene (m.p.:
112°C) has been obtained from the corresponding dodecahydrofuran by
treatment with sulfur (Le Guillanton, 1966).

$C_4S–C_5–C_6–C_6$

Acenaphthothiophenes, benzindenothiophenes, cyclopentanaphthothiophenes and fluorenothiophenes belong to this class of thiaarenes some of which were detected in petroleum.

Five different acenaphthothiophenes of the molecular formula $C_{14}H_8S$
(m.w.: 208) are known, the [3,4-*b*]- and the [4,3-*b*]-isomer of which were
found in petroleum fractions (Lumpkin, 1964; Lyapina *et al.*, 1980*a,b*).

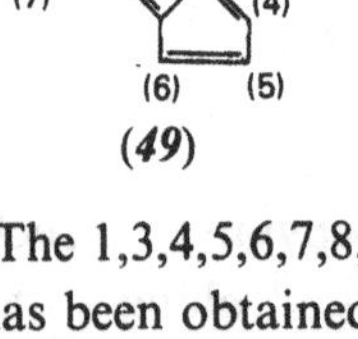

acenaphtho[1,2-*b*]thiophene
(**50**)

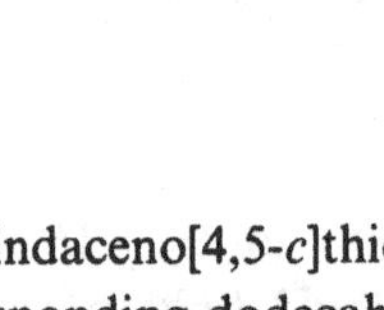

acenaphtho[1,2-*c*]thiophene
(**51**)

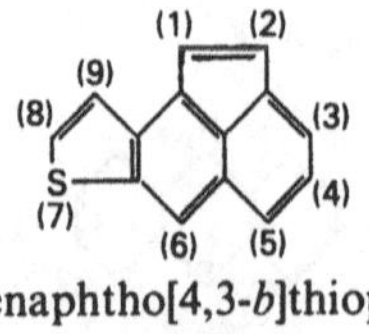

acenaphtho[4,3-*b*]thiophene
(**52**)

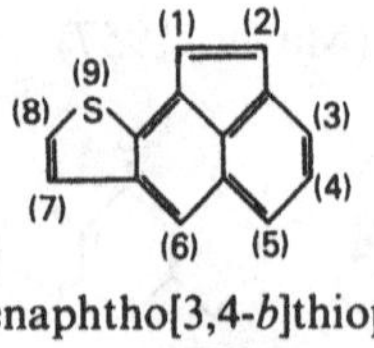

acenaphtho[3,4-*b*]thiophene
(**53**)

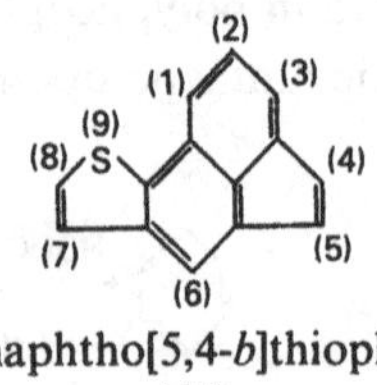

acenaphtho[5,4-*b*]thiophene
(**54**)

Acenaphtho[1,2-b]thiophene

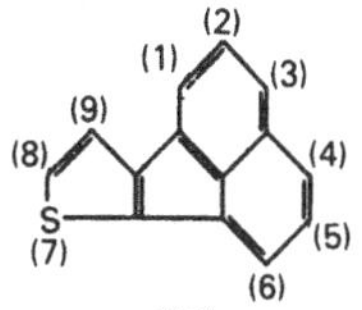

(50)

m.w.: 208
m.p.: 63°C

Acenaphtho[1,2-*b*]thiophene was prepared by treatment of 1-chloro-2-formylacenaphthylene with ethylthioglycolate and subsequent decarboxylation of the free acid (Hauptmann *et al.*, 1969):

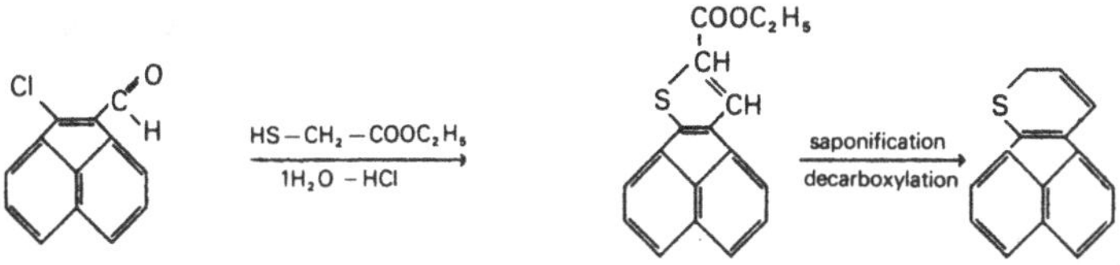

Its synthesis by sulfurization of alkylacenaphthylenes (Morel and Mollier, 1965) or by Vilsmayer-Haack formylation of tetrahydroaromatic ketones and condensation of the chloroformyl derivatives with Na_2S/bromopropionic ethyl ester and subsequent aromatization (Cagniant and Kirsch, 1975) was also described. The latter method also has been applied for the preparation of acenaphtho[5,4-*b*]thiophene (*54*). ^{1}H-NMR spectra of acenaphtho[1,2-*b*]thiophene were recorded by Bartle *et al.* (1971*b*) and MO calculations have been carried out by various authors (Scholz and Heidrich, 1967; Mallion, 1973; Bartle, 1973; Scholz *et al.*, 1973).

Acenaphtho(1,2-c)thiophene

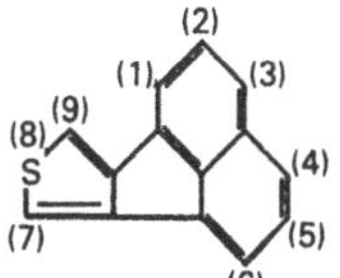

(51)

m.w.: 208
m.p.: 98.5°C

This system has been synthesized by condensation of acenaphthene-quinone and thiodiglycolic ester, aromatization with acetic anhydride and subsequent heating with copper in quinoline:

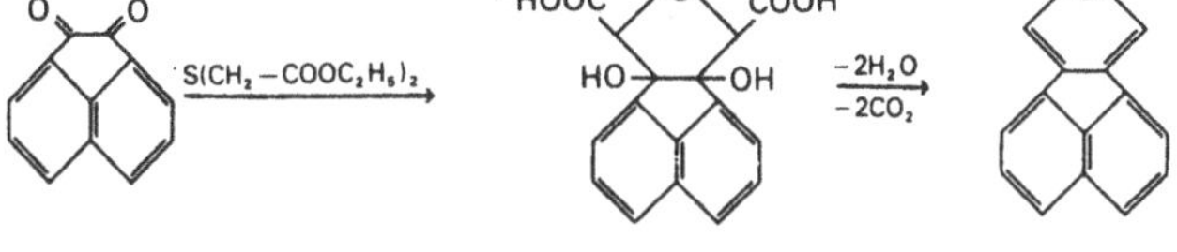

MO calculations and NMR-spectra have been recorded (Scholz and Heidrich, 1967; Bartle *et al.*, 1971*b*; Scholz *et al.*, 1973; Bartle, 1973; Mallion, 1973).

Except 1*H*-benz[*b*]indeno[5,6-*d*]thiophene, among the benz[*b*]indeno- and cyclopentanaphthothiophenes, some of which are known as thiasteroids, none was found to occur in environmental matter. Syntheses of the following systems or derivatives thereof have been published (references are given in parentheses).

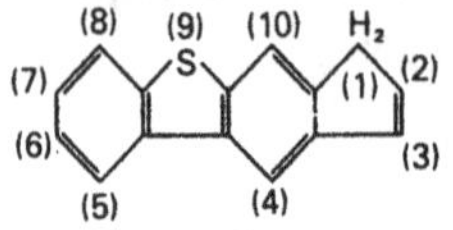

(*55*)

1*H*-benz[*b*]indeno[5,6-*b*]thiophene
m.w.: 222 ($C_{15}H_{10}S$)
(Mel'nikova *et al.*, 1981; Iglamova *et al.*, 1982)

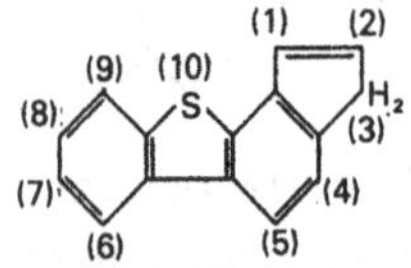

(*56*)

3*H*-benz[*b*]indeno[5,4-*d*]thiophene
m.w.: 222 ($C_{15}H_{10}S$)
(Mitra and Tilak, 1956*a,b*;
Crenshaw and Luke, 1969)

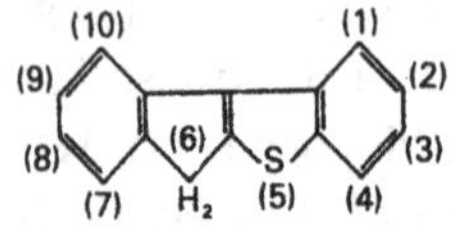

(*57*)

6*H*-benz[*b*]indeno[1,2-*d*]thiophene
m.w.: 222 ($C_{15}H_{10}S$)
(Sauter and Dzerovicz, 1969)

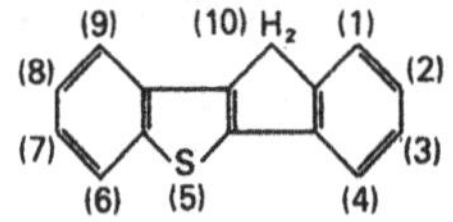

(*58*)

10*H*-benz[*b*]indeno[2,1-*d*]thiophene
m.w.: 222 ($C_{15}H_{10}S$)
(Barton *et al.*, 1972; Iddon *et al.*, 1974)

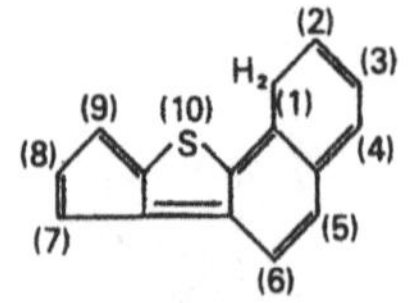

(*59*)

1*H*-cyclopenta[*b*]naphtho[2,1-*d*]thiophene
m.w.: 222 ($C_{15}H_{10}S$)
(Schultz *et al.*, 1978)

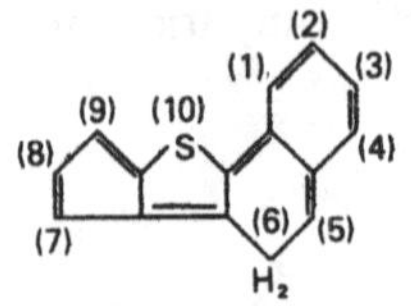

(*60*)

6*H*-cyclopenta[*b*]naphtho[2,1-*d*]thiophene
m.w.: 222 ($C_{15}H_{10}S$)
(Van Hes *et al.*, 1968)

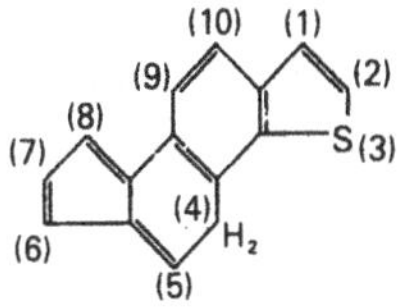

(*61*)

4*H*-cyclopenta[5,6]naphtho[1,2-*b*]thiophene
m.w.: 222 (C$_{15}$H$_{10}$S)
(Corvers *et al.*, 1977)

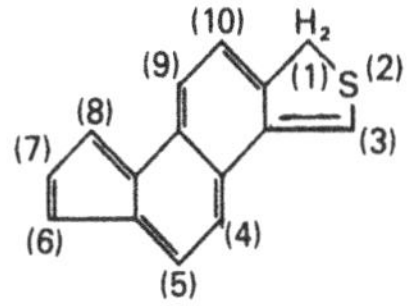

(*62*)

1*H*-cyclopenta [5,6]naphtho[1,2-*c*]thiophene
m.w.: 222 (C$_{15}$H$_{10}$S)
(Wolff *et al.*, 1970;
Wolff and Zanati, 1970*a,b*)

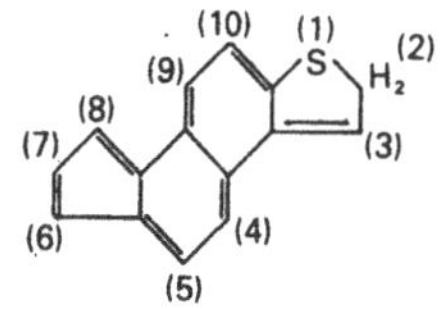

(*63*)

2*H*-cyclopenta[5,6]naphtho[2,1-*b*]thiophene
m.w.: 222 (C$_{15}$H$_{10}$S)
(Kishi and Komeno, 1971)

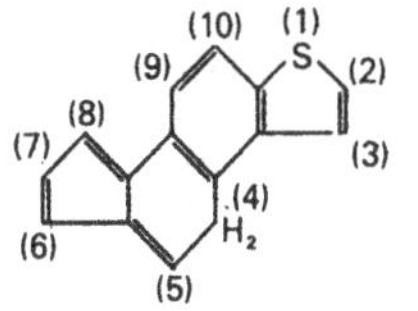

(*64*)

4*H*-cyclopenta[5,6]naphtho[2,1-*b*]thiophene
m.w.: 222 (C$_{15}$H$_{10}$S)
(Kishi and Komeno, 1971)

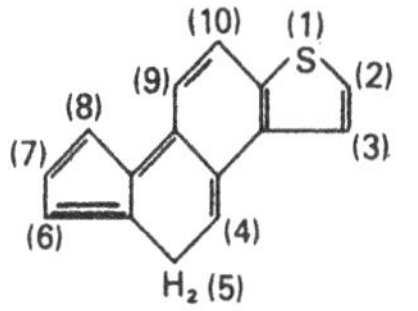

(*65*)

5*H*-cyclopenta[5,6]naphtho[2,1-*b*]thiophene
m.w.: 222 (C$_{15}$H$_{10}$S)
(Jacob and Cagniant, 1969)

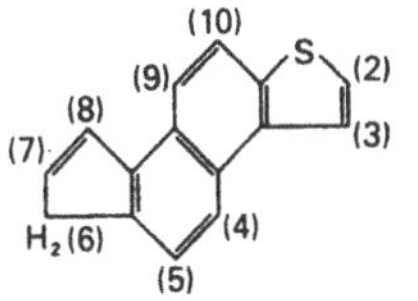

(*66*)

6*H*-cyclopenta[5,6]naphtho[2,1-*b*]thiophene
m.w.: 222 (C$_{15}$H$_{10}$S)
(Bhide and Jogdeo, 1974;
Jacob and Cagniant, 1969, 1977)

Out of the isomers of fluorenothiophenes only the 9*H*-fluoreno[2,3-*b*]thiophene (*67*) has been found in petroleum distillates (Lyapina *et al.*,

1980*b*; Mel'nikova *et al.*, 1981). Another isomeric system, 6*H*-fluoreno[4,3-*b*]thiophene (*68*) has been synthesized by Stobbe condensation of formylthiophenes with succinic ester (El-Rayyes and Al-Salman, 1975).

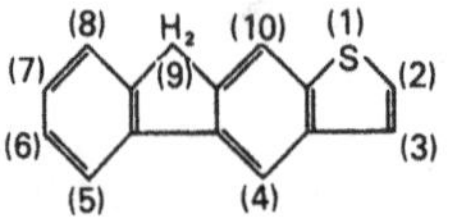

9*H*-fluoreno[2,3-*b*]thiophene
m.w.: 222 ($C_{15}H_{10}S$)

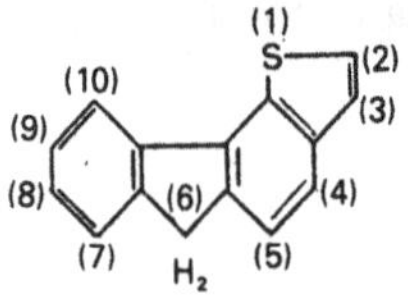

(*67*)

6*H*-fluoreno[4,3-*b*]thiophene
m.w.: 222 ($C_{15}H_{10}S$)

(*68*)

$C_4S–C_6–C_6–C_6$

Tetracyclic thiophenes with three benzene rings are the most abundant thiaarenes in the environment. By far the highest concentrations are found for the isomeric benzonaphthothiophenes, but also various anthra- and phenanthrothiophenes have been detected, whereas no definite hints are available for the environmental relevance of phenalenothiophenes.

Anthra[1,2-b]thiophene

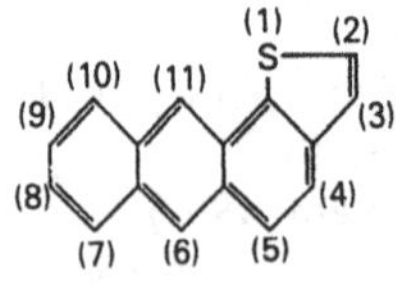

m.w.: 234 ($C_{16}H_{10}S$)
m.p.: 121°C

(*69*)

This compound has been identified in coal tar (Nishioka *et al.*, 1985*a*), coal oil and solvent-refined coal materials (Nakamura, 1983; Wise *et al.*, 1983). It has been synthesized by Diels-Alder condensation of naphtho-1,4-quinone and 3-vinylthiophene giving 4,5,6,11-tetrahydro-anthra[1,2-*b*]thiophene-6,11-quinone which upon chloranil treatment, subsequent reduction and aromatization yields the thiaarene (Faller, 1968). Other synthetic routes as well as IR-, UV- and NMR-spectral data have been reported (Faller, 1968; Maruyama *et al.*, 1980; Tominaga *et al.*, 1981*a*).

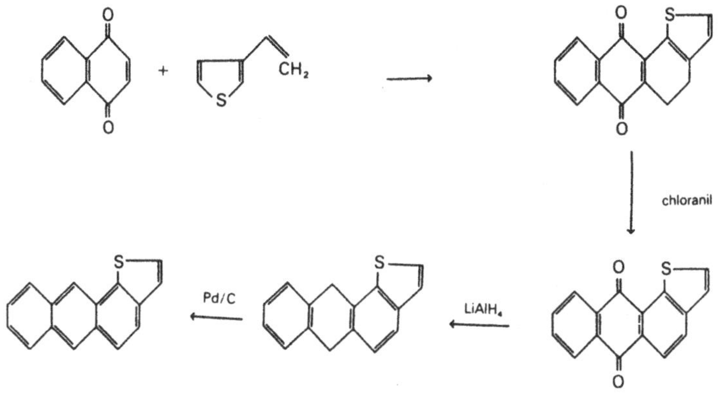

Anthra[2,1-b]thiophene

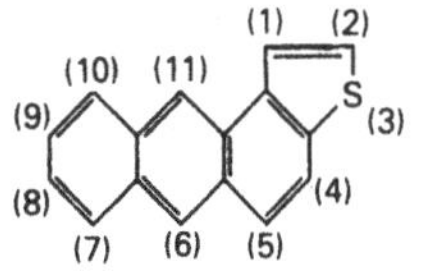

m.w.: 234 ($C_{16}H_{10}S$)
m.p.: 196°C

(70)

This isomer is present in coal oil (Nakamura, 1983; Wise *et al.*, 1983). It has been synthesized analogously to its [1,2-*b*]isomer **(69)** from naphtho-1,4-quinone and 2-vinylthiophene (Faller, 1968). The 4-phenyl derivative has been prepared by photochemical reaction of 2-bromo-3-methoxy-1,4-naphthoquinone with 1-phenyl-1-(2-thienyl)ethylene and subsequent reduction of the 6,11-quinone (Maruyama *et al.*, 1977, 1980):

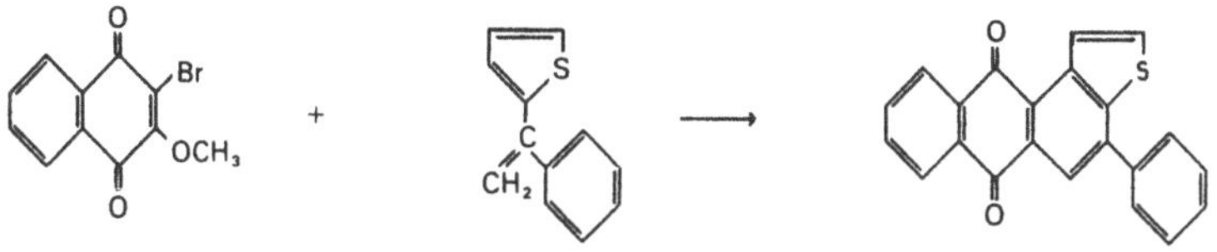

Anthra[2,3-b]thiophene

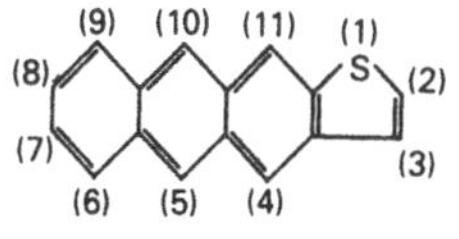

m.w.: 234 ($C_{16}H_{10}S$)
m.p.: 330°C

(71)

Anthra[2,3-*b*]thiophene was found to be present in coal liquids and in shale oil (Wise *et al.*, 1983; Kong *et al.*, 1984). Its synthesis has been described by Tominaga *et al.*, (1981*a*) and by Faller (1968). It may be obtained from naphthalene-2,3-dicarboxylic acid anhydride by Friedel-Crafts reaction with thiophene, reduction to 3-(2-thenyl)-2-naphthalenecarboxylic acid and subsequent reduction to the corresponding alcohol. The latter, after CrO_3-oxidation to the aldehyde, is cyclized to the above thiaarene:

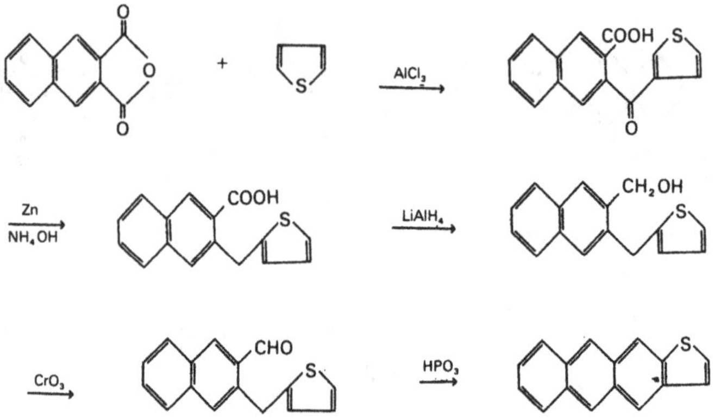

The electron structure has been calculated by DasGupta and Birss (1980).

Phenanthro[1,2-b]thiophene

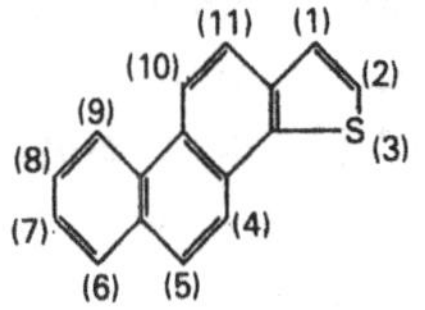

m.w.: 234 ($C_{16}H_{10}S$)
m.p.: 168–170°C

(72)

Along with other isomers this thiaarene has been detected in coal tar (Nishioka *et al.*, 1985*a*), in coal oil (Nakamura, 1983; Castle *et al.*, 1983) and in marine organisms (Vassilaros *et al.*, 1982*a*). It has been synthesized by different routes (Cagniant and Kirsch, 1975; Iwao *et al.*, 1980). Iwao *et al.* (1980) reported a synthesis with about 24% total yield by condensation of 1-naphthaldehyde with 3-thenylphosphonate followed by photocylization in the presence of oxygen and iodine:

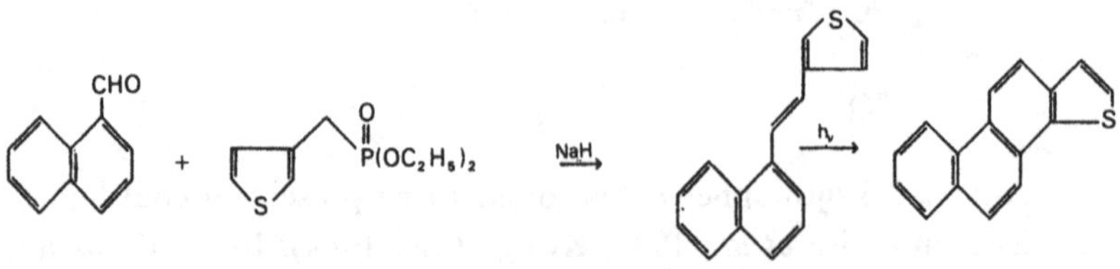

The ^{1}H- and ^{13}C–NMR-spectra have been published by Martin *et al.* (1983).

Phenanthro[2,1-b]thiophene (synonym: thiopheno-2,3:2',1'-phenanthrene)

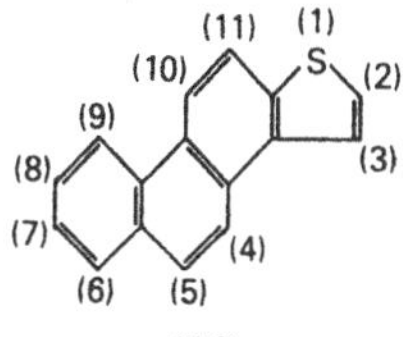

(11) (1)
(10) S (2)
(9) (3)
(8)
(7) (4)
(6) (5)

(*73*)

m.w.: 234 ($C_{16}H_{10}S$)
m.p.: 237–238°C

Phenanthro[2,1-*b*]thiophene was found in coal oil (Nakamura, 1983; Wise *et al.*, 1983) and in petroleum (Payzant *et al.*, 1983). Analogously to the [1,2-*b*]-isomer Iwao *et al.* (1980) have synthesized this system in a 75% total yield starting with 2-thenylphosphonate:

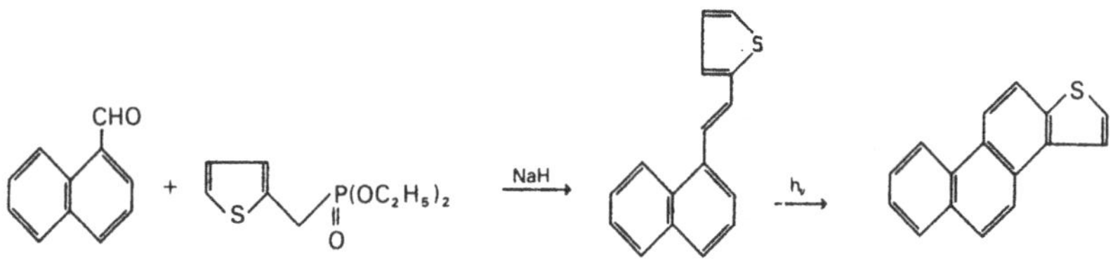

CHO + S P(OC$_2$H$_5$)$_2$ →(NaH) →(hν)
O

Phenanthro[2,3-b]thiophene (synonym: thiopheno-2,3:2',3'-phenanthrene)

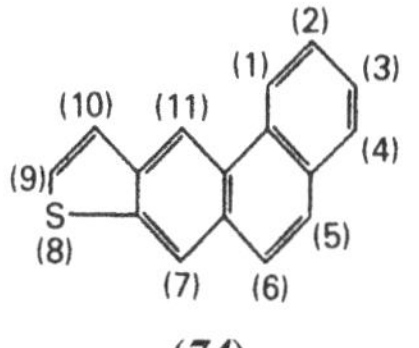

(2)
(1) (3)
(10) (11) (4)
(9) (5)
S
(8)
(7) (6)

(*74*)

m.w.: 234 ($C_{16}H_{10}S$)
m.p.: 161–161.5°C

Phenanthro[2,3-*b*]thiophene has been detected in coal oil (Nakamura, 1983; Wise *et al.*, 1983) and in coal tar (Nishioka *et al.*, 1986*b*). The system has been synthesized by Sandin and Fieser (1940) and Newman and Ihrman (1958). Iwao *et al.* (1980) more recently used a route starting with thienyloxazolidine which after lithiation was condensed with 2-naphthaldehyde. After hydrolysis, cyclization and Pd/H$_2$-reduction, 2-(2-naphthylmethyl)-3-thiophenecarboxylic acid was obtained which upon LiAlH$_4$-reduction, subsequent CrO$_3$-oxidation in pyridine and final cyclization with polyphosphoric acid gives the above compound in an overall yield of about 22%:

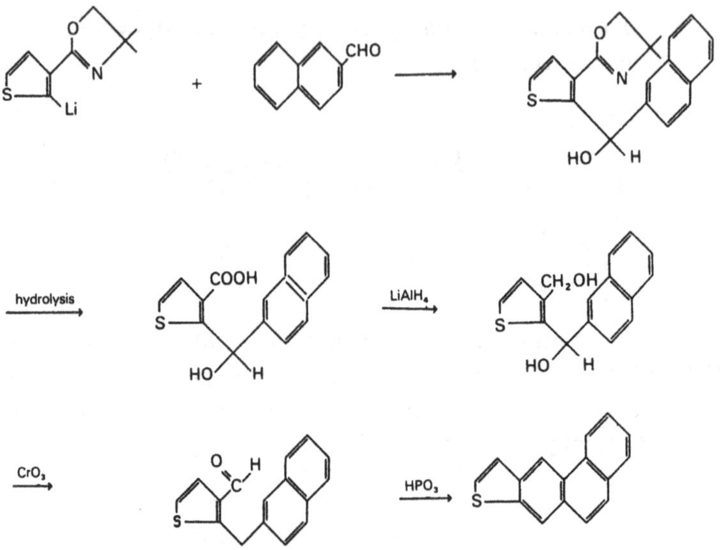

NMR- and UV-spectral data have been published (Carruthers and Crowder, 1957; Iwao *et al.*, 1980) and MO-studies were carried out by Zahradnik and Parkanyi (1965).

Phenanthro[3,2-b]thiophene (synonym: thiopheno-2,3:3',2'-phenanthrene)

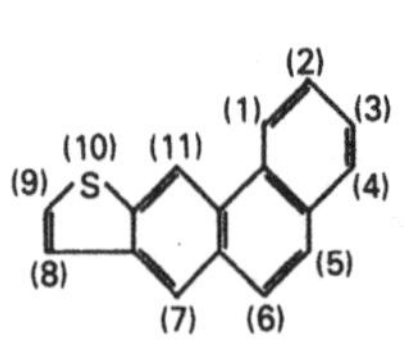

m.w.: 234 ($C_{16}H_{10}S$)
m.p.: 121–122°C

(75)

This thiaarene, which occurs in coal tar (Nishioka *et al.*, 1986*b*) and in coal oil (Nakamura, 1983; Wise *et al.*, 1983), has been synthesized in analogy to the above [2,3-*b*]-isomer (Iwao *et al.*, 1980), with 1-naphth-aldehyde as starting material and in an overall yield of about 13%. NMR-spectra (Iwao *et al.*, 1980) and MO calculation (Zahradnik and Parkanyi, 1965) have been presented.

Phenanthro[3,4-b]thiophene (synonym: thiopheno-2,3:3',4'-phenanthrene)

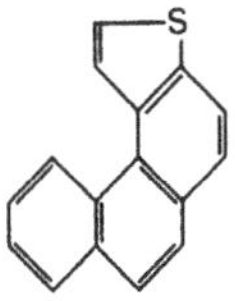

m.w.: 234 ($C_{16}H_{10}S$)
m.p.: 82.5–83.5°C

(76)

Phenanthro[3,4-*b*]thiophene, occurring in coal oil (Nakamura, 1983; Wise *et al.*, 1983) and in coal tar (Nishioka *et al.*, 1985*a*), has been prepared by cyclization of 3-phenanthrylthioglycolic acid (Paresh and Chaudhury, 1951), by Diels-Alder reaction of 1-(2-thienyl)-3,4-dihydro-naphthalene with maleic anhydride and subsequent dehydrogenation and decarboxylation (Szmuszkovicz and Modest, 1950), and more recently by Iwao *et al.* (1980) in total yield of 15% by Wadsworth-Emmons reaction between 2-naphthaldehyde and 2-thenylphosphonate giving 1-(2-thienyl)-2-(2-naphthyl)ethene which then is photocyclized:

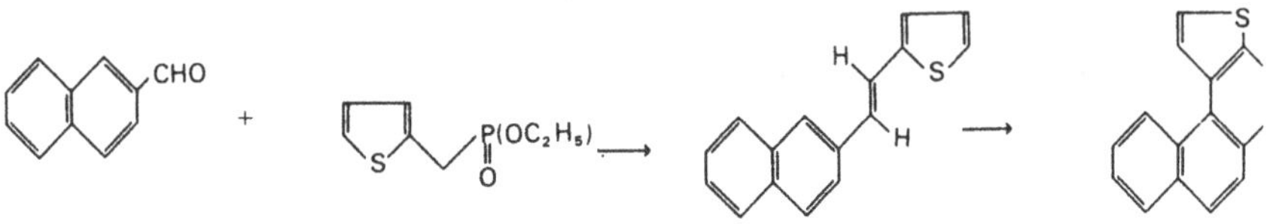

The authors also presented NMR- and UV-data on this compound.

Phenanthro[4,3-b]thiophene

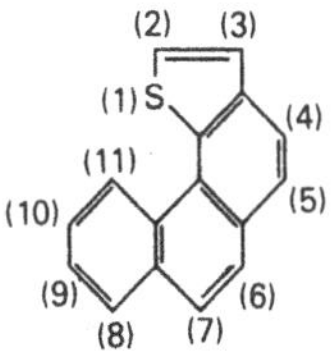

m.w.: 234 ($C_{16}H_{10}S$)
m.p.: 94–95°C

(77)

Along with other isomers this thiaarene has been detected in coal oils (Nakamura, 1983; Wise *et al.*, 1983) and in coal tars (Nishioka *et al.*, 1985*a*). Several syntheses have been reported (Szmuszkovicz and Modest, 1950; Cagniant and Kirsch, 1975; Iwao *et al.*, 1980; Castle *et al.*, 1983), among which the Wadsworth-Emmons reaction between 2-naphthalde-hyde and 3-thenylphosphonate with a subsequent photocyclization in analogy to the above route seems to be the most elegant one (54% yield). NMR- and UV-spectra were recorded by Iwao *et al.* (1980).

Phenanthro[9,10-b]thiophene (synonym: thiopheno-2,3:9′,10′-phenanthrene)

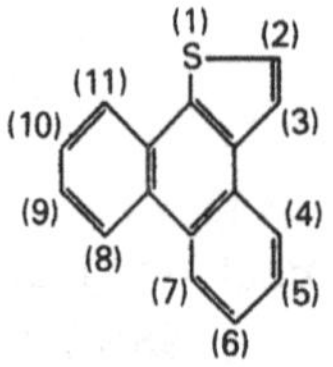

m.w.: 234 ($C_{16}H_{10}S$)
m.p.: 151–152°C

(*78*)

Phenanthro[9,10-*b*]thiophene was found in coal oil (Nakamura, 1983; Wise *et al.*, 1983) and in coal tar (Nishioka *et al.*, 1985a). For its synthesis several routes have been published. Wynberg *et al.* (1967) obtained phenanthro[9,10-*b*]thiophene by photocyclization of 2,3-diphenylthiophene in the presence of air:

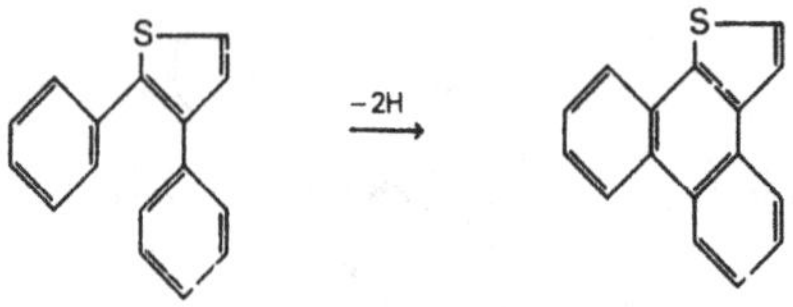

Iwao *et al.* (1980) synthesized it by Grignard reaction of 9-bromophenanthrene with β,β-diethoxyethyldisulfide resulting in 9-phenanthrylthioethanal diethylacetale which was cyclized with polyphosphoric acid to the orange-coloured phenanthro[9,10-*b*]thiophene in a total yield of 25%:

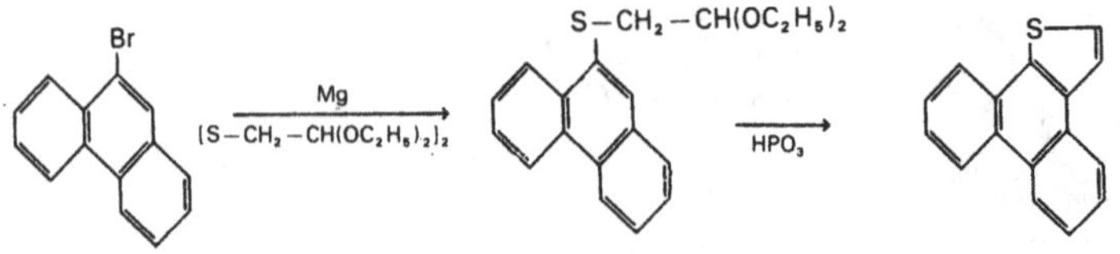

Sidorenko *et al.* (1983*b*) prepared this isomer by arylation of acrylic acid with 9-bromophenanthrene. The 9-phenanthreneacrylic acid was cyclocondensed with thionylchloride in the presence of $(C_2H_5)_3N;CH_2-C_6H_5X^-$, and the product then hydrolysed. After decarboxylation and dechlorination, phenanthro[9,10-*b*]thiophene was obtained in a total yield of 23%:

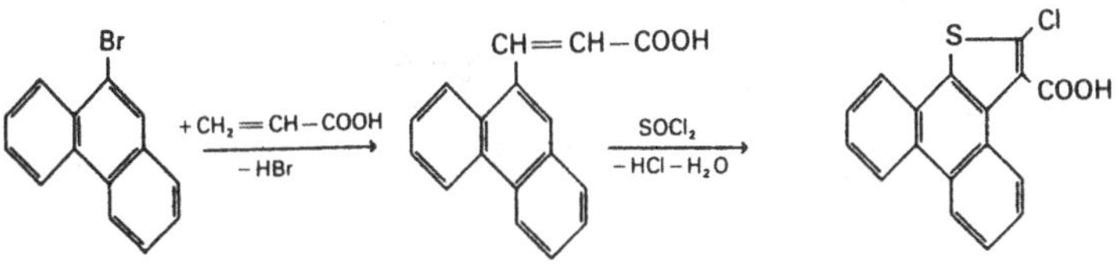

NMR- and UV-spectral data were presented by Iwao *et al.* (1980).

Phenanthro[9,10-c]thiophene (synonym: thiopheno-3,4:9'10'-phenanthrene)

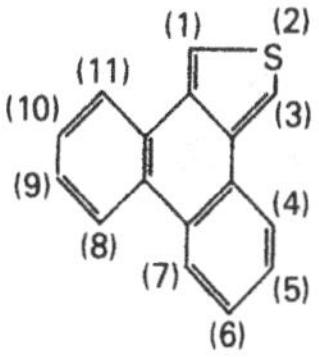

m.w.: 234 ($C_{16}H_{10}S$)
m.p.: 169°C

(79)

This isomer has not yet been detected in environmental matter. It has been synthesized by reaction of 9-bromomethyl-10-chloro-methylphenanthrene with alcoholic sodium sulfide (Stille and Foster, 1963; Millar and Wilson, 1964; Shields *et al.*, 1975):

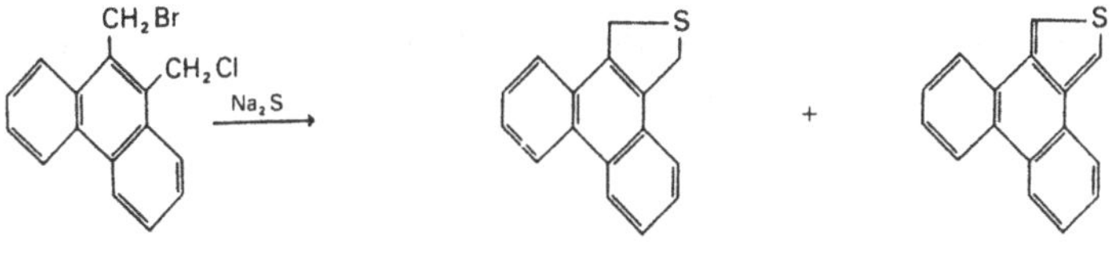

This system can also be obtained by treatment of 2,2-di-(phenylethinyl)-diphenyl with tris(triphenylphosphine)rhodium(I)chloride and reaction with sulfur (Müller *et al.*, 1971):

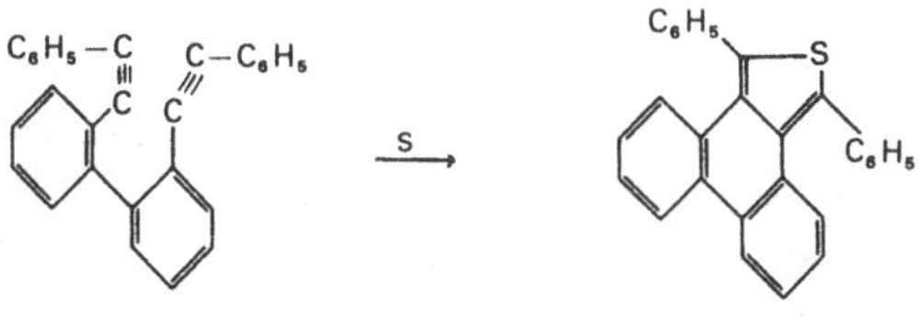

The sulfone of this compound was obtained by SO_2-insertion under ring enlargement into the following cyclobutene derivative (Cava and Mangold, 1964):

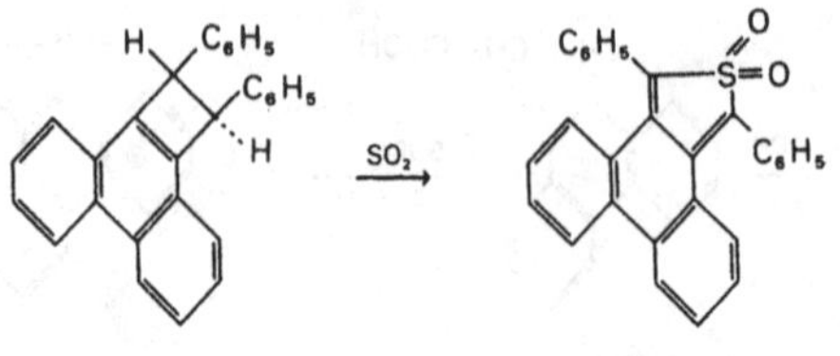

Another route starts with phenanthrene-9,10-quinone which after reaction with thioglycolic ester (Kochkanyan *et al.*, 1974) and subsequent decarboxylation (Hauptmann *et al.*, 1969) gives phenanthro[9,10-*c*]thiophene in an overall yield of 9%:

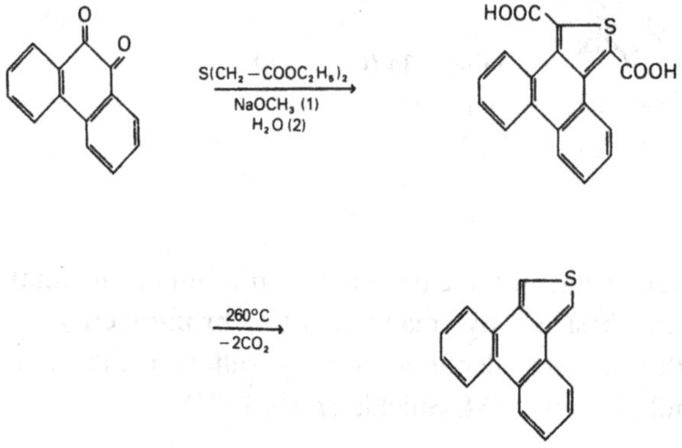

π-Electron calculations of this thiaarene have been carried out by DasGupta and Birss (1980).

Phenanthro[4,5-bcd]thiophene

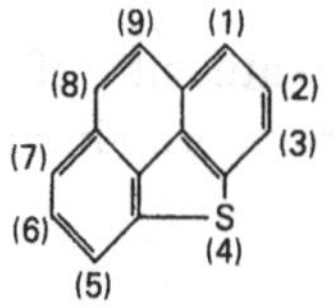

m.w.: 208 ($C_{14}H_8S$)
m.p.: 135°C

(*80*)

This compound is a common environmental thiaarene often associated with pyrene. It has been found in coal (White and Lee, 1980; Chiu *et al.*, 1983), in coal tar (Borwitzky *et al.*, 1977; Borwitzky and Schomburg, 1979; Burchill *et al.*, 1982*a*; Nishioka *et al.*, 1985*a*, 1986*ab*), in pitch (Burchill *et al.*, 1982*a*), in coal derived products, especially in synfuels (Lee *et al.*, 1980; Walsh *et al.*, 1983; Nakamura, 1983; Willey *et al.*, 1981*b*; Later *et al.*, 1981; Kong *et al.*, 1984; Nishioka *et al.*, 1986*b*; Lee *et al.*, 1980; White and Lee, 1980; Burchill *et al.*, 1982*b*), in anthracene oil (Burchill *et al.*, 1982*a*, 1983) and accordingly in coal combustion effluents (Lee *et al.*, 1980). It was found and separated from commercially available polycyclic aromatic hydrocarbons (Karcher *et al.*, 1979, 1981) and was also detected in various carbon blacks (Lee and Hites, 1976; Fitch *et al.*, 1978; Locati *et al.*, 1979; Alsberg *et al.*, 1982; Colmsjö and Östman, 1982), in Diesel exhaust (Tong and Karasek, 1984) and in air particulates (Howard and Mills, 1983; Grimmer *et al.*, 1985; Chiu *et al.*, 1983). Phenanthro[4,5-*bcd*]thiophene was detected in the aquatic environment (Vassilaros *et al.*, 1982*a*), especially in fish (Vassilaros *et al.*, 1982*b*; Lee *et al.*, 1982; Baumann *et al.*, 1982; Vassilaros *et al.*, 1982*a*; West *et al.*, 1985), in mussels (Kveseth *et al.*, 1982), in sewage discharge (Kveseth *et al.*, 1982; Vassilaros *et al.*, 1982*a*), in tap water (Kveseth *et al.*, 1982) and in minerals (West *et al.*, 1985). Furthermore, it is a minor compound in fossil fuels such as crude oil (Grimmer *et al.*, 1983*a*), shale oil (Chiu *et al.*, 1983; Willey *et al.*, 1981*a,b*; Kong *et al.*, 1984) and accordingly also in motor oil (Grimmer *et al.*, 1981*a*).

The compound was synthesized by Klemm and coworkers (Klemm *et al.*, 1970; Klemm and Hsin, 1976) by H_2S-treatment of phenanthrene on an alumina catalyst at 630°C. Tedjamulia *et al.* (1983*a*) have described the synthesis of phenanthro[4,5-*bcd*]thiophene and four of its monomethyl derivatives (1-, 2-, 3- and 8-isomer) by cyclization of 2-(1-dibenzothiophenyl) acetaldehyde:

None of the four phenalenothiophenes [m.w.: 222 ($C_{15}H_{10}S$)] described in the literature has been definitely identified in environmental matter.

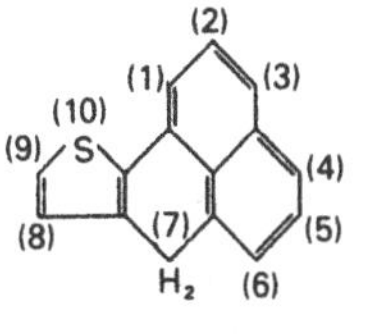

7*H*-phenaleno[1,2-*b*]thiophene

(*81*)

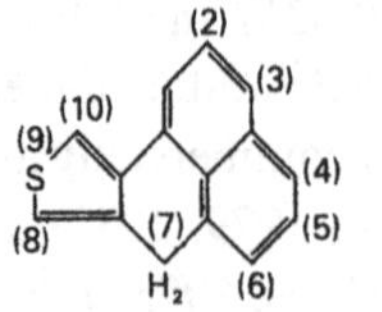

7*H*-phenaleno[1,2-*c*]thiophene

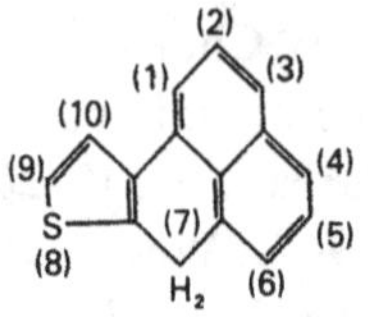

(82)

7*H*-phenaleno[2,1-*b*]thiophene

(83)

The above isomers were synthesized by reduction of the phenalenothio-phenones which were obtained by condensation of the corresponding quinones with glycerol and sulfuric acid (MacDowell *et al.*, 1971):

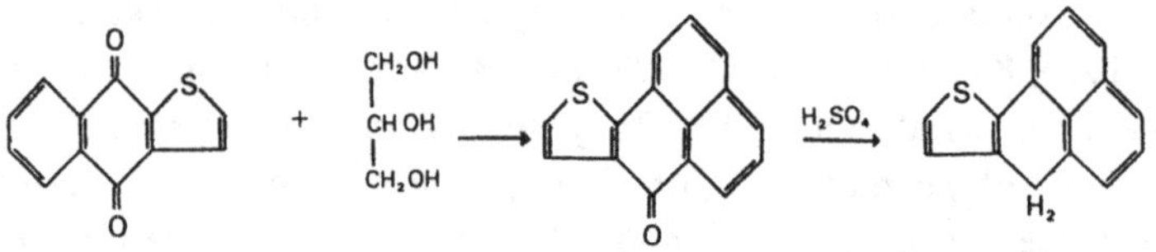

Phenaleno[1,9-bc]thiophene (synonym: phenaleno[6,7-*bc*]-thiophene)

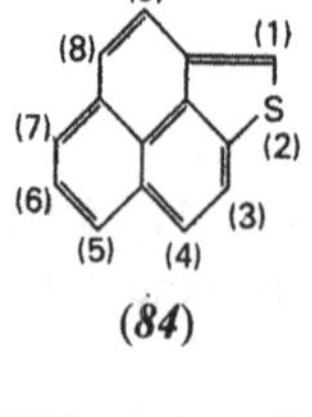

m.w.: 208 (C$_{14}$H$_8$S)
m.p.: 156°C

(84)

This system has been found in heavy oil and in tars (Nishioka *et al.*, 1985*a*). Its synthesis has been described by Tominaga *et al.* (1981*b*). 1-Methylnaphtho[2,1-*b*]thiophene, after bromination with N-bromo-succinimide and subsequent KCN-treatment, resulted in 1-cyanomethylnaphtho[2,1-*b*]thiophene which after conversion into the corresponding aldehyde was cyclized with polyphosphoric acid to phenaleno[1,9-*bc*]thiophene in an overall yield of 7%:

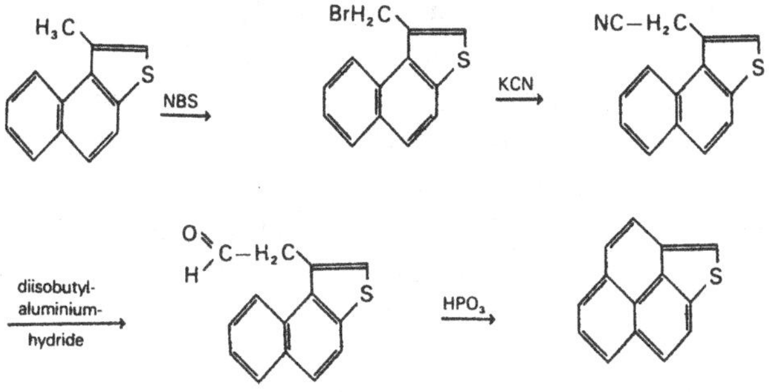

Benzonaphthothiophenes

The two isomers, benzo[*b*]naphtho[1,2-*d*]- and -[2,1-*d*]thiophene, are the most abundant thiaarenes in the environment, whereas the [2,3-*d*]-isomer is significantly lower in concentration.

Benzo[b]*naphtho[1,2-*d]*thiophene* (synonyms: 1,2-benzodiphenylene sulfide; 7-thiabenzo[*c*]fluorene; naphtho[2,1-*b*]benzothiophene; 3,4-benzo-9-thiafluorene)

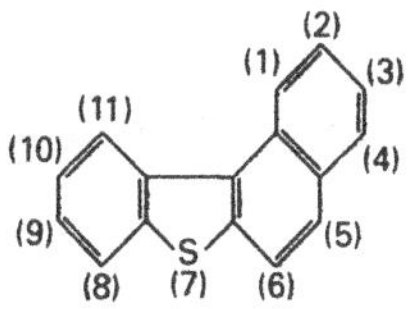

m.w.: 234 ($C_{16}H_{10}S$)
m.p.: 102°C

Benzo[*b*]naphtho[1,2-*d*]thiophene and occasionally also various methyl derivatives of it have been found in crude oil (Grimmer *et al.*, 1983*a*), in shale oil (Willey *et al.*, 1981*b*; Kong *et al.*, 1984), in petroleum fractions (Oshima *et al.*, 1966; Carruthers and Stewart, 1967), in coal liquids and coal products (Kong *et al.*, 1982, 1984; Wise *et al.*, 1983; Lucke *et al.*, 1985; Nishioka *et al.*, 1986*b*; Willey *et al.*, 1981*b*), in flue gases from coal-fired power plants (Nielsen, 1984), in hard coal (Grimmer *et al.*, 1985; Schmidt *et al.*, 1986, 1987) and brown-coal emission (Grimmer *et al.*, 1983*b*), in carbon black (Silva *et al.*, 1982) in coal tar and pitch (Shultz *et al.*, 1965; Nishioka *et al.*, 1985*a*, 1986*b*; Burchill *et al.*, 1982*a*), in Diesel exhaust (Hites *et al.*, 1981; Howard and Mills, 1983), in motor oils (Grimmer *et al.*, 1981*a*), and in air particulate matter (Lee *et al.*, 1982; Nielsen, 1984). Accordingly, it was found secondarily in the aquatic environment (Vassilaros *et al.*, 1982*a*), in river water (Grimmer *et al.*, 1981*c*), in sediments (Lee *et al.*, 1982) and in fish (Vassilaros *et al.*, 1982*a,b*; Lee *et al.*, 1982).

Various routes for the synthesis of benzo[*b*]naphtho[1,2-*d*]thiophene have been employed. Rabindran and Tilak (1953*b*) and Campaigne and Osborn (1968) have synthesized it by condensation of 2-bromocyclohexanone with β-thionaphthol in NaOH. The product was cyclized with phosphorous pentoxide and the resulting 8,9,10,11-tetrahydrobenzo[*b*]naphtho[1,2-*d*]thiophene aromatized with selenium. This method was also applied recently for the preparation of a highly purified product (Karcher *et al.*, 1983):

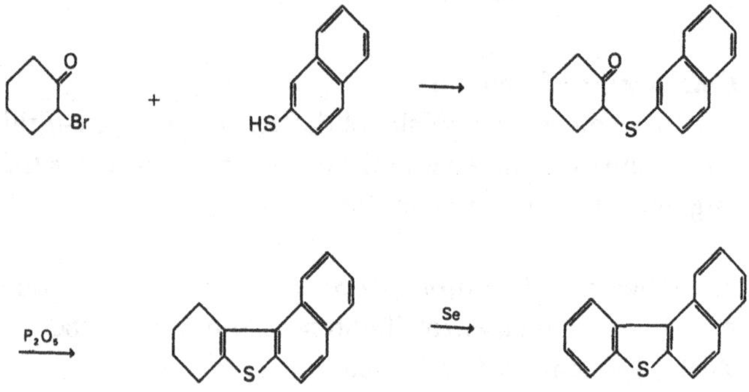

Its formation by pyrolysis from 6a,11b-dihydrobenzo[*b*]naphtho[1,2-*d*]thiophene-7,7-dioxide has been reported (Davies *et al.*, 1968; Taylor *et al.*, 1968). Tominaga *et al.* (1982*a,c*) synthesized benzo[*b*]naphtho[1,2-*d*]thiophene by condensation of benzo[*b*]thiophene-2-aldehyde with diethyl benzylphosphonate and subsequent photocyclization:

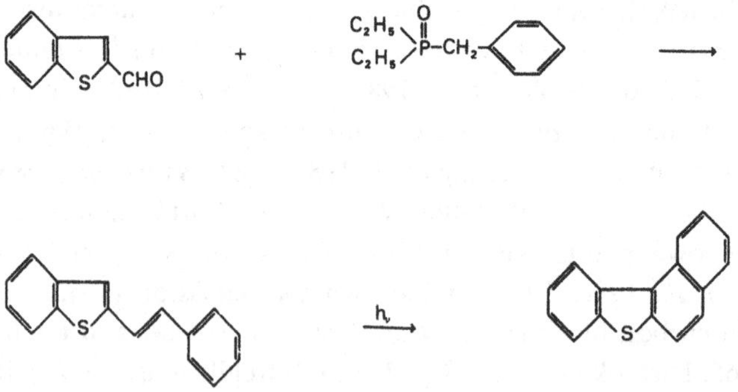

These authors also described the synthesis of all of the ten isomeric monomethyl derivatives which were obtained by Wadsworth-Emmons reaction of *o*-, *p*-, or *m*-methylbenzaldehyde with diethyl 2-benzo[*b*]thenylphosphonate which resulted in *o*-, *p*-, or *m*-methylstyrylbenzo[*b*]thiophenes in 60–70% yield. Subsequent photocyclization gave the corresponding monomethylbenzo[*b*]naphtho-[1,2-*d*]thiophenes (yields: 1- (10%); 2- (45%); 3- (22%); 4-methyl derivative (42%)):

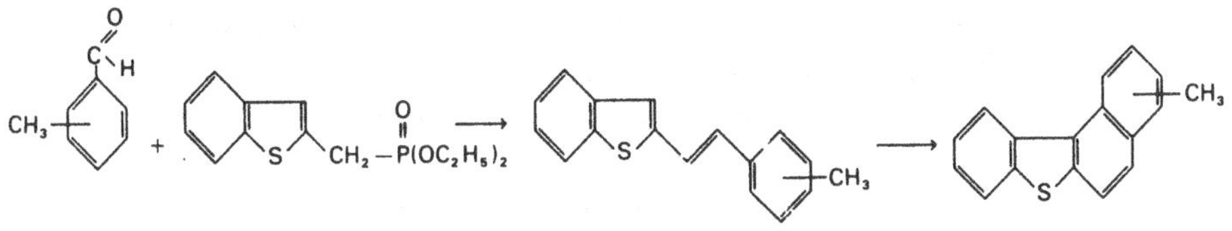

Similarly, the 8-, 9-, and 10-methyl derivatives were obtained from 5-, 6-, or 7-methyl-2-styrylbenzo[*b*]thiophene in a total yield of 36%, 32%, and 32%, respectively. The synthesis of the 5- and the 11-isomers was also described by the above working group (Tominaga *et al.*, 1982*a,c*; Castle *et al.*, 1984).

An interesting entrance to this thiaarene system is provided by H_2O_2-treatment of benzo[*b*]thiophene giving the sulfone which then is heated in tetralin at 180–200°C yielding 6a,11b-dihydrobenzo[*b*]naphtho[1,2-*d*]thiophene-7,7-dioxide through an intermediate product (Bordwell *et al.*, 1951; Davies *et al.*, 1952*a,b*; Taylor and Wallace, 1968). The dioxide then is aromatized with Pd/C and the resulting sulfone reduced to the thiaarene:

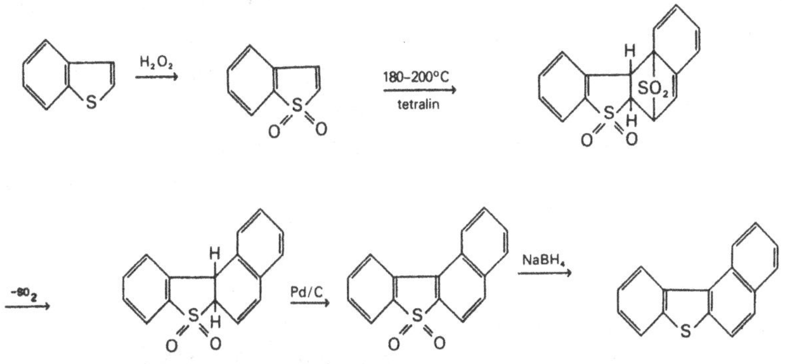

Apart from these routes other syntheses for the benzo[*b*]naphtho[1,2-*d*]thiophene system have been published (Davies and Porter, 1957*b*; Schultz, 1974; Blatt *et al.*, 1976).

UV- (Badger and Christie, 1956*b*; Campaigne and Osborn, 1968; Karcher *et al.*, 1982, 1985), fluorescence- (Karcher *et al.*, 1985), Shpol'skii fluorescence- (Colmsjö *et al.*, 1984; Karcher *et al.*, 1985), mass- (Meyerson and VanderHaar, 1962), ^{1}H- and ^{13}C–NMR- (Karcher *et al.*, 1985), and IR-spectral data (Karcher *et al.*, 1985) have been published and theoretical studies on the π-electron structure have been carried out (Campaigne and Osborn, 1968; Momicchioli and Rastelli, 1970).

When tested for mutagenicity (McFall *et al.*, 1984) and carcinogenicity (Dannenberg, 1960), benzo[*b*]naphtho[1,2-*d*]thiophene was found to be inactive. However, it was found to be a weak monooxygenase inducer (Jacob *et al.*, 1983; Norpoth *et al.*, 1984). Application to the human skin caused allergic reaction upon irradiation (Wulf *et al.*, 1963).

Benzo[b]*naphtho*[2,1-d]*thiophene* (synonyms: naphtho[1,2-*b*]-benzothiophene; 1,2-benzo-9-thiofluorene; 9-thia-1,2-benzo-fluorene; 11-thiabenzo[*a*]fluorene)

m.w.: 234 ($C_{16}H_{10}S$)
m.p.: 186°C

(*86*)

This thiaarene is ubiquitous in the environment. It has been detected in coal tar and derivatives (Kruber and Grigoleit, 1954; Lang and Eigen, 1967; Lee and Hites, 1976; Karcher *et al.*, 1979; Lee *et al.*, 1980; Kong *et al.*, 1982, 1984; Nakamura, 1983; Wise *et al.*, 1983; Wilson *et al.*, 1984; Lucke *et al.*, 1985; Willey *et al.*, 1981*b*; Nishioka *et al.*, 1985*a*; Burchill *et al.*, 1982*a*; Nishioka *et al.*, 1986*b*), in carbon black (Lee and Hites, 1976), in shale oil (Chiu *et al.*, 1983; Willey *et al.*, 1981*b*; Kong *et al.*, 1984), in crude oil (Ho *et al.*, 1975; Grimmer *et al.*, 1983*a*), in petroleum products (DGMK, 1983; Grimmer *et al.*, 1983*a*), in fresh and used motor oil (Grimmer *et al.*, 1981*ab*), in metal working oil (Eyres, 1981), in Diesel oil (Kaishev *et al.*, 1961), in Diesel exhaust and Diesel engine soot (Yu and Hites, 1981; Kaschani, 1983; Tong and Karasek, 1984), in brown coal emissions (Grimmer *et al.*, 1983*b*), and in smoke condensate of tobacco and related materials (Bhide *et al.*, 1984). Accordingly, it was also detected in air (Grimmer *et al.*, 1980*b*) and air particulate matter (Lee *et al.*, 1982; Spitzer and Danneker, 1984), in river sediments (Grimmer, 1979; Lee *et al.*, 1982; Vassilaros *et al.*, 1982*a*), in water (Grimmer and Naujack, 1979), in fish (Vassilaros *et al.*, 1982*a,b*; Lee *et al.*, 1982), and in sewage sludge (Grimmer *et al.*, 1978*a*, 1980*a*).

Klemm *et al.* (1978) described the insertion of sulfur into 2-phenylnaphthalene by H_2S-treatment of the latter at 450–630°C catalyzed by a sulfided cobaltous oxide–molybdic oxide–alumina mixture:

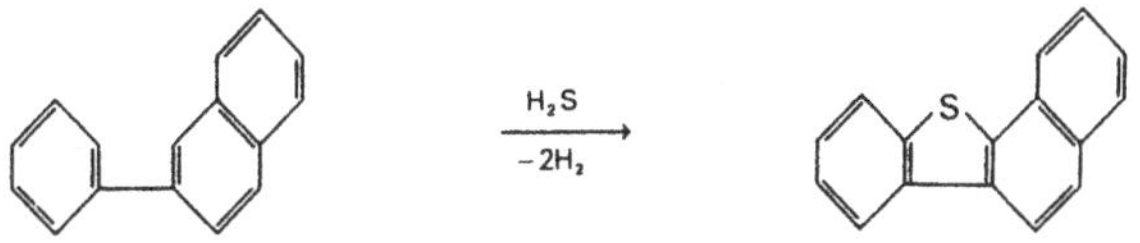

Croisy *et al.* (1975, 1984) obtained benzo[*b*]naphtho[2,1-*d*]thiophene by Elbs cyclodehydration of 3-(2-methylbenzoyl)benzo[*b*]thiophene or of benzoylmethylbenzo[*b*]thiophene, although the formation of the [2,3-*d*]-isomer was to be expected:

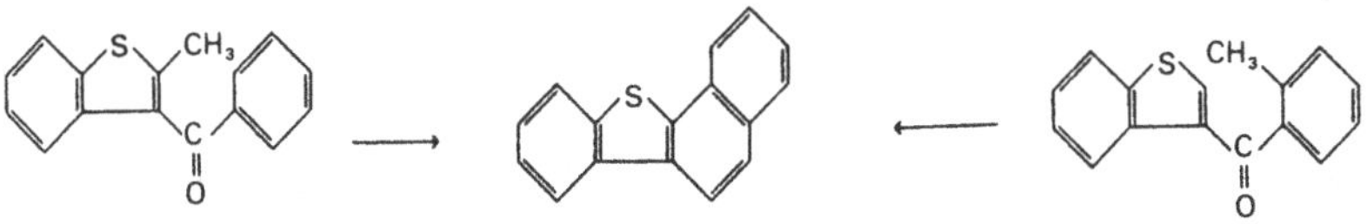

Rabindran and Tilak (1951*a*) as well as Campaigne and Osborn (1968) obtained it by condensation of 2-bromo-1-tetralone with benzene thiol, P_2O_5-treatment and subsequent aromatization with Pd/C. In a similar way a highly purified (>99.0%) product used as reference material was synthesized by condensation of 2-bromocyclohexanone with 1-naphthalenethiol, P_2O_5-treatment and Se-dehydrogenation:

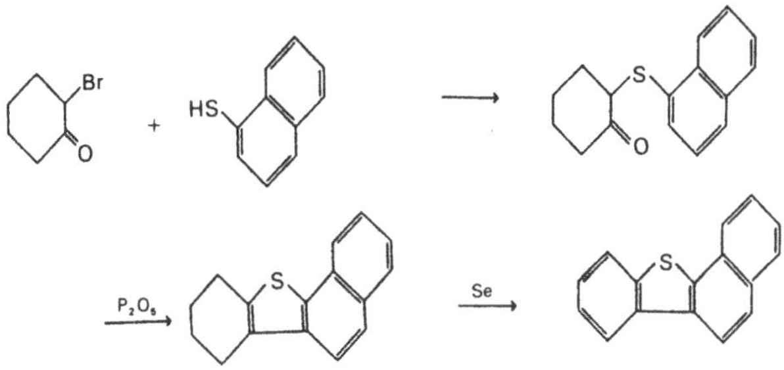

Benzo[*b*]naphtho[2,1-*d*]thiophene was prepared by Wadsworth-Emmons reaction and subsequent photocyclization (Davies *et al.*, 1957; Campaigne and Osborn, 1968) starting with (i) benzo[*b*]thiophene-3-aldehyde or (ii) with 3-benzo[*b*]thenylphosphonate with overall yields of 55% or 52%:

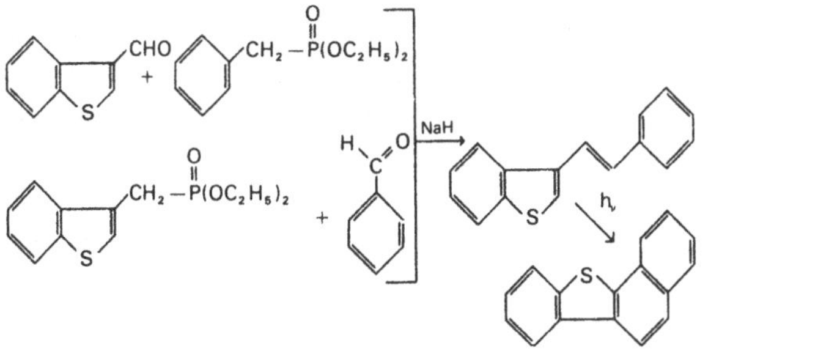

Various other approaches to obtain this thiaarene system have been made, e.g. conversion of dibenzothiophene in several steps to the 4-(4'-methylpenten-1'-yl)dibenzothiophene which was cyclized by BF_3 to 2,4-dimethyl-1,2,3,4-tetrahydrobenzo[*b*]naphtho[2,1-*d*]thiophene which upon Pd/C-treatment gave the aromatic system (Gourier and Canonne, 1973):

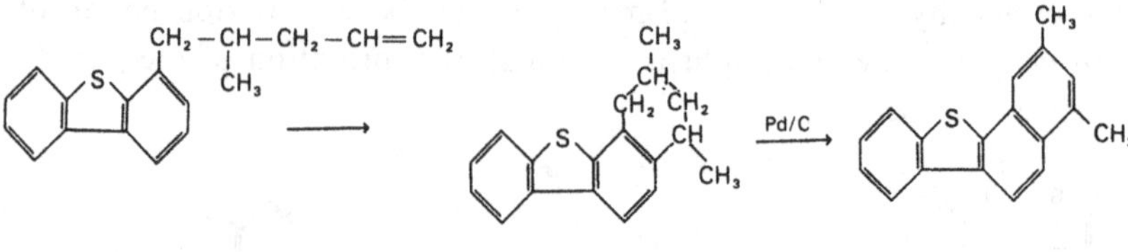

Pschorr cyclization of 2-amino-1-naphthyl-*p*-tolyl sulfide results in the formation of the 8-methyl-benzo[*b*]naphtho[2,1-*d*]thiophene, whereas *o*-tolyl sulfide gives the 10-methyl- and *m*-tolyl sulfide a mixture of the 7- and 9-methyl isomers (Campbell and Keen, 1964); however, other routes have also been described for the synthesis of all isomeric monomethylbenzo[*b*]naphtho[2,1-*d*]thiophenes (Carruthers and Stewart, 1965*a,b*; Tominaga *et al.*, 1982*b*) and for this thiaarene system (Carruthers and Douglas, 1959).

Formylation (Buu-Hoi, 1969) and other electrophilic substitution reactions occur in the 5-position (Dacka and Janczewski, 1980):

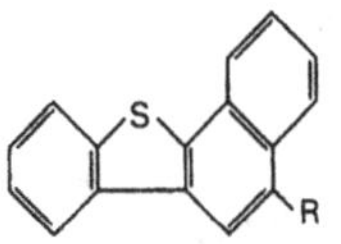

$R = -SO_3H; -Br; -NO_2$
$-CH_2Cl; -COCH_3$

The UV- (Badger and Christie, 1965*b*; Karcher *et al.*, 1982, 1985), fluorescence- (Karcher *et al.*, 1985), low temperature fluorescence/phosphorescence- (Karcher *et al.*, 1985), mass- (Meyerson and VanderHaar, 1962; Riepe and Zander, 1979; Karcher *et al.*, 1985), IR- (McDonald and Cook, 1967; Karcher *et al.*, 1985), and ^{1}H- and ^{13}C-NMR-spectra (Karcher *et al.*, 1985) have been recorded.

Benzo[*b*]naphtho[2,1-*d*]thiophene (Karcher *et al.*, 1981; Pelroy *et al.*, 1983; McFall *et al.*, 1984) and its methyl derivatives (McFall *et al.*, 1984) have been tested for mutagenicity and found positive. In recent studies (Croisy *et al.*, 1984; Brune and Deutsch-Wenzel, 1986) it was found to be carcinogenic and also to be a moderate monooxygenase inducer (Jacob *et al.*, 1983; Norpoth *et al.*, 1984) which may be of biological importance since this thiaarene is bioaccumulated in marine organisms and ubiquitous in the human environment.

Benzo[b]*naphtho*[*2,3*-d]*thiophene* (synonyms: 2,3-benzo-9-thiofluorene; naphtho[2,3-*b*]benzothiophene; 9-thia-2,3-benzofluorene)

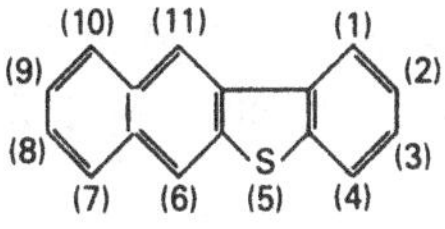

(10) (11) (1)
(9) (2)
(8) (3)
(7) (6) (5) (4)

(*87*)

m.w.: 234 ($C_{16}H_{10}S$)
m.p.: 158.7°C

Benzo[*b*]naphtho[2,3-*d*]thiophene has been detected in crude oil (Grimmer *et al.*, 1978*b*), in shale oil (Willey *et al.*, 1981*b*; Kong *et al.*, 1984), in various petroleum fractions (Mel'nikova *et al.*, 1981; Melikadse and Gverdtsiteli, 1975; Brodskii *et al.*, 1977; Lyapina *et al.*, 1980*a,b*; Teplitskaya *et al.*, 1981; Smith *et al.*, 1983; Katti *et al.*, 1984), in coal tar and pitch (Kruber and Rappen, 1940; Lang and Eigen, 1967; Mlochowski and Skrzywan, 1969; Burchill *et al.*, 1982*a*; Nishioka *et al.*, 1985*a*, 1986*b*), in coal liquids and related products (Kong *et al.*, 1982, 1984; Nakamura, 1983; Wise *et al.*, 1983; Grimmer *et al.*, 1985; Lucke *et al.*, 1985; Willey *et al.*, 1981*b*; Nishioka *et al.*, 1986*b*, Karcher *et al.*, 1981) and in coking plant effluents (Burchill *et al.*, 1978). According to its occurrence in coal tar, it was found in trace amounts in some commercially available polycyclic aromatic hydrocarbons (Karcher *et al.*, 1981). Benzo[*b*]naphtho[2,3-*d*]thiophene also has been detected in aquatic biota (Vassilaros *et al.*, 1982*a,b*) and in the emissions of hard-coal (Grimmer *et al.*, 1985) and brown-coal-fired residential stoves (Grimmer *et al.*, 1983*b*).

The compound was synthesized by ring closure of 4-(2-dibenzothienyl)butyric acid as obtained by succinoylation of dibenzothiophene and subsequent reduction (Campaigne *et al.*, 1969; Gverdtsiteli and Litvinov, 1970*a*):

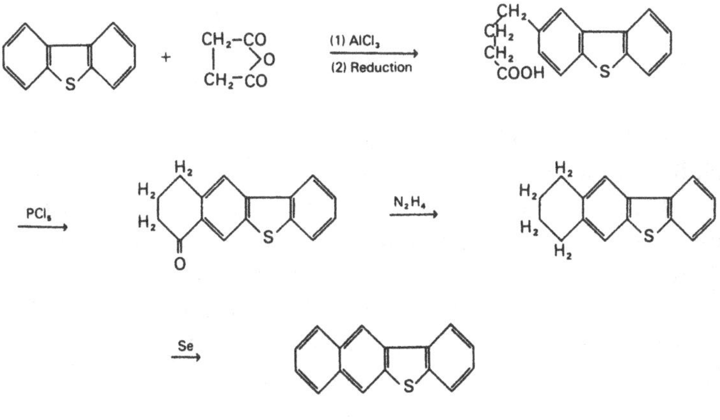

The 7-methyl derivative can be obtained by reaction of the above ketone with CH_3MgI (Gverdtsiteli and Litvinov, 1970a).Some other methyl derivatives can be synthesized from the methyl-substituted dibenzothiophenes following the above route. Another way to obtain benzo[b]naphtho[2,3-d]thiophene is the Elbs cyclodehydration of o-methylated aroylbenzo[b]thiophene or aroyl-3-methylbenzo[b]thiophene (Akhobadze et al., 1975d):

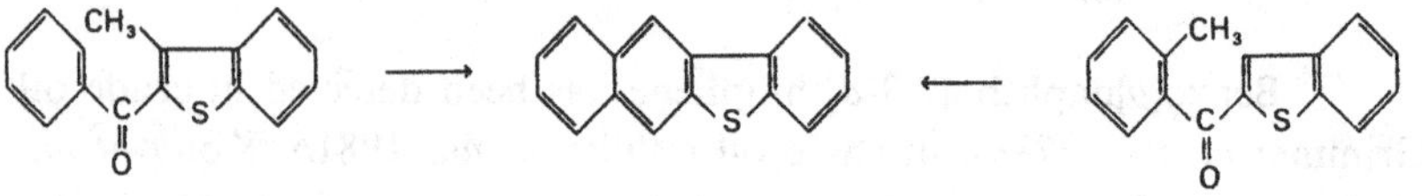

Pd/C-reduction of 2-benzo[b]thienyl-o-hydroxymethylbenzoic lactone to o-(2-benzo[b]thienyl)benzoic acid, subsequent reduction to the corresponding alcohol, oxidation to the aldehyde with CrO_3 and ring closure with polyphosphoric acid yielded also benzo[b]naphtho[2,3-d]thiophene (Akhobadze et al., 1975b):

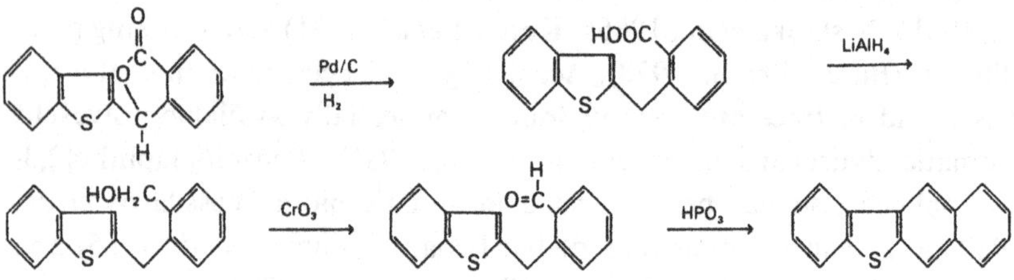

This thiaarene system also can be prepared by thermal decomposition of 2-alkyl-3-(α-hydroxybenzyl)benzo[b]thiophenes (Utkina et al., 1976b):

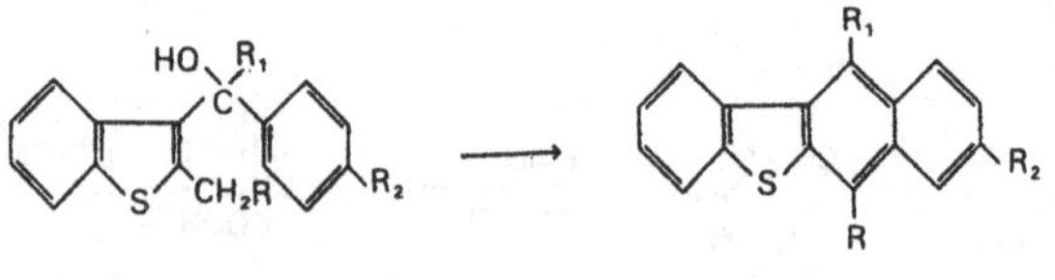

Benzo[b]naphtho[2,3-d]thiophene is formed during the pyrolysis of phthalic anhydride in the presence of thiophene (Akhobadze et al., 1975a). Apart from the above routes other routes have been described (Akhobadze et al., 1975c; Badger and Christie, 1956b) and various methyl derivatives were also synthesized, e.g. by Campaigne et al. (1969).

UV-(Karcher et al., 1982, 1985; Badger and Christie, 1956b; Nikitina et al., 1972), fluorescence- (Nikitina et al., 1972; Karcher et al., 1982, 1985), low temperature fluorescence/phosphorescence (Akhobadze et al.,

1975*a,b,c,d*, 1977; Utkina *et al.*, 1976*b*; Karcher *et al.*, 1985), IR-(Akhobadze *et al.*, 1975*c*; Karcher *et al.*, 1985), mass- (Smith *et al.*, 1983; Karcher *et al.*, 1985) and ^{1}H- and ^{13}C–NMR-spectra (Karcher *et al.*, 1985) have been recorded.

Benzo[*b*]naphtho[2,3-*d*]thiophene was found to be very weakly muta-genic in *S. typhimurium* TA 100, whereas no such effect could be verified with strain TA 98 (Pelroy *et al.*, 1983; McFall *et al.*, 1984). Among all of the isomeric monomethylbenzo[*b*]naphtho[2,3-*d*]thiophenes only the 4-isomer exhibited mutagenic activity in TA 98 (McFall *et al.*, 1984). Evidence also has been presented that pretreatment of rats with benzo[*b*]naphtho[2,3-*d*]thiophene does not influence the metabolic activity of the S-9-mix with regard to the mutagenic activity of polycyclic aromatic hydrocarbons such as benz[*a*]anthracene (Norpoth *et al.*, 1984).

C_4S–C_4S–C_6–C_6

Various benzothienobenzothiophenes and naphthodithiophenes belong to this class of compounds, but only two of them have been found in petroleum fractions.

*[1]Benzothieno[2,3-*b*][1]benzothiophene* (synonym: 2,3-bis-benzo[*b*]thiophene)

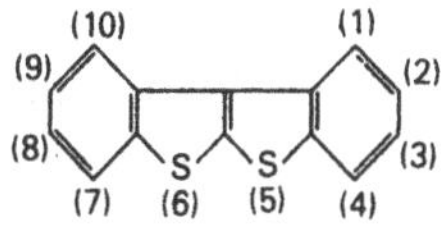

m.w.: 240 ($C_{14}H_8S_2$)
m.p.: 142°C

(*88*)

This system was detected in petroleum fractions (Drushel and Sommers, 1966; Hunt and Shabanowitz, 1982) and in coal-related products (Kong *et al.*, 1982). It has been synthesized by Murthy *et al.* (1961) by sulfur insertion into 3-phenylbenzo[*b*]thiophene:

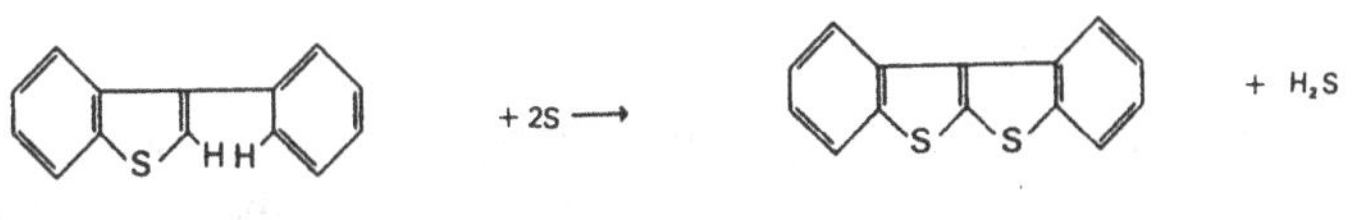

The system also was obtained by sulfur-bridging of (i) 2-halo-3-phenylbenzothiophenes or (ii) 1,1,1-trichloro-2,2-diphenylethane (*Inst. org. synth.*, 1966; Voronkov and Udre, 1968; Geering, 1966):

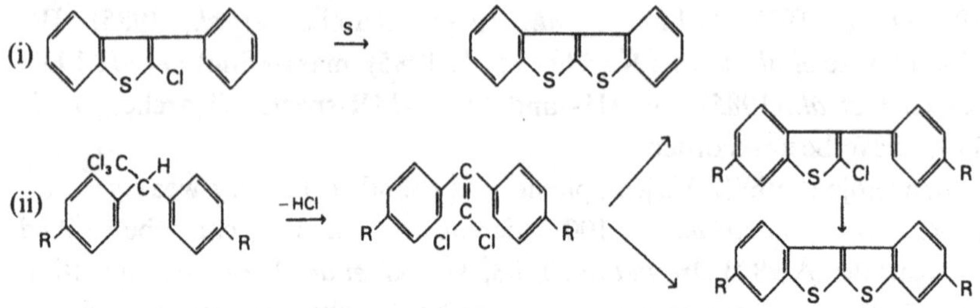

(i)

(ii)

Reaction of 1,1-diphenylethene with sulfur has also been reported to give [1]benzo[2,3-*b*][1]benzothiophene (Dayagi *et al.*, 1970), and Mitra *et al.* (1957) reported a synthesis starting with benzo[*b*]thiophene-2-thiol and 2-bromocyclohexanone:

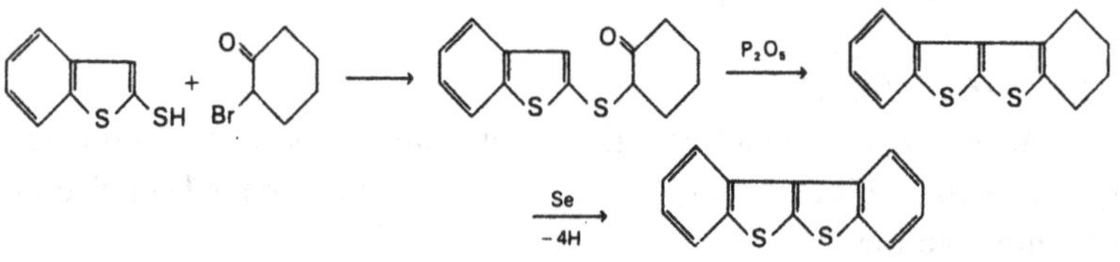

Treatment of [1]benzo[2,3-*b*][1]benzothiophene with peracetic acid results in the formation of mono- (m.p.: 235°C) and disulfone (m.p.: 315°C).

MO-calculations have been carried out (Deward and Trinajstic, 1970; Parkanyi and Herndon, 1978; DasGupta and Birss, 1980) and NMR-spectral data have been presented by Dayagi *et al.* (1970).

[*1*]*Benzothieno*[*3,2*-b][*1*]*benzothiophene* (synonym: thianaphtheno[3,2-*b*]-thianaphthene)

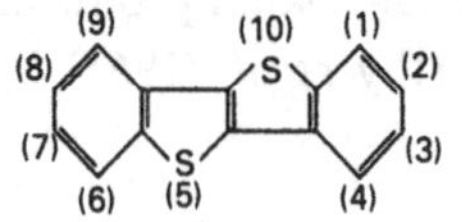

(89)

m.w.: 240 ($C_{14}H_8S_2$)
m.p.: 215.5°C

[1]Benzothieno[3,2-*b*][1]benzothiophene has been detected in petroleum (Drushel and Sommers, 1966). It can be synthesized from 1,2,2-trichloro-1,2-diphenylethane through 1,2-dichloro-1,2-diphenylethylene and subsequent treatment with sulfur (Geering, 1969):

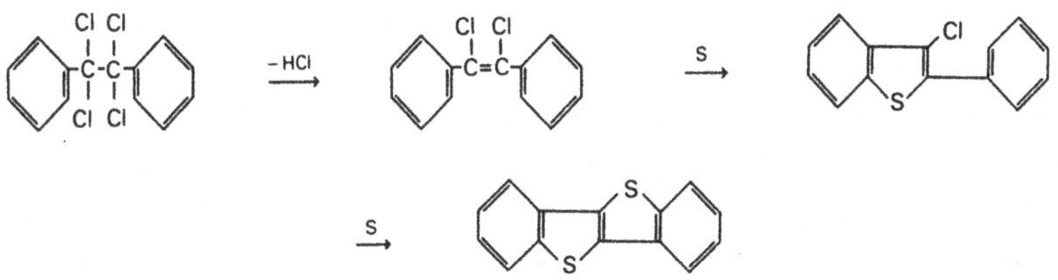

Thermal treatment of trichlorophenylmethane with sulfur at 400°C also resulted in the formation of this sytem (Geering, 1966; Voronkov *et al.*, 1983), which was furthermore obtained from isophorone after treatment with sulfur through an intermediary product by heating and Wolff-Kishner reduction (Ebel *et al.*, 1963; Voronkov and Khokhlova, 1974):

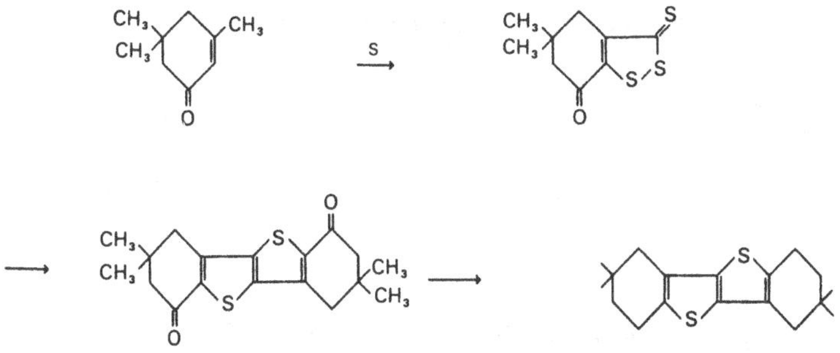

Ricci *et al.* (1972) described a synthesis by succinylation of thieno[3,2-*b*]benzothiophene and subsequent cyclization to the tetrahydroketone which upon heating in vacuo leads directly to [1]benzothieno[3,2-*b*][1]benzothiophene:

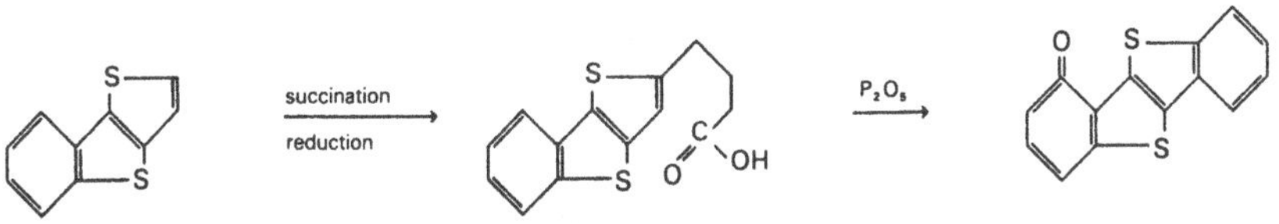

Analogous to the [2,3-*b*]-isomer Ghaisas and Tilak (1957) synthesized it starting with benzo[*b*]thiophene-3-thiol and 2-bromocyclohexanone. Zherdeva *et al.* (1980) obtained this system from stilbene-2,2′-disulfonylchloride by HI-reduction, and heating of dichlorophenylmethane with sulfur (1:1) for 10 h at 250–300°C has also been reported to give this compound (Voronkov and Udre, 1972). However, additional routes were also reported (Behringer and Meinetsberger, 1981). Recently, Barudi *et al.* (1980a,b) obtained [1]benzothieno[3,2-*b*][1]benzothiophene by heating stilbene-2,2′-dithiols.

Nitration of [1]benzothieno[3,2-*b*][1]benzothiophene occurs at C-2 and C-4 (Barudi *et al.*, 1980*a*,*b*). IR- (Voronkov and Pereferkovich, 1969), UV- (Voronkov and Pereferkovich, 1969), NMR- (Voronkov and Khokhlova, 1974) and mass spectra (Voronkov and Khokhlova, 1974) have been recorded. Some derivatives of this thiaarene were found to be of commercial interest because they exhibit pesticidal activities against *Alternaria solani* and *Pythium* species (Voronkov and Udre, 1972).

Kudo *et al.* (1984) synthesized the following four benzothienobenzothiophenes by condensation of 2- or 3-benzo[*b*]thenylphosphonate with 3- or 2-thiophenealdehyde or by condensation of 2- or 3-thenylphosphonate with 3- or 2-benzothiophenealdehyde and subsequent photocyclization of the resulting olefins (yields in parentheses):

*[1]benzothieno[4,5-*b*][1]benzothiophene* (**90**):

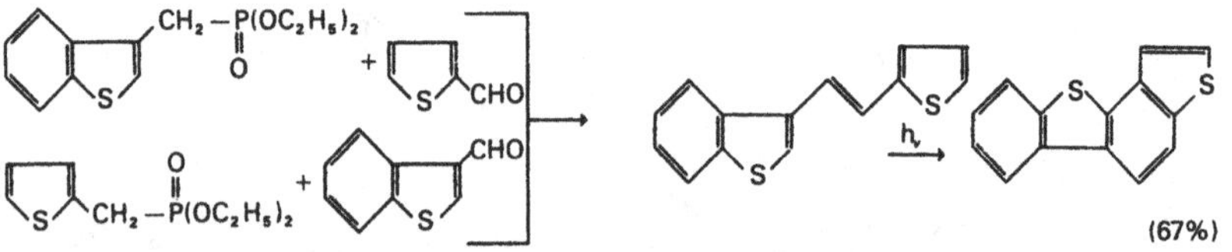

(67%)

*[1]benzothieno[5,4-*b*][1]benzothiophene* (**91**):

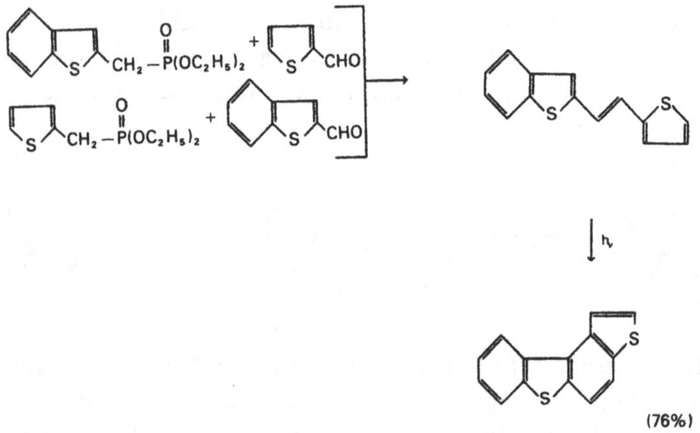

(76%)

[*1*]benzothieno[6,7-b][*1*]benzothiophene (**92**):

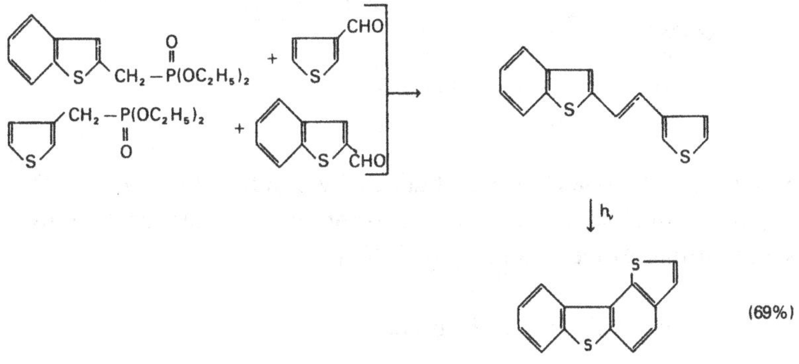

(69%)

[*1*]benzothieno[7,6-b][*1*]benzothiophene (**93**)

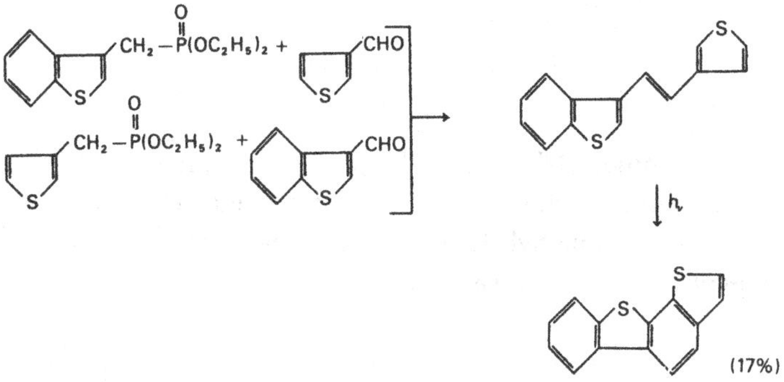

(17%)

Syntheses have also been described for [1]benzothieno[5,6-*b*][1]-benzothiophene (**94**) (Ahmed *et al.*, 1973), its [6,5-*b*]-isomer (**95**) (Ghaisas and Tilak, 1955), and for [2]benzothieno[5,6-*b*][1]benzothiophene (**96**) (Müller *et al.*, 1975).

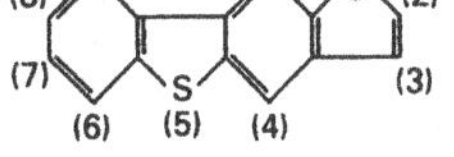

m.w.: 240 ($C_{14}H_8S_2$)

[1]benzothieno[5,6-*b*][1]benzothiophene
(**94**)

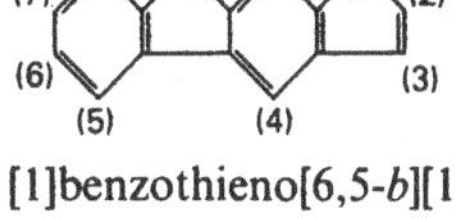

m.w.: 240 ($C_{14}H_8S_2$)

[1]benzothieno[6,5-*b*][1]benzothiophene
(**95**)

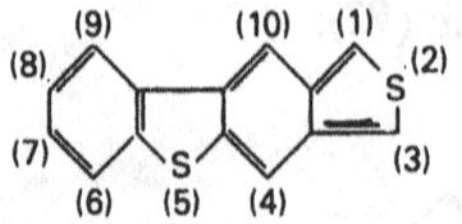
(9)
(10)
(1)
(8)
(2)
S
(7)
S
(3)
(6)
(5)
(4)

m.w.: 240 ($C_{14}H_8S_2$)

[2]benzothieno[5,6-*b*]benzothiophene
(*96*)

Some naphthodithiophenes were obtained by condensation of naphthalenedithiols with either α-chloroacetone or bromoacetaldehyde dimethylacetale according to Desai and Tilak (1961).

*Naphtho[1,2-*b*:3,4-*b'*]dithiophene*

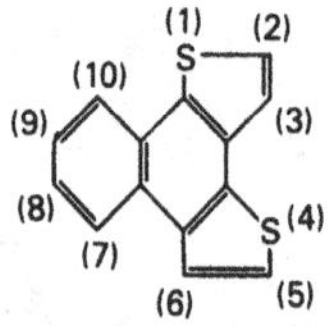
(1)
(2)
S
(10)
(9)
(3)
(8)
S
(4)
(7)
(6)
(5)

m.w.: 240 ($C_{14}H_8S_2$)
m.p.: 134°C

(*97*)

Naphtho[1,2-*b*:3,4-*b'*]dithiophene was prepared by condensation of naphthalene-1,3-dithiol with bromoacetaldehyde dimethylacetal, whereas its 3,6-dimethyl derivative could be obtained by condensation with α-chloroacetone (Desai and Tilak, 1961):

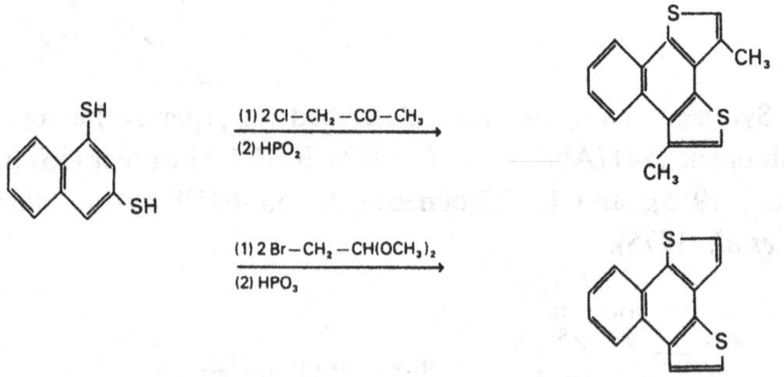
SH
SH
(1) 2 Cl–CH₂–CO–CH₃
(2) HPO₃
S
CH₃
S
CH₃
(1) 2 Br–CH₂–CH(OCH₃)₂
(2) HPO₃
S
S

*Naphtho[1,2:4,3-*b'*]dithiophene*

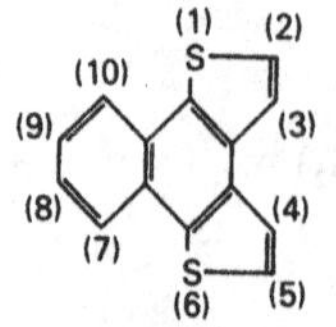
(1)
(2)
S
(10)
(9)
(3)
(8)
(4)
(7)
S
(6)
(5)

m.w.: 240 ($C_{14}H_8S_2$)
m.p.: 169°C

(*98*)

Naphtho[1,2-*b*:4,3-*b*']dithiophene was obtained by Desai and Tilak (1961) who condensed naphthalene-1,4-dithiol with bromoacetaldehyde dimethylacetal. Subsequent cyclization was achieved with polyphosphoric acid.

Naphtho[1,2-b:5,6-b']dithiophene

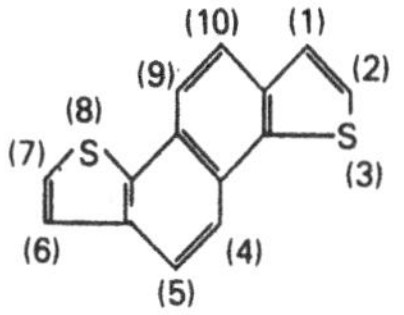

m.w.: 240 ($C_{14}H_8S_2$)
m.p.: > 360°C (?)

(*99*)

In analogy to the aforementioned isomer this thiaarene system was prepared from naphthalene-1,5-dithiol and α-chloroacetone by Desai and Tilak (1961).

Naphtho[1,2-b:8,7-b']dithiophene

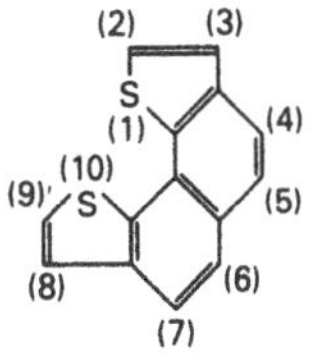

m.w.: 240 ($C_{14}H_8S_2$)
m.p.: 126°C

(*100*)

This compound was synthesized by Muller *et al.* (1977) in a 12-step synthesis starting with the condensation of thiophene-2-aldehyde with malonic ester.

Naphtho[2,1-b:6,5-b']dithiophene

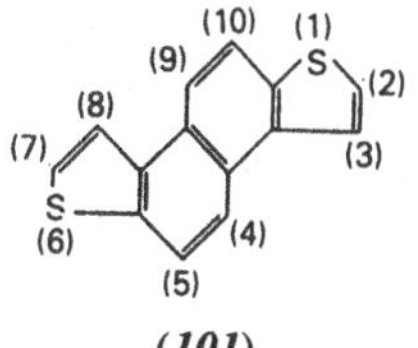

m.w.: 240 ($C_{14}H_8S_2$)
m.p.: 265°C

(*101*)

This thiaarene system, being a heterocyclic steroid analogue, has been synthesized by Jogdeo and Bhide (1979) by condensation of a isothiouronium acetate with 2-methyl-3-oxothiophane-1,1-dioxide giving the seco-dithiaandrostatriene system. Cyclization of the latter and isomerization with polyphosphoric acid yielded 2,3,3a,9,10,10a-hexahydro-10a-methylnaphtho[2,1-*b*:6,5-*b'*]dithiophene-1,1-dioxide (synonym: 3,17-dithio-A-nor-14β-estra-1,5,6,8-tetraene-17-dioxide):

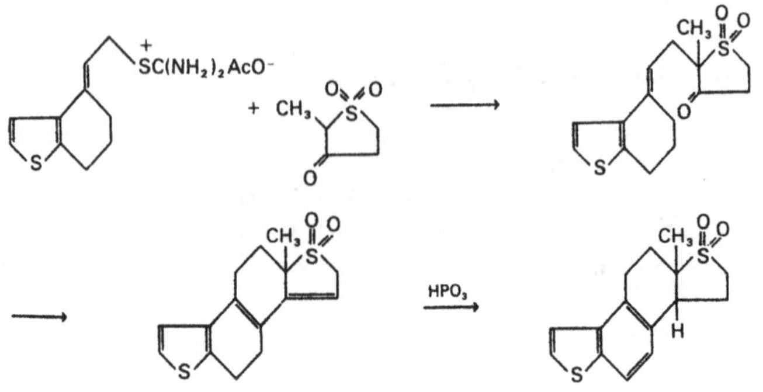

*Naphtho[2,1-*b*:7,8-*b'*]dithiophene*

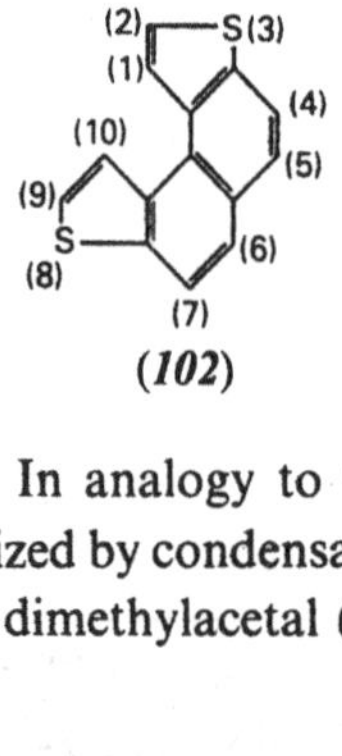

m.w.: 240 (C$_{14}$H$_8$S$_2$)
m.p.: 163°C

(102)

In analogy to the aforementioned isomers this compound was synthesized by condensation of naphthalene,2,7-dithiol with bromoacetaldehyde dimethylacetal (Desai and Tilak, 1961):

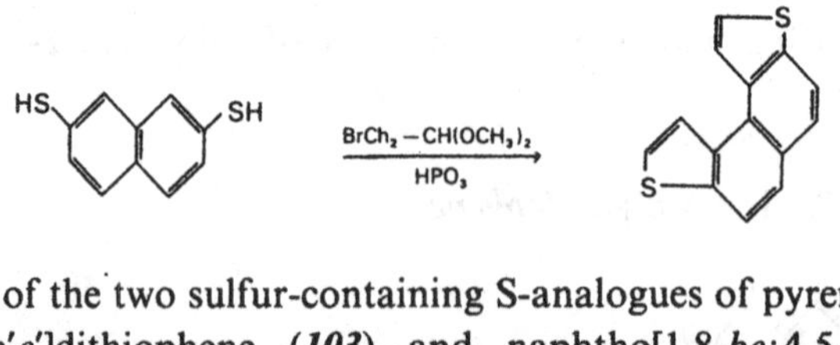

Both of the two sulfur-containing S-analogues of pyrene, naphtho[1,8-*bc*:5,4-*b'c'*]dithiophene (103) and naphtho[1,8-*bc*:4,5-*b'c'*]dithiophene (104) have not yet been synthesized. However, molecular orbital calculations for them have been carried out by Hess and Schaad (1973).

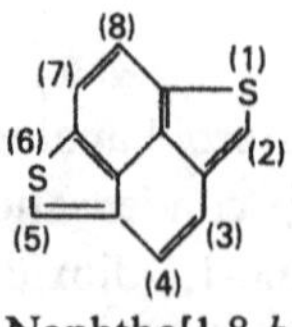

m.w.: 214 (C$_{12}$H$_6$S$_2$)

Naphtho[1,8-*bc*:4,5-*b'c'*]dithiophene
(103)

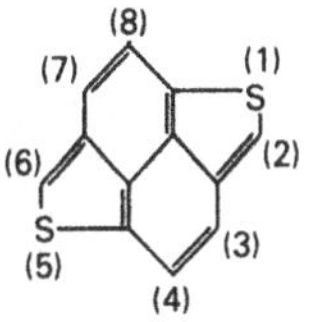

m.w.: 214 ($C_{12}H_6S_2$)

Naphtho[1,8-*bc*:5,4-*b'c'*]dithiophene
(104)

$C_5S-C_6-C_6-C_6$

Benzo[kl]*thiaxanthene* (synonyms: benzothioxanthene; benzothiaxanthene; 1,10-benzothiaxanthene; 1,10-benzo-5-thiaxanthene; 7-thiabenzanthrene)

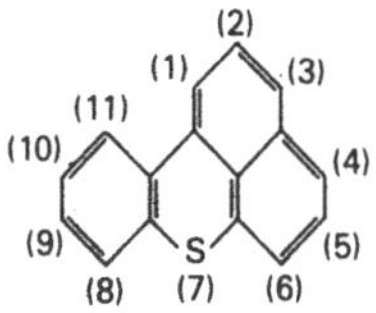

m.w.: 234 ($C_{16}H_{10}S$)
m.p.: 78–79°C

(105)

This quasi-aromatic thiaarene has not been definitely identified in environmental matter. It has been synthesized by various routes, e.g. starting with 2,4-dichloronaphthalenethiol and *o*-nitrochlorobenzene (Davies *et al.*, 1957) or with α-(*o*-bromophenylthio)naphthalene which upon Kharasch reaction gave benzo[*kl*]thiaxanthene (Nespoli and Tiecco, 1966; Tiecco, 1968). This system was also obtained from 1,8-dehydronaphthalene and diphenyldisulfide in dichloromethane at room temperature (De Luca *et al.*, 1983). Davies *et al.* (1968) reported the formation of its 7,7-dioxide from solvent-free heating of 6a,11b-dihydrobenzo[*b*]naphtho[1,2-*d*]thiophene-7,7-dioxide. In this reaction also benzo[*b*]naphtho[1,2-*d*]thiophene and *o*-(1-naphthyl)benzenesulfonic acid are formed:

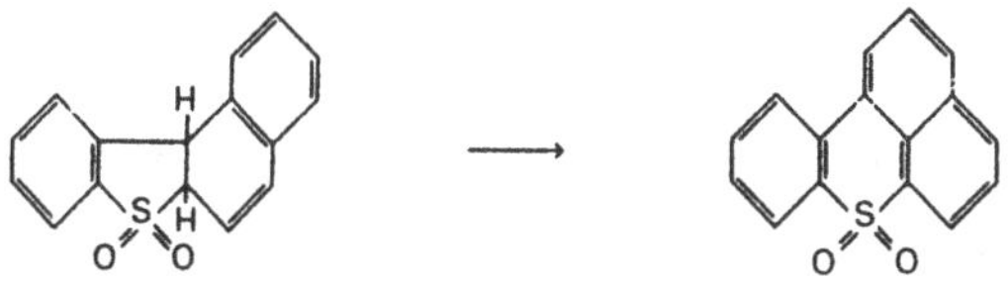

6-Methyl-8,9,10,11-tetrahydrobenzo[*kl*]thiaxanthene has been made by condensation of 2-methyl-napthalene-1-thiol with 2-chlorocyclohexanone and subsequent ring closure with polyphosphoric acid (Muller and Cagniant, 1968):

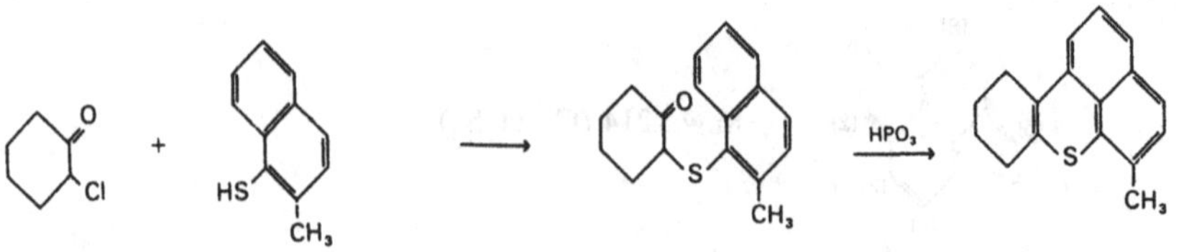

Partially or completely hydrogenated derivatives of three compounds belonging to this class have been detected in petroleum, namely 2*H*-anthra[2,3-*b*]thiopyran (Lyapina *et al.*, 1980*b*), 2*H*-phenaleno[1,9-*bc*]thiopyran (Lyapina *et al.*, 1982), and 2*H*-phenanthro[4,5-*bcd*]thiopyran (Lyapina *et al.*, 1980*a*).

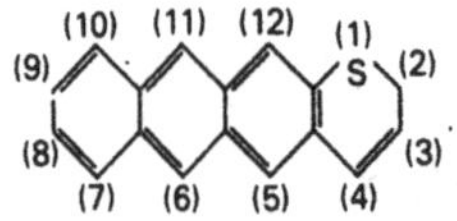

m.w.: 248 (C$_{17}$H$_{12}$S)

2*H*-anthra[2,3-*b*]thiopyran (synonym: 1-thia-2*H*-naphthacene)
(*106*)

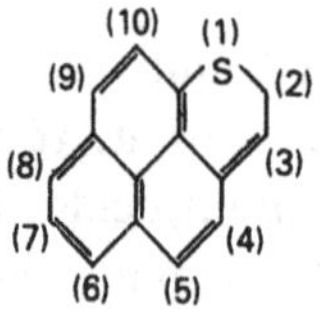

m.w.: 222 (C$_{15}$H$_{10}$S)

2*H*-phenaleno[1,9-*bc*]thiopyran (synonym: 1-thia-2*H*-pyrene)
(*107*)

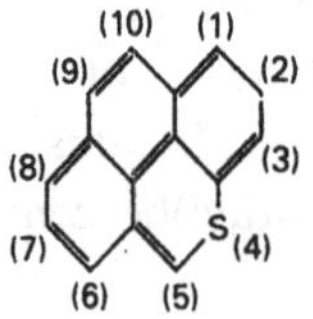

m.w.: 222 (C$_{15}$H$_{10}$S)

2*H*-phenanthro[4,5-*bcd*]thiopyran (synonym: 4-thia-2*H*-pyrene)
(*108*)

Some thiaarene systems isosteric to chrysene, benz[*a*]anthracene, naphthacene, and benzo[*c*]chrysene such as the following benzonaphthothiopyrans, phenanthrothiopyrans and benzothiaxanthenes have been synthesized and physical data reported (references in parentheses).

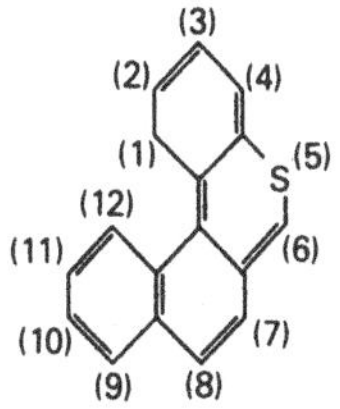

m.w.: 248 ($C_{17}H_{12}S$)

1*H*-benzo[*b*]naphtho[1,2-*d*]thiopyran
(synonym: 1*H*-5-thiabenzo[*c*]phenanthrene)
(Tilak *et al.*, 1969)
   (*109*)

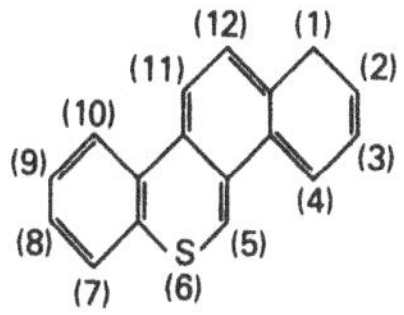

m.w.: 248 ($C_{17}H_{12}S$)

1*H*-benzo[*b*]naphtho[2,1-*d*]thiopyran
(synonym: 1*H*-6-thiachrysene)
(Koenst *et al.*, 1970)
   (*110*)

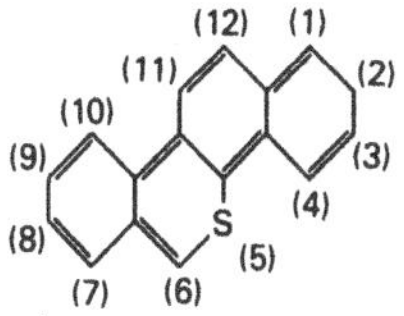

m.w.: 248 ($C_{17}H_{12}S$)

2*H*-benzo[*d*]naphtho[1,2-*b*]thiopyran
(synonym: 2*H*-5-thiachrysene)
(Tilak *et al.*, 1969)
   (*111*)

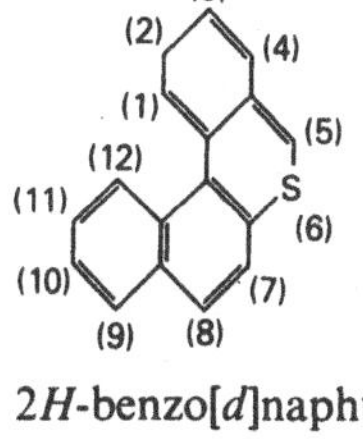

m.w.: 248 ($C_{17}H_{12}S$)

2*H*-benzo[*d*]naphtho[2,1-*b*]thiopyran
(synonym: 2*H*-6-thiabenzo[*c*]phenanthrene)
(Tilak *et al.*, 1969)
   (*112*)

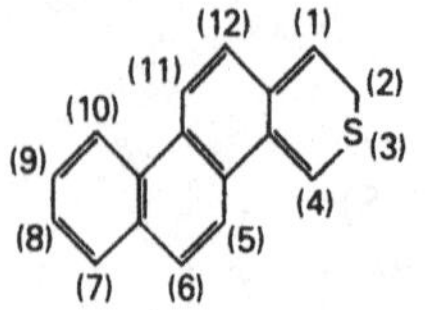

m.w.: 248 ($C_{17}H_{12}S$)

2*H*-phenanthro[1,2-*c*]thiopyran
(synonym: 2*H*-3-thiachrysene)
(Shiro *et al.*, 1982)

(113)

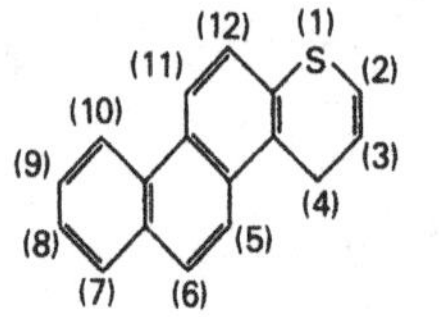

m.w.: 248 ($C_{17}H_{12}S$)

4*H*-phenanthro[2,1-*b*]thiopyran
(synonym: 4*H*-1-thiachrysene)
(Nazarov *et al.*, 1953*a,b*)

(114)

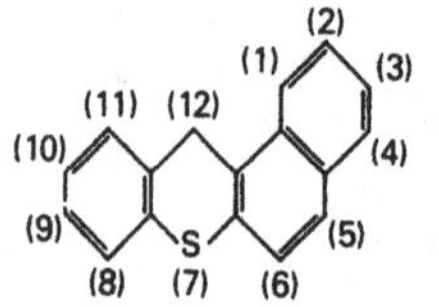

m.w.: 248 ($C_{17}H_{12}S$)

12*H*-benzo[*a*]thiaxanthene
(synonym: 12*H*-7-thiabenz[*a*]anthracene)
(Drozd and Pak, 1970; Drozd *et al.*, 1969*a,b*)

(115)

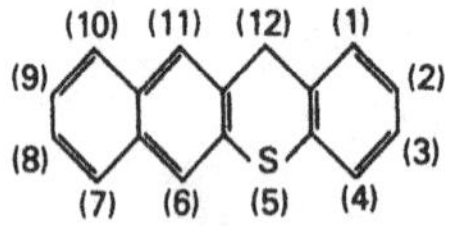

m.w.: 248 ($C_{17}H_{12}S$)

12*H*-benzo[*b*]thiaxanthene
(synonym: 12*H*-5-thianaphthacene)
(Drozd *et al.*, 1969*a*)

(116)

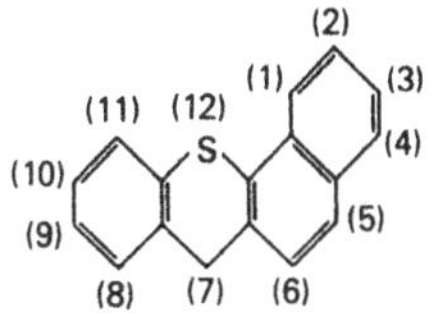

m.w.: 248 ($C_{17}H_{12}S$)

7*H*-benzo[*c*]thiaxanthene
(synonym: 7*H*-12-thiabenz[*a*]anthracene)
(Pelz and Protiva, 1963; Drozd *et al.*, 1969*a,b*;
Drozd and Pak, 1970)
(*117*)

$C_5S–C_5S–C_6–C_6$ and $C_5S–C_5S–C_6–C_6–C_6$

Recently two peri-condensed systems, 1,6-dithiapyrene (*118*) and 3,10-dithiaperylene (*119*), and their diphenyl derivatives belonging to this class have been synthesized by Nakasuji *et al.* (1986).

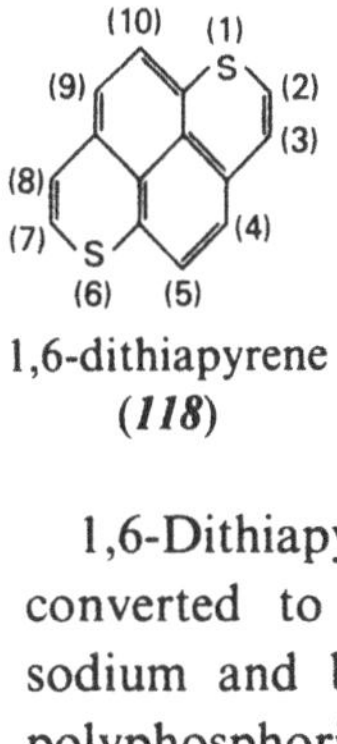

m.w.: 240 ($C_{14}H_8S_2$)
m.p.: 228–229°C

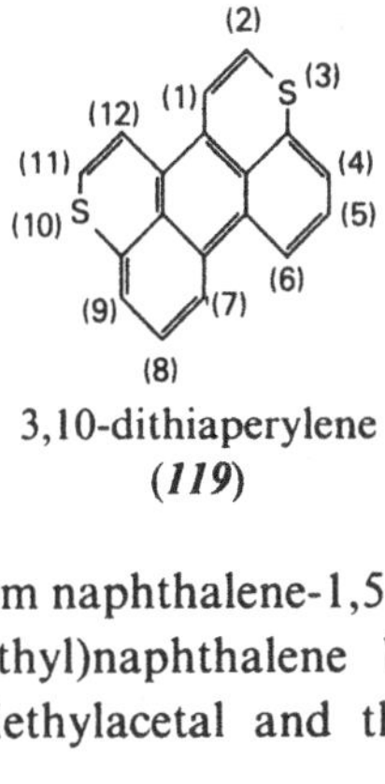

m.w.: 290 ($C_{18}H_{10}S_2$)
m.p.: 228–230°C

1,6-dithiapyrene
(*118*)

3,10-dithiaperylene
(*119*)

1,6-Dithiapyrene was prepared from naphthalene-1,5-dithiol which was converted to 1,5-bis(thiodiethoxyethyl)naphthalene by reaction with sodium and bromoacetaldehyde diethylacetal and then cyclized with polyphosphoric acid:

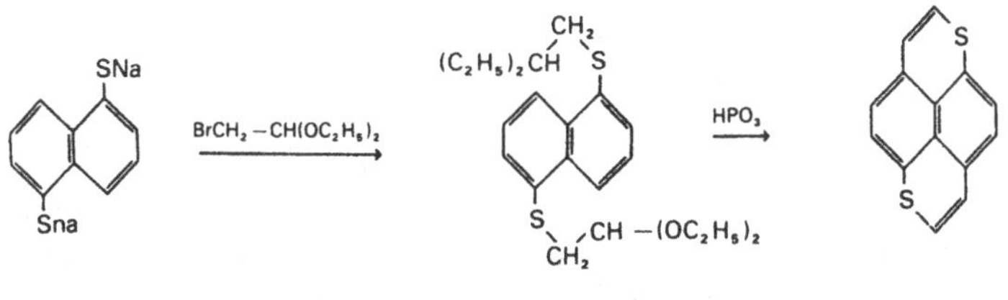

Reductive coupling of benzothiapyranone with $TiCl_4/Zn$, subsequent photocyclization and dehydrogenation of the resulting 1,2,11,12-tetrahydro-3,10-dithiaperylene yielded 3,10-dithiaperylene:

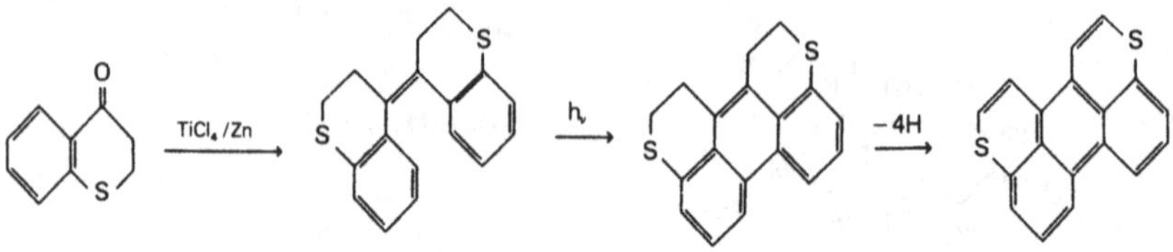

UV-, NMR-and mass spectral data for both of the above compounds have been reported by Nakasuji *et al.* (1986).

2.4   Pentacyclic compounds
$C_4S–C_5–C_5–C_6–C_6$

Three diindenothiophenes have been described:

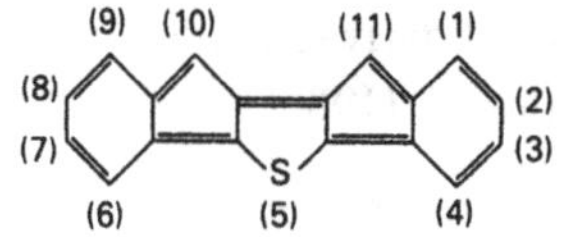

m.w.: 258 ($C_{18}H_{10}S$)

diindeno[1,2-*b*:2′,1′-*d*]thiophene
(*120*)

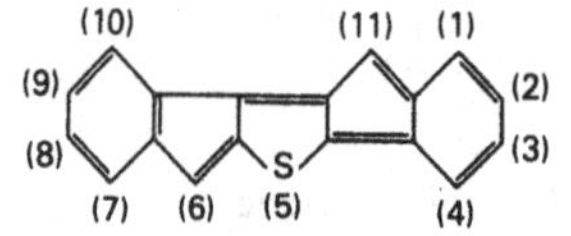

m.w.: 258 ($C_{18}H_{10}S$)

diindeno[1,2-*b*:1′,2′-*d*]thiophene
(*121*)

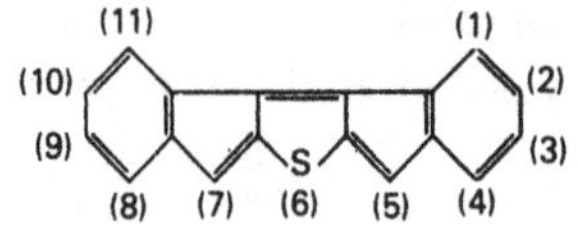

m.w.: 258 ($C_{18}H_{10}S$)

diindeno[2,1-*b*:1′,2′-*d*]thiophene
(*122*)

Synthetic approaches to obtain diindeno[1,2-*b*:2′,1′-*d*]thiophene (*120*) were summarized by Konar (1984). A synthesis for the diindeno[1,2-*b*:1′,2′-*d*]thiophene (*121*) system was reported by Poirier and Lozac'h (1966); they reported that base-catalyzed self-condensation of 1-indanone gave 2-(1-indanylidene)-1-indanone which upon sulfurization yielded 6*H*-diindeno[1,2-*b*:1′,2′-*d*]thiophene-11-one:

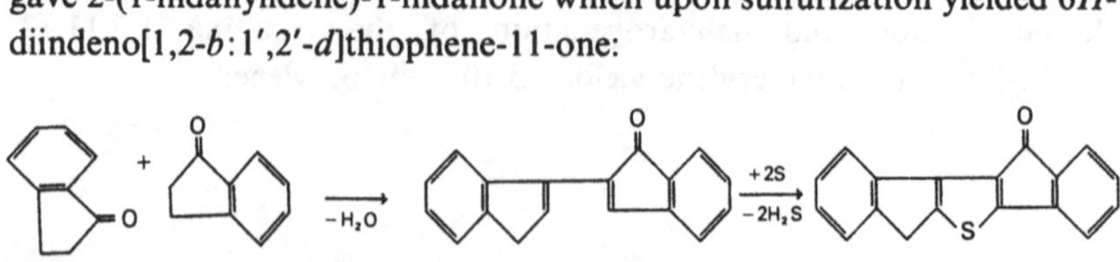

Diindeno[2,1-*b*:1',2'-*d*]thiophene (*122*) has been prepared by LiAlH$_4$/AlCl$_3$ reduction of 5*H*,7*H*-bis-indeno[2,3-*b*:3',2'-*d*]thiophene-5,7-dione (MacDowell and Patrick (1967*b*).

The mass spectra of all three isomers have been studied by Glinzer *et al.* (1983*a*).

$C_4S–C_5–C_6–C_6–C_6$

The following systems belong to this class, some of which have been found in petroleum: acenaphthobenzothiophenes, aceanthryleno-thiophenes, acephenanthrylenothiophenes, benzindenobenzothiophenes, benzofluorenothiophenes, cyclopentaphenanthrothiophenes, cyclopen-tanthrathiophenes, fluoranthenothiophenes and indenonaph-thothiophenes.

*Acenaphtho(3,4-*b]benzo[d]*thiophene*
(synonym: benzo[*b*]acenaphtho[4,3-*d*]thiophene)

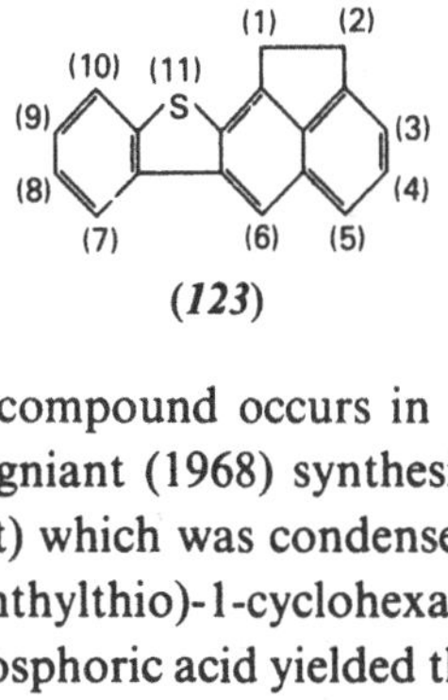

m.w.: 260 (C$_{18}$H$_{12}$S)
m.p.: 165°C

(*123*)

This compound occurs in petroleum (Lyapina *et al.*, 1980*a,b*). Faller and Cagniant (1968) synthesized this system from acenaphthene-3-thiol (Na-salt) which was condensed with 2-chlorocyclohexanone to give 2-(3-acenaphthylthio)-1-cyclohexanone which then upon cyclization with polyphosphoric acid yielded the 7,8,9,10-tetrahydro derivative. Treatment with Pd/CaCO$_3$ gave acenaphtho[3,4-*b*]benzo[*d*]thiophene:

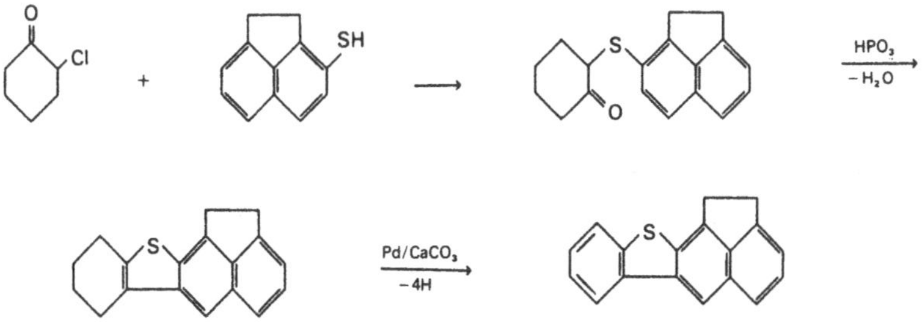

Campaigne *et al.* (1970) synthesized it by Reformatzky reaction of 7-oxo-7,8,9,10-tetrahydrobenzo[*b*]naphtho[2,3-*d*]thiophene with bromoacetic ester, dehydration with formic acid and subsequent hydrolysis.

Cyclization of the product under Friedel-Crafts conditions gave 1-oxo-acenaphtho[3,4-*b*]benzo[*d*]thiophene which can be reduced to the base compound:

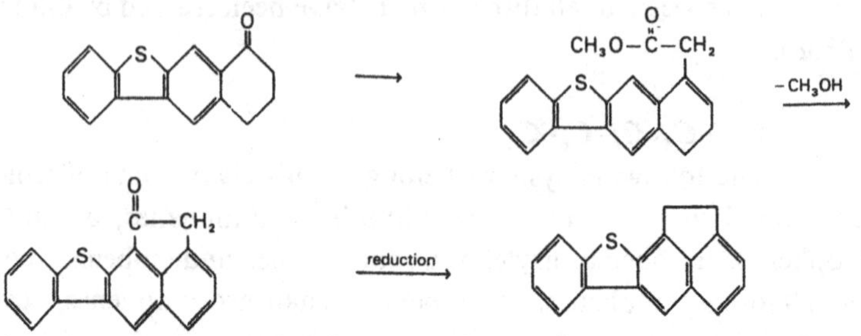

In a series of papers Faller (1961*a,b*, 1966*a*) described additional methods for the preparation of this system and its methyl derivatives. He also presented UV- and NMR-spectra of this thiaarene (Faller, 1967).

Acenaphtho[4,3-b]benzo[d]*thiophene*
(synonym: benzo[*b*]acenaphtho[3,4-*d*]thiophene)

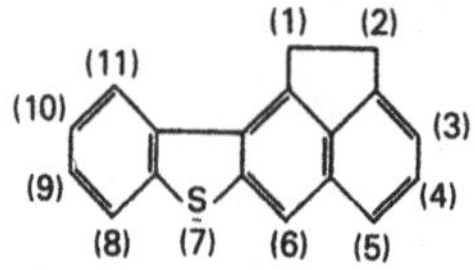

m.w.: 260 ($C_{18}H_{12}S$)
m.p.: 197°C

(*124*)

This compound was synthesized by Faller (1965) from in-danylbenzothiophene ketone by cyclization; he also observed its formation as a side product during the synthesis of the [7,8-*b*]isomer. NMR- and UV-spectra of this system were recorded (Faller, 1967).

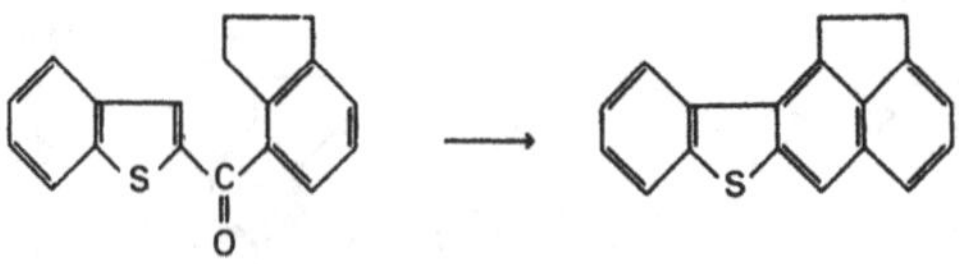

Acenaphtho[5,4-b]benzo[d]*thiophene*
(synonym: benzo[*b*]acenaphtho[4,5-*d*]thiophene)

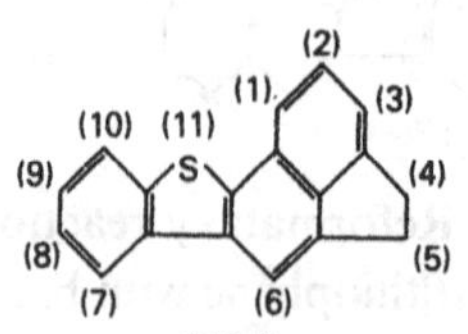

m.w.: 260 ($C_{18}H_{12}S$)
m.p.: 145.5°C

(*125*)

Faller and Cagniant (1968) have synthesized this system from 2-chlorocyclohexanone and acenaphthene-5-thiol. NMR- and UV-spectra of this thiaarene have been recorded (Faller, 1966*b*).

Several dihydro-aceanthrylenothiophenes (= aceanthrenothiophenes) have been synthesized by the Faller group, e.g. the [7,8-*b*]-; [8,7-*b*]-; [9,10-*b*]- and the [10,9-*b*]-isomer.

*Aceanthreno[7,8-*b]*thiophene*
(synonym: 6,7-dihydroaceanthryleno[7,8-*b*]thiophene)

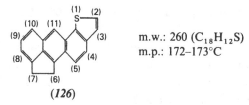

m.w.: 260 ($C_{18}H_{12}S$)
m.p.: 172–173°C

(*126*)

Aceanthreno[7,8-*b*]thiophene was prepared by reaction of 4-cyanoindane and 7-bromobenzo[*b*]thiophene (Faller, 1966*a,b*) who recorded its UV- and NMR-spectrum (Faller, 1967). He also synthesized aceanthreno[8,7-*b*]-, [9,10-*b*]- and [10,9-*b*]-thiophene (Faller 1966*a,b* 1967) for all of which he has published also UV- and NMR-spectral data.

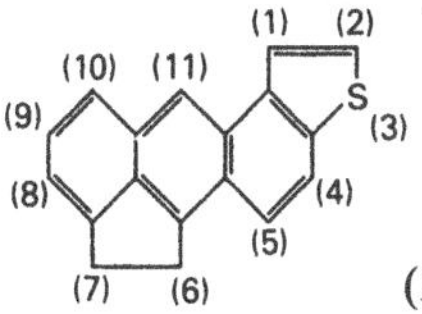

m.w.: 260 ($C_{18}H_{12}S$)
m.p.: 190°C

(*127*)

Aceanthreno[8,7-*b*]thiophene (synonym: 6,7-dihydroaceanthryleno[8,7-*b*] thiophene)

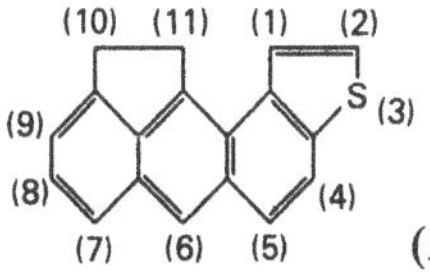

m.w.: 260 ($C_{18}H_{12}S$)
m.p.: 212°C

(*128*)

Aceanthreno[9,10-*b*]thiophene (synonym: 10,11-dihydroaceanthryleno-[9,10-*b*]thiophene)

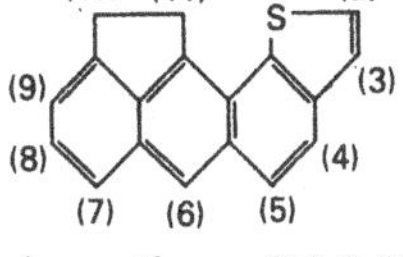

m.w.: 260 ($C_{18}H_{12}S$)
m.p. of the 2,3,4-trimethyl derivative 149–150°C

(*129*)

Aceanthreno[10,9-*b*]thiophene (synonym: 10,11-dihydroaceanthryleno-[10,9-*b*]thiophene)

Acephenanthreno[7,8-b]thiophene
(synonym: 9,10-dihydroacephenanthryleno[7,8-*b*]thiophene)

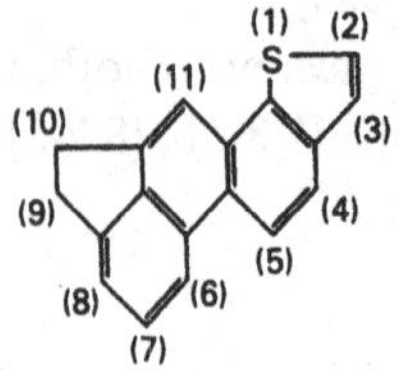

m.w.: 260 ($C_{18}H_{12}S$)

(130)

The synthesis of the 2-methyl derivative (m.p.: 169.5°C) could be achieved by starting with the tetrahydroacephenanthrenone which upon Vilsmeier-Haack formylation and condensation of the chloroformyl product was treated with sodium sulfide and subsequently condensed with ethyl α- bromopropionate. The resulting product was cyclized and then dehydrogenated (Cagniant and Kirsch, 1975).

The preparation of some benzo[*b*]fluorenothiophenes has been reported by Bergamasco and Porter (1977). The following systems were described:

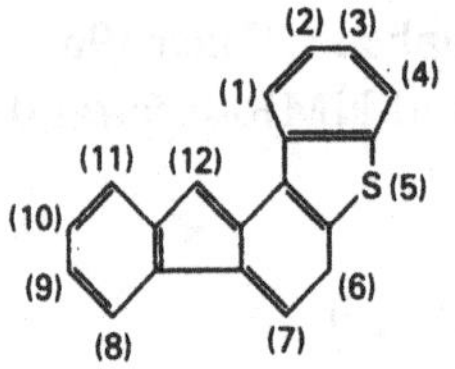

m.w.: 272 ($C_{19}H_{12}S$)

6*H*-benzo[*b*]fluoreno[1,2-*d*]thiophene
(131)

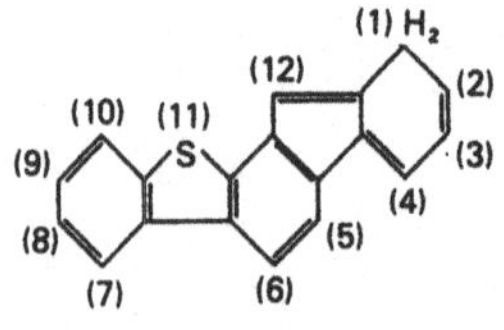

m.w.: 272 ($C_{19}H_{12}S$)

1*H*-benzo[*b*]fluoreno[2,1-*d*]thiophene
(132)

7H-8,9-Dihydrocyclopent[5,6]anthra[1,2-b]thiophene

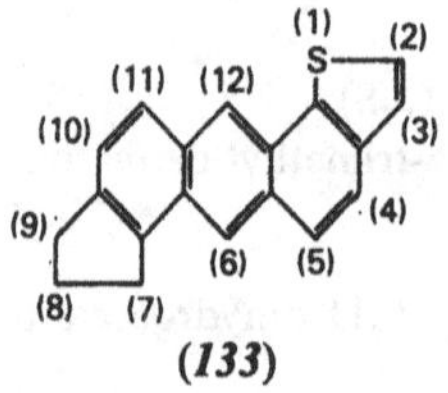

m.w.: 274 ($C_{19}H_{14}S$)

(133)

The 2,3-dimethyl derivative of this system is formed in trace amounts during the synthesis of 2,3,4-trimethylaceanthreno[10,9-*b*]thiophene (Faller, 1966*a*).

Due to their structural relation to steroids, some cyclopentaphenanthrothiophenes have been synthesized and the following systems have been described in the literature (Jaeger and Karrer, 1963; Komeno, 1964; Takeda and Komeno, 1964; Manhas and Rao, 1969). They have not been detected in environmental matter.

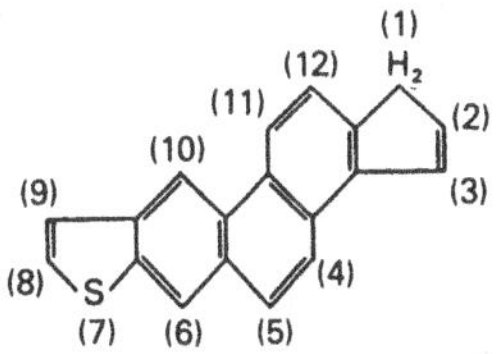

m.w.: 272 ($C_{19}H_{12}S$)

1*H*-cyclopenta[7,8]phenanthro[2,3-*b*]thiophene
(**134**)

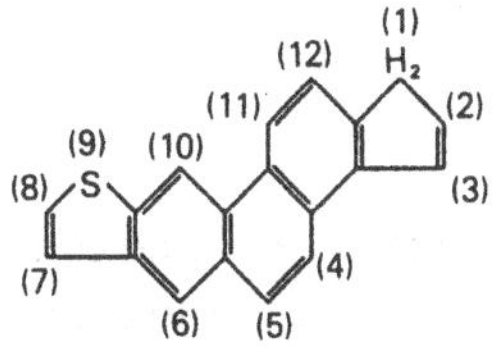

m.w.: 272 ($C_{19}H_{12}S$)

1*H*-cyclopenta[7,8]phenanthro[3,2-*b*]thiophene
(**135**)

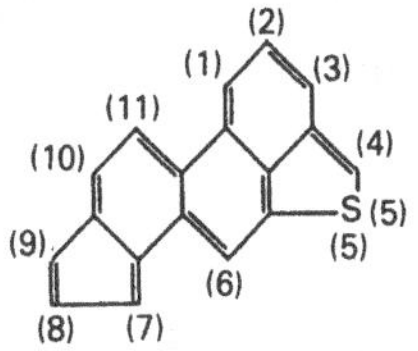

m.w.: 272 ($C_{19}H_{12}S$)

cyclopenta[7,8]phenanthro[10,1-*bc*]thiophene
(**136**)

*Fluorantheno[3,2-*b*]thiophene*

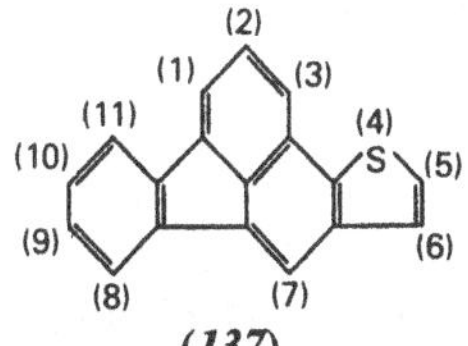

m.w.: 258 ($C_{18}H_{10}S$)

(**137**)

The base component has not yet been synthesized. However, attempts to cyclize 4-fluoranthenethioglycolic acid under Friedel-Crafts conditions resulted in the formation of a dimeric ketone (Shenbor and Tsaberyabyi, 1969):

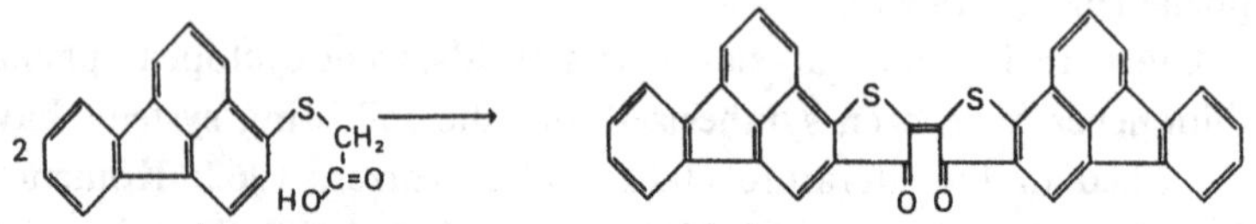

The formation of an indenonaphthothiophene after photochemical ring closure of 2-naphthyl-3-indenylsulfide was observed (Schultz and DeTar, 1976; Herkstroeter and Schultz, 1984):

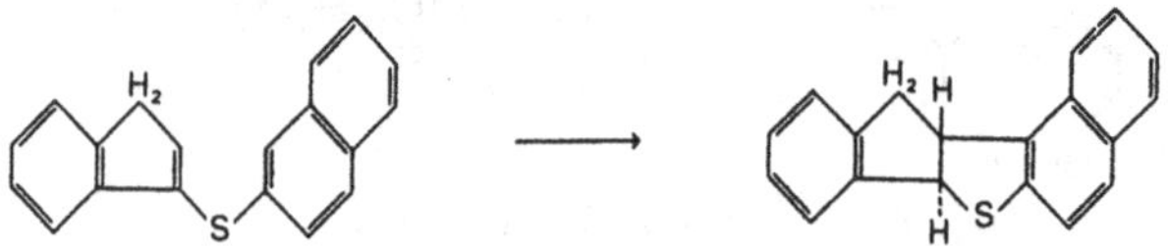

7a-12a-dihydro-12*H*-indeno[1,2-*b*]
naphtho[1,2-*d*]thiophene
(*138*)

$C_4S-C_6-C_6-C_6-C_6$

Several environmentally abundant isomers are found in this class of compounds many of which are isosteric to carcinogenic and/or mutagenic carbocyclic systems. The following parent thiaarene systems are discussed in this section: anthrabenzothiophenes, benzophenaleno-thiophenes, benzanthrathiophenes, benzophenanthrothiophenes, chry-senothiophenes, dinaphthothiophenes, naphthacenothiophenes, pyr-enothiophenes, and triphenylenothiophenes.

Anthra[1,2-b]benzo[d]thiophene
(synonyms: naphthothiafluorene; naphtho[2,3-*a*]-9-thiafluorene)

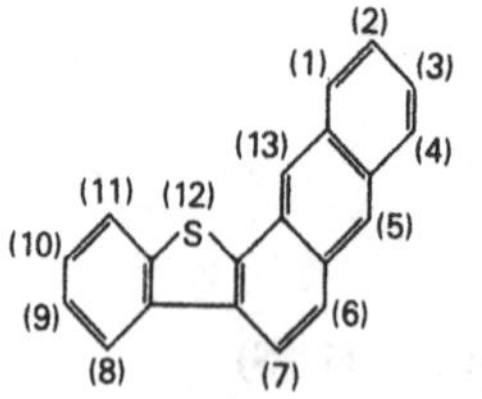

m.w.: 284 ($C_{20}H_{12}S$)
m.p.: 227°C

(*139*)

This thiaarene has been detected in coal oil (Nakamura, 1983; Wise *et al.*, 1983). It can be obtained by a multistep synthesis starting with 4-dibenzothiophene-aldehyde in an overall yield of 27% (Tedjamulia *et al.*, 1983c):

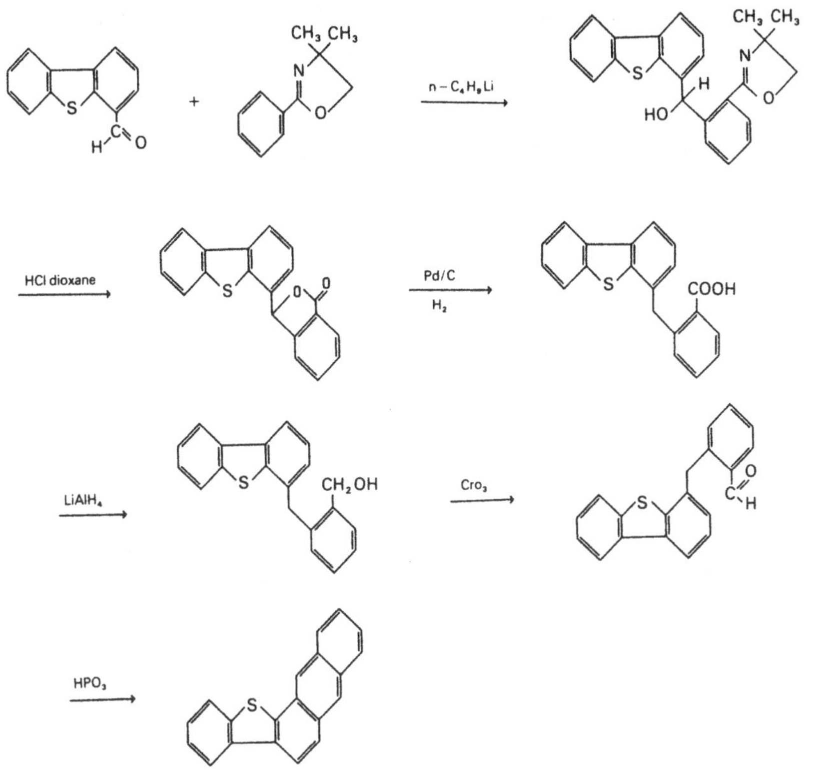

In mixture with benzo[*b*]phenanthro[3,4-*d*]thiophene it can also be prepared by Wadsworth-Emmons reaction of benzo[*b*]thenyl-3-phosphonate and 2-naphthaldehyde and subsequent photocyclization of the 3-(2-naphthylethenyl)benzo[*b*]thiophene (Croisy *et al.*, 1975; Pratap *et al.*, 1982*b*):

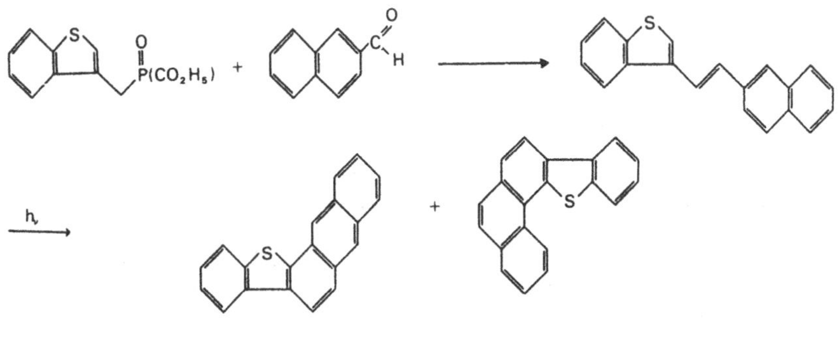

The system previously was synthesized from 3-vinylthianaphthene (Davies and Porter, 1957*c*) and later from 2-oxo-1,2,4a,5,6,11bhexahydrobenzo[*b*]naphtho[2,1-*d*]thiophene by ring extension through Michael-addition (Sastry and Tilak, 1961).

*Anthra[2,1-*b]*benzo*[d]*thiophene*
(synonym: naphtho[2,3-*c*]-9-thiafluorene)

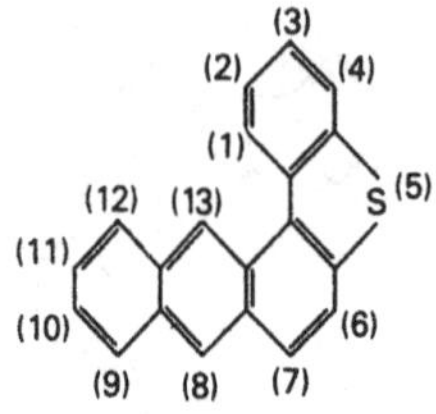

m.w.: 284 ($C_{20}H_{12}S$)

(140)

In mixture with anthra[2,3-*b*]benzo[*d*]thiophene, this compound may be obtained from dibenzothiophene by acylation with phthalic anhydride, cyclization with polyphosphoric acid and subsequent reduction with Sn/HCl (Gverdtsiteli and Litvinov, 1970*b*,*c*):

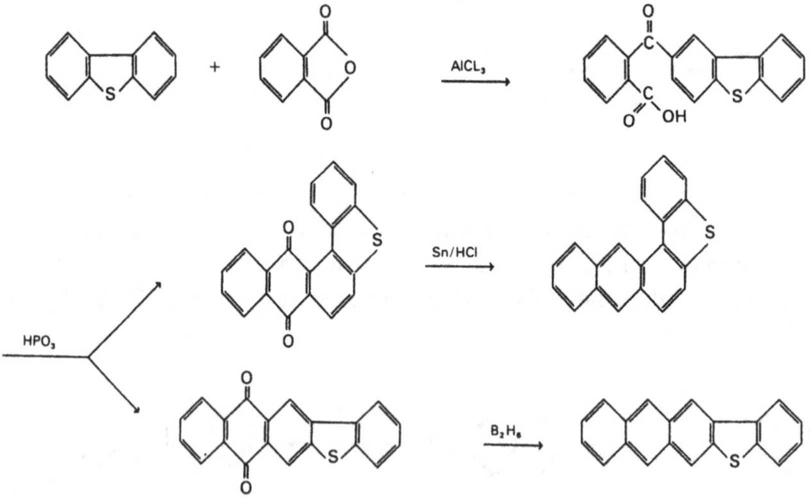

A similar route has been described by Tedjamulia *et al.* (1983*c*) also resulting in a mixture of the two isomers which, however, can be separated by HPLC or column chromatography. In this case the keto group of the condensation product is first reduced and the cyclization is carried out with the aldehyde:

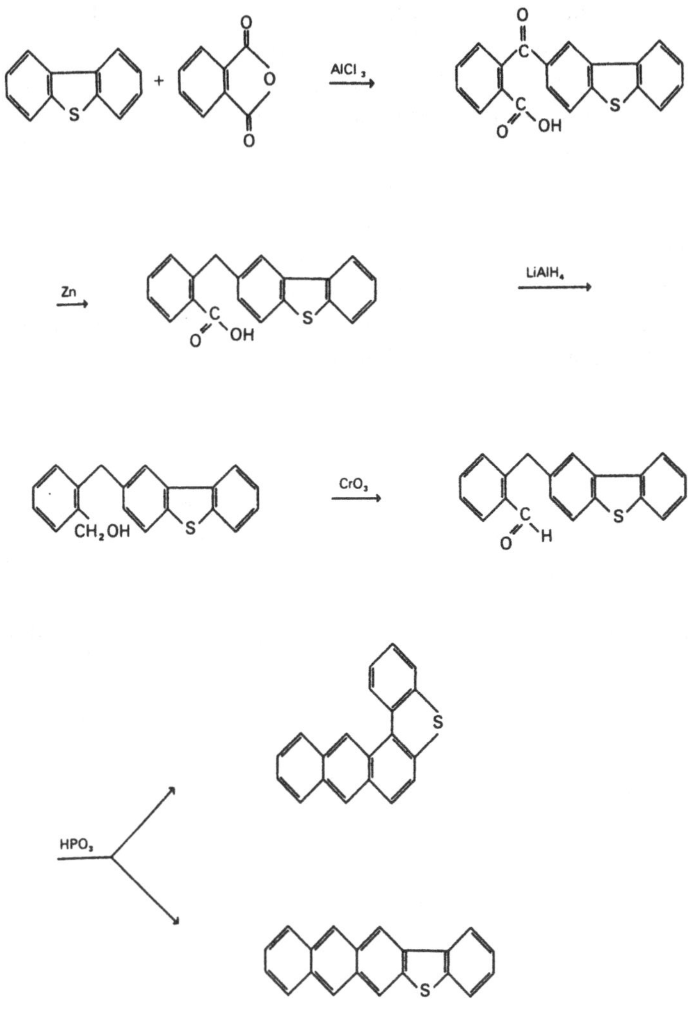

Gas chromatographic behaviour has been studied (Litvinov *et al.*, 1973). Fluorescence and luminescence spectra were recorded (Nikitina *et al.*, 1972; Akhobadze *et al.*, 1976, 1977).

Anthra[2,3-b]benzo[d]thiophene
(synonym: naphtho[2,3-*b*]-thiafluorene)

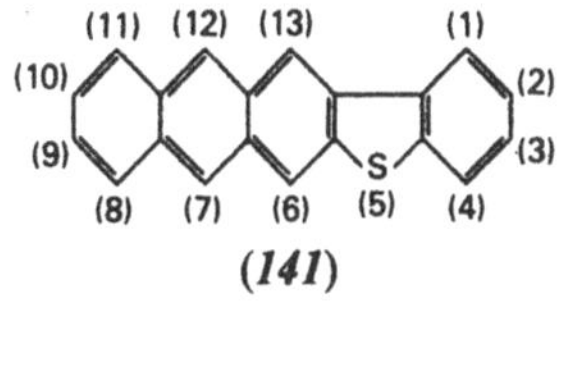

m.w.: 284 ($C_{20}H_{12}S$)
m.p.: 250°C

(141)

Anthra[2,3-*b*]benzo[*d*]thiophene can be detected by quasilinear luminescence spectroscopy in petroleum and in petroleum products (Akhobadze *et al.*, 1977; Teplitskaya *et al.*, 1981). Its gas chromatographic behaviour has been studied by Litvinov *et al.* (1973), and luminescence spectra have been recorded by Akhobadze *et al.* (Akhobadze *et al.*, 1976, 1977; Teplitskaya *et al.*, 1981). Fluorescence, quasiluminar fluorescence and absorption spectra at 77°K have also been measured (Nikitina *et al.*, 1972; Utkina *et al.*, 1976*a*).

Syntheses for anthra[2,3-*b*]benzo[*d*]thiophene during which its [2,1-*b*]isomer (*140*) also is formed are described under the latter compound (Gverdtsiteli and Litvinov, 1970*b*; Tedjamulia *et al.*, 1983*c*). Cherry *et al.* (1967) reported on its formation from dibenzothienyl-*o*-tolyl-ketone by cyclization:

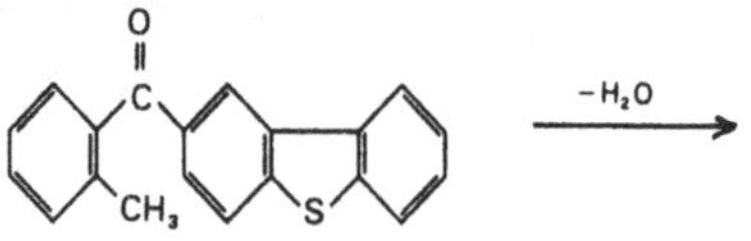

An approach to this sytem by Pschorr reaction has been published by Peters and Tenny (1977):

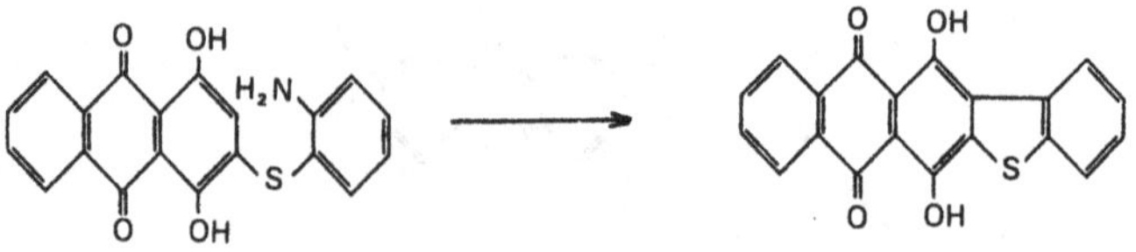

A potential technical use as a glass-reinforced plastic may arise from polyoxoarenes of the following structure:

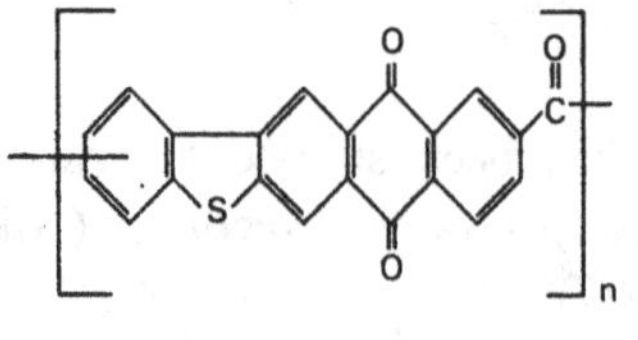

which are formed in a reaction of dibenzothiophene with trimellithic acid trichloride in nitrobenzene or 1,1,2,2-tetrachloroethane (Messerle and Musina, 1976).

Benzo[4,5]phenaleno[1,9-bc]thiophene

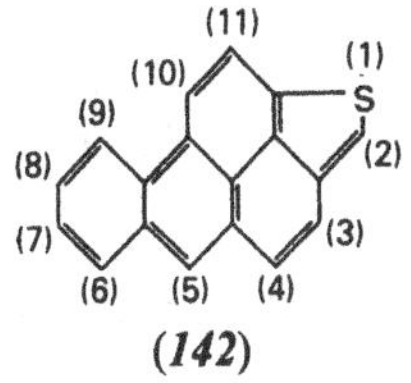

(**142**)

m.w.: 258 ($C_{18}H_{10}S$)

and

Benzo[4,5]phenaleno[9,1-bc]thiophene

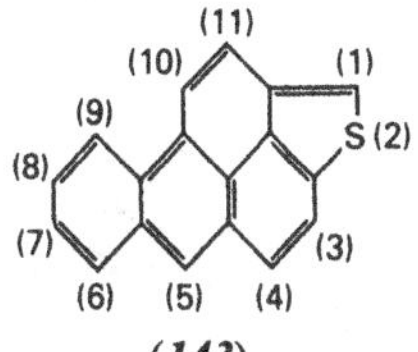

(**143**)

m.w.: 258 ($C_{18}H_{10}S$)

Gas chromatographic and HPLC retention times and separation conditions for both compounds have been provided by Nakamura (1983) and Wise *et al.* (1983). Tominaga *et al.* (1982*a*) published their synthesis; the [1,9-*bc*]-isomer was prepared by reaction of 4-methyl-thiophene-2-aldehyde with diethyl 1-naphthylmethylphosphonate giving 1-(4-methyl-2-thienyl)-2-(1-naphthyl)ethene which upon photocyclization gives 3-methylphenanthro[2,1-*b*]thiophene. This is brominated with N-bromo-succinimide to the 3-bromomethyl derivative and then is converted with KCN into the 3-cyanomethyl compound. Reduction leads to the corresponding aldehyde which is cyclized by means of polyphosphoric acid treatment (overall yield: 6%):

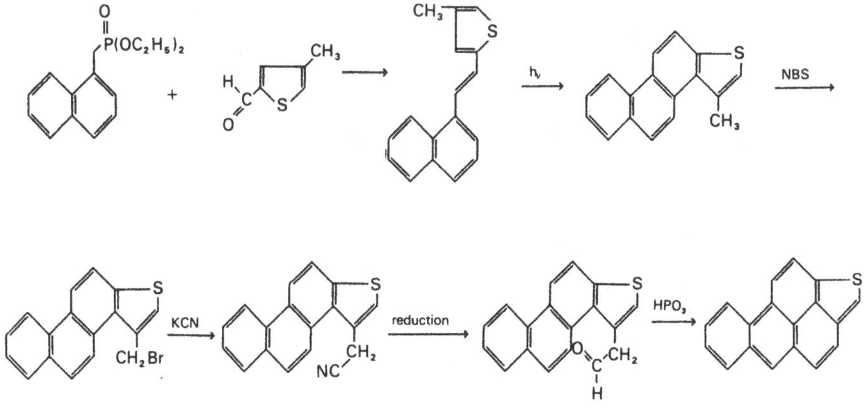

The [9,1-*bc*]-isomer was synthesized by the same authors in 8 steps with an overall yield of about 1% using the following route:

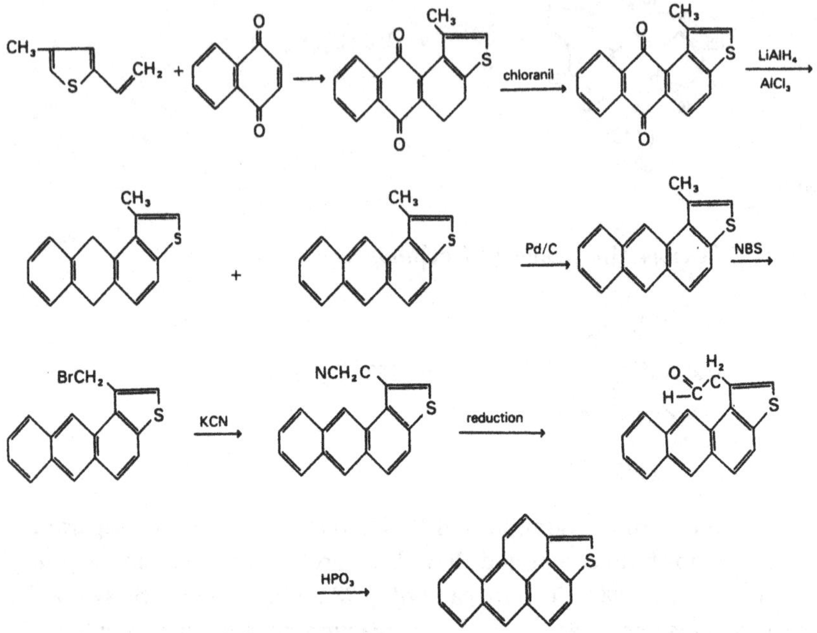

*Benzo[1,2]phenaleno[4,3-*bc*]thiophene*
(synonym: benz[4,10]anthra[1,9-*bc*]thiophene)

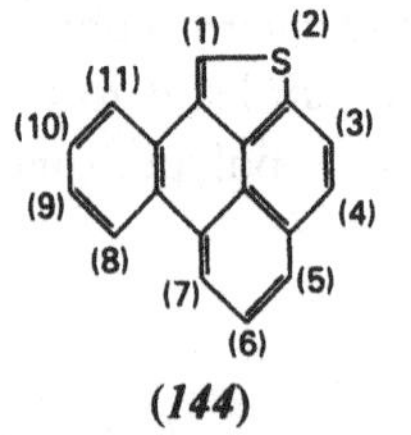

m.w.: 258 ($C_{18}H_{10}S$)

(144)

*Benzo[1,2]phenaleno[3,4-*bc*]thiophene*
(synonym: benz[4,10]anthra[9,1-*bc*]thiophene)

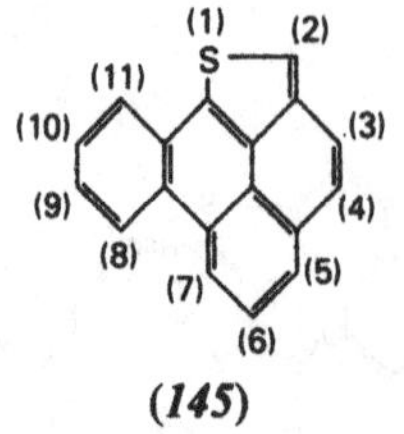

m.w.: 258 ($C_{18}H_{10}S$)

(145)

Both compounds have been tentatively identified in coal oil (Nakamura, 1983) and GC as well as HPLC retention times have been recorded (Nakamura, 1983; Wise *et al.*, 1983). Their syntheses have been described by Pratap *et al.* (1982*a*) according to the following scheme:

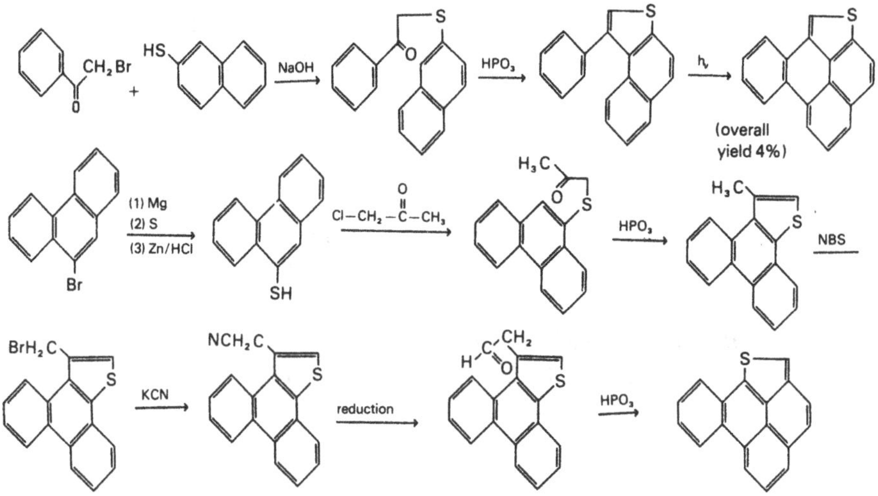

Benzo[b]*phenanthro*[*1,2-d*]*thiophene* (synonyms: naphtho[1′,2′,3,4]-9-thiafluorene; naphtho[1,2-*c*]-9-thiafluorene)

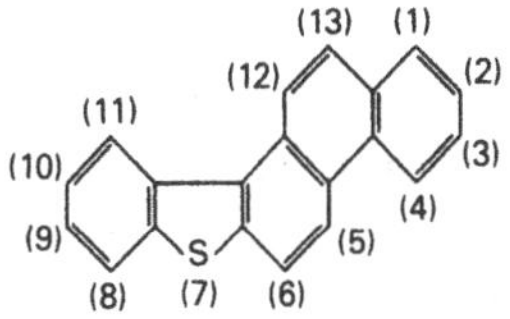

m.w.: 284 ($C_{20}H_{12}S$)
m.p.: 169°C

(*146*)

This compound was detected in particulate emissions of aluminium smelters (Murayama and Moriyama, 1982). It was synthesized first by Davies and Porter (1957*a*) by condensation of benzo[*b*]thiophene-1,1-dioxide with 1-vinylnaphthalene and subsequent reduction of the sulfone formed and selenium dehydrogenation of the dihydro product:

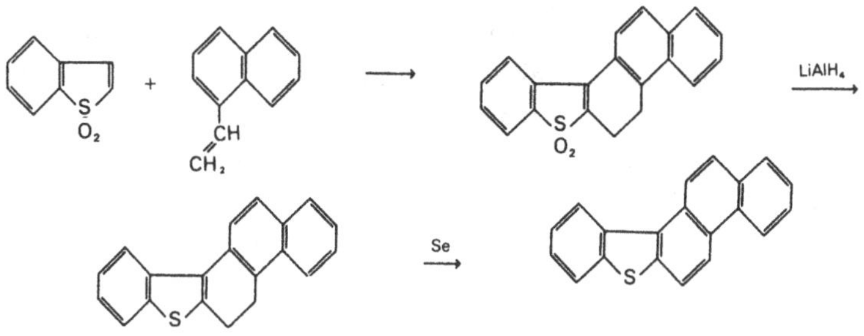

It was also synthesized by Pratap *et al.* (1982*b*) and by Castle *et al.* (1983) from benzo[*b*]thiophene-2-aldehyde and 1-naphthyl diethylphosphonate followed by photocyclization of the condensation product:

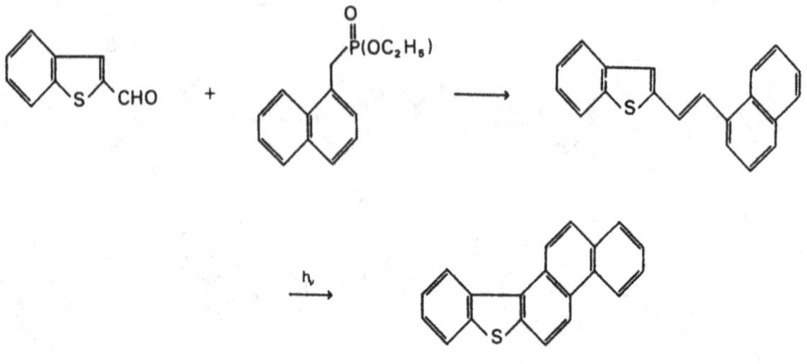

Benzo[b]*phenanthro*[2,1-d]*thiophene*
(synonym: naphtho[2,1-*a*]-9-thiafluorene)

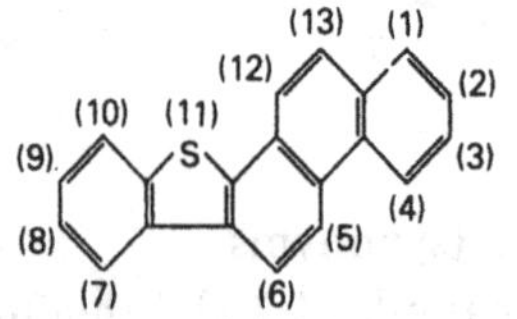

m.w.: 284 ($C_{20}H_{12}S$)
m.p.: 331°C

(*147*)

This system is present in coal oil and related materials (Nakamura, 1983; Wise *et al.*, 1983; Kong *et al.*, 1984). It has been prepared by Croisy *et al.* (1975) by photochemical cyclization of 1-(1-naphthyl)-2-(3-thienyl)ethene prepared by condensation of α-naphthylacetic acid and 3-formylbenzo[*b*]thiophene in acetic anhydride followed by decarboxylaton:

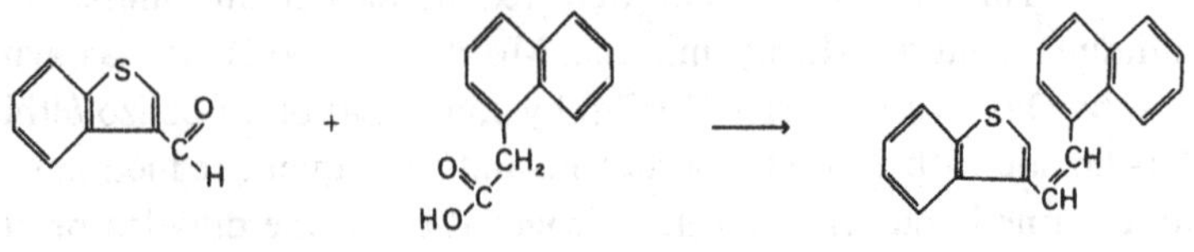

They later described a general synthesis for benzonaphthothiophenes and benzophenanthrothiophenes through Elbs cyclodehydration of ortho-methylated aroyl-benzo[*b*]thiophenes by which the above thiaarene was also obtainable (Croisy *et al.*, 1984). The authors also published UV- and NMR-data:

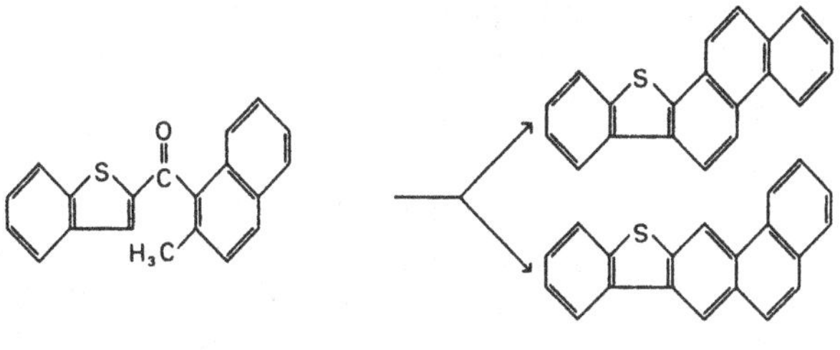

Two synthetic routes were described by Lee's group (Pratap *et al.*, 1982*b*; Tedjamulia *et al.*, 1983*c*; Castle *et al.*, 1983):

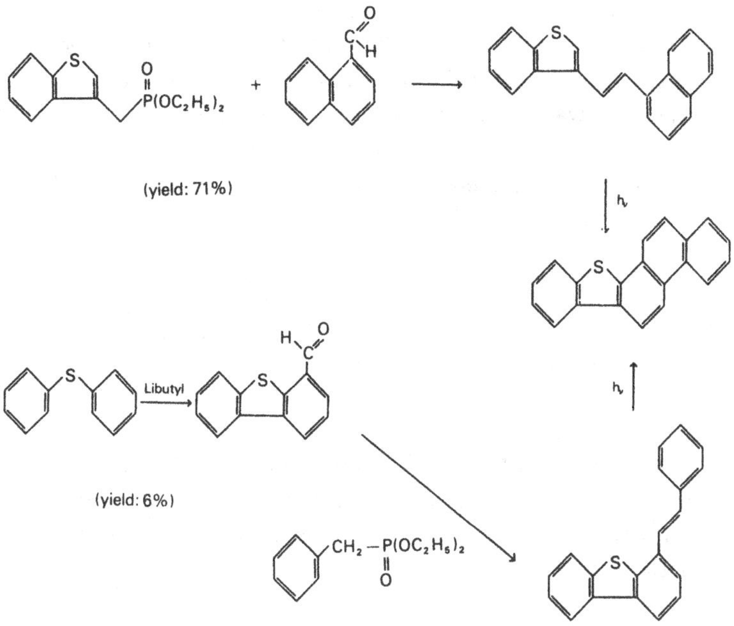

(yield: 71%)

(yield: 6%)

Lamberton and Paine (1976) reported on the synthesis of 5-hydroxy-benzo[*b*]phenanthro[2,1-*d*]thiophene by Friedel-Crafts ring closure of 2-(2-naphthyl)benzo[*b*]thiophene-3-propionic acid:

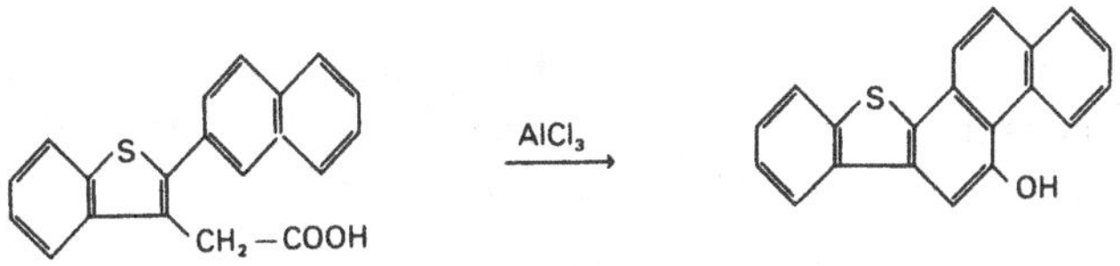

Benzo[b]*phenanthro[2,3-*d]*thiophene* (synonyms: 2,3:7,8-dibenzothiophanthrene; naphtho[1,2-*b*]-9-thiafluorene; 9-thianaphtho[1',2':2,3]fluorene)

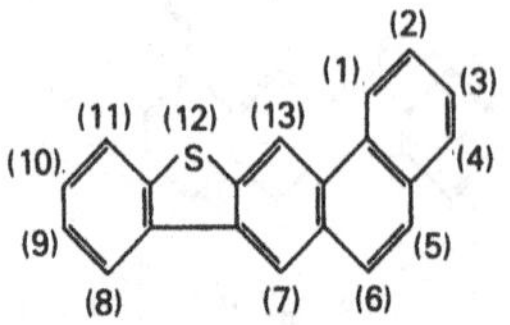

m.w.: 284 ($C_{20}H_{12}S$)
m.p.: 327°C (Tedjamulia *et al.*, 1983*c*)
328°C (Pillai *et al.*, 1963)
323°C (Badger and Christie, 1958)
245°C (Croisy *et al.*, 1984)

(148)

Benzo[*b*]phenanthro[2,3-*d*]thiophene was found to be present in coal oil (Nakamura, 1983). GC and HPLC retention times have been reported (Nakamura, 1983; Wise *et al.*, 1983, Wise and May, 1983). The compound was prepared from 2-(1-naphthoyl)benzo[*b*]thiophene-3-carboxylic acid which upon reduction to 2-(1-naphthyl-methyl)benzo[*b*]thiophene-3-carboxylic acid was cyclized with $Zn/ZnCl_2/NaCl$:

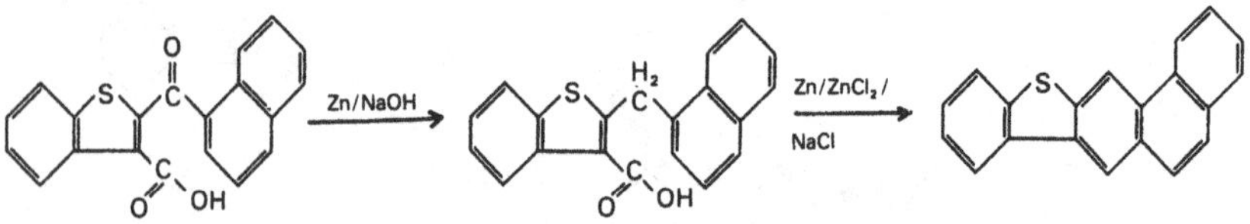

Badger and Christie (1958) obtained it through Elbs cyclodehydrogenation of 3-(1-methyl-2-naphthoyl)benzo[*b*]thiophene, whereas Croisy *et al.* (1984) used (2-(1-naphthoyl)-3-methylbenzo[*b*]thiophene as starting material:

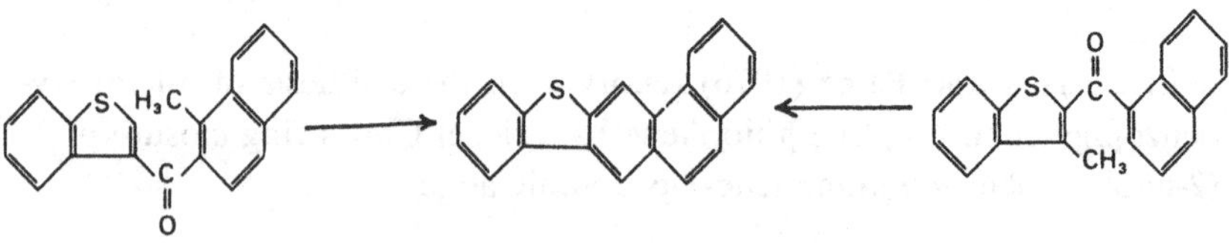

Tedjamulia *et al.* (1983*c*) reported two different ways to synthesize benzo[*b*]phenanthro[2,3-*d*]thiophene, one leading to a separable mixture of isomers (overall yield 24%), and another more specific one (overall yield 41%):

(a)

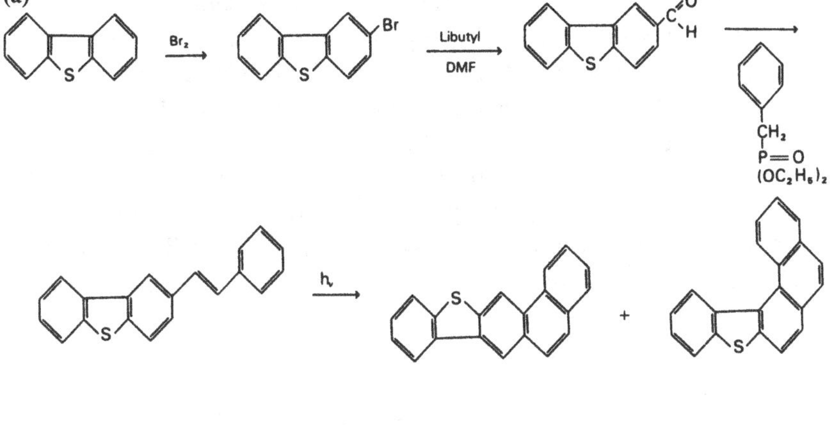

(b)

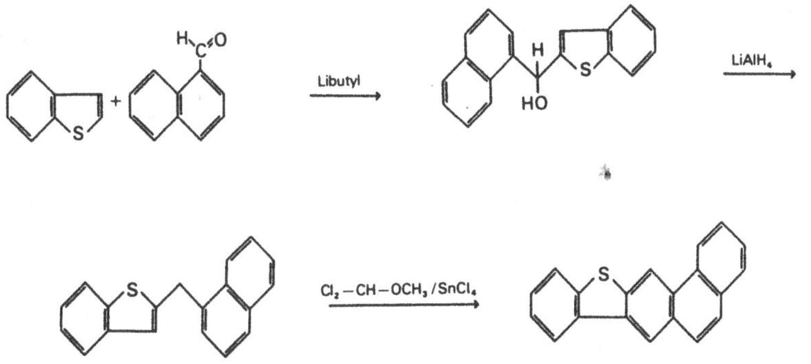

UV- and NMR-spectral data have been provided by Croisy *et al.* (1984) and MO-calculations on benzo[*b*]phenanthro[2,3-*d*]thiophene have been carried out by Zahradnik and Parkanyi (1965). The compound was found to be carcinogenic and even more potent than the very potent PAH-isoster dibenz[*a,h*]anthracene.

> *Benzo*[b]*phenanthro*[*3,2*-d]*thiophene* (synonyms: 2,3,5,6-dibenzothiophenanthrene; naphtho[2,1-*b*]-9-thiafluorene; 9-thianaphtho[2′,1′-2,3]fluorene)

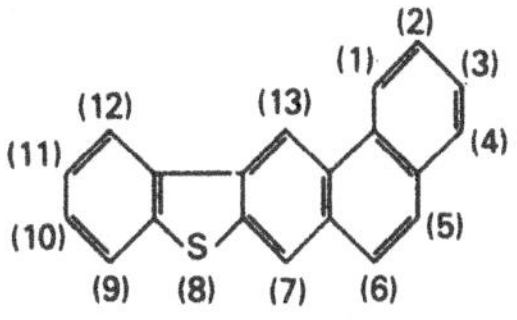

(149)

m.w.: 284 ($C_{20}H_{12}S$)
m.p.: 184°C (Croisy *et al.*, 1984)
     142°C (Badger and Christie, 1958)
     115°C (Pillai *et al.*, 1963)

The compound was detected in coal oil (Nakamura, 1983). GC and HPLC retention data have been published (Nakamura, 1983; Wise *et al.*, 1983; Wise and May, 1983). It was synthesized by Badger and Christie (1958) from 3-(2-methyl-1-naphthoyl)benzo[*b*]thiophene. Croisy *et al.* (1984), however, found that by partial rearrangement mainly benzo[*b*]phenanthro[3,4-*d*]thiophene is formed. They obtained the [3,2-*d*]-isomer in 67% yield by Elbs pyrolysis of 3-(1-naphthoyl)2-methylbenzo[*b*]thiophene accompanied by 16–17% of the [2,3-*d*]- and the [3,2-*d*]-isomer, respectively:

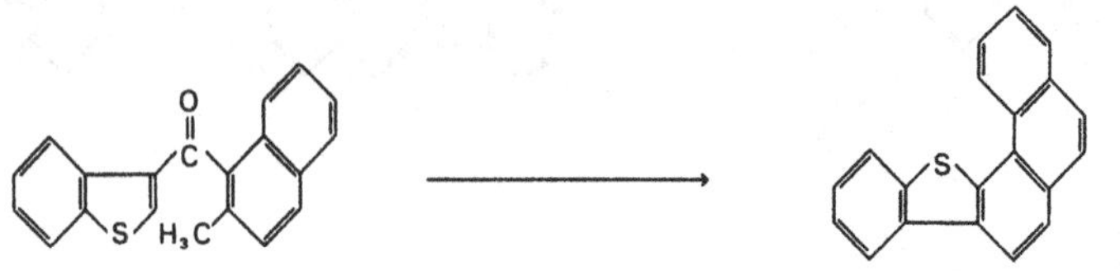

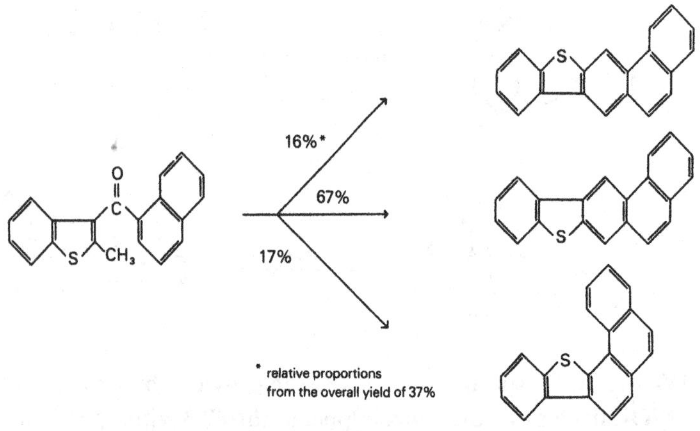

16%*
67%
17%
* relative proportions from the overall yield of 37%

Consequently, Croisy *et al.* (1984) doubted that the synthesis described by Pillai *et al.* (1963) actually yielded the [3,2-*d*]-isomer and they observed rather that the [3,4-*d*]-isomer is formed.

Later Tedjamulia *et al.* (1983*c*) described a synthetic access to this thiaarene starting from benzo[*b*]thiophene and naphthalene-2-aldehyde:

Libutyl
AlCl3 / LiAlH4
Cl2CHOCH3
SnCl4

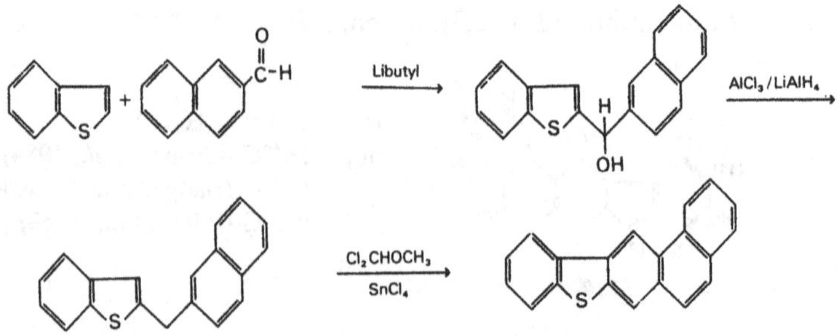

Cylization of 2-(2-naphthylmethyl)benzo[*b*]thiophene with acetic anhydride and stannic tetrachloride resulted in the 13-methyl derivative:

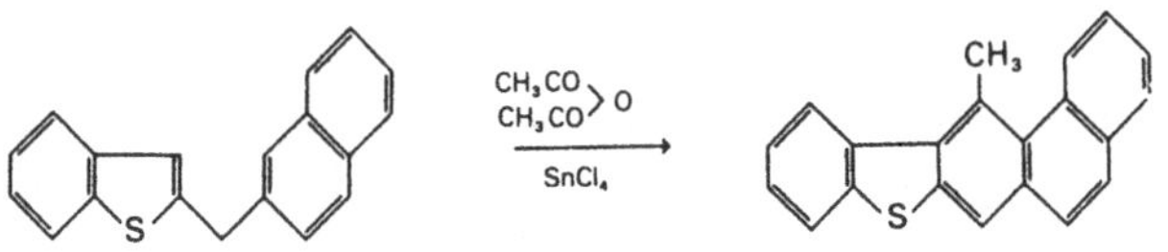

NMR- and UV-spectral data of benzo[*b*]phenanthro[3,2-*d*]thiophene have been published by Croisy *et al.* (1984) and MO-calculations were carried out by Zahradnik and Parkanyi (1965).

Carcinogenicity for this thiaarene in mice following subcutaneous injection was found to be more pronounced than with the carbocyclic isoster dibenz[*a,j*]anthracene (Croisy *et al.*, 1984).

Benzo[b]*phenanthro*[3,4-d]*thiophene* (synonyms:
9-thianaphtho[1',2'-1,2]fluorene: naphtho[1,2-*a*]-9-thiafluorene

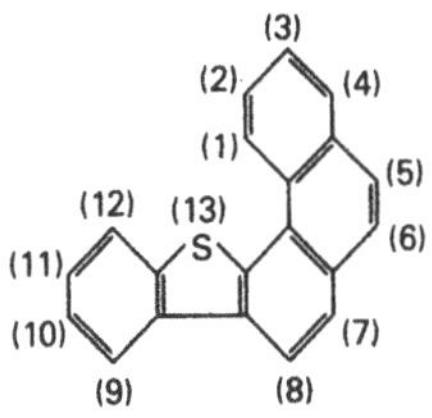

m.w.: 284 ($C_{20}H_{12}S$)
m.p.: 127°C

(*150*)

The compound was found in coal oil (Nakamura, 1963). GC and HPLC retention data have been published (Nakamura, 1983; Wise *et al.*, 1983; Wise and May, 1983). The synthesis has been described by Pratap *et al.* (1982*b*) starting with benzo[*b*]thenyl-3-phosphonate and naphthalene-2-aldehyde which gives 3-(1-naphthylethenyl)benzo[*b*]thiophene. The latter was photocyclized resulting in a mixture of benzo[*b*]phenanthro[3,4-*d*]thiophene and anthra[1,2-*b*]benzo[*d*]thiophene (for reaction scheme see under the latter). Croisy *et al.* (1984) presented evidence that the above system can be obtained by Elbs pyrolysis of 3-(2-methyl-1-naphthoyl)benzo[*b*]thiophene:

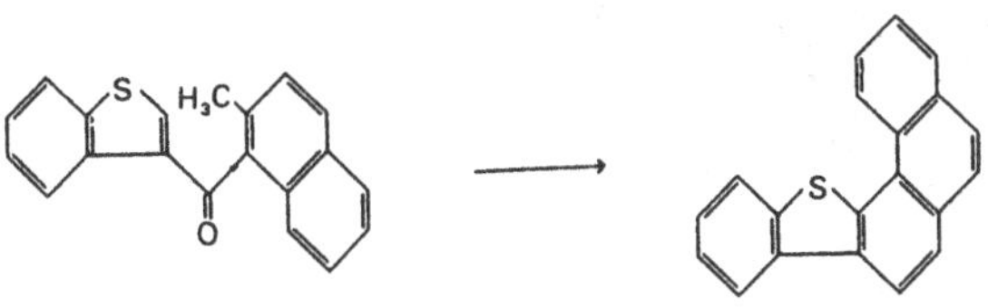

Benzo[*b*]phenanthro[3,4-*d*]thiophene was found to be a very potent carcinogen for mice after subcutaneous injection and may be compared to benzo[*a*]pyrene in this respect (Croisy *et al.*, 1984).

Benzo[b]*phenanthro[4,3-d]thiophene* (synonyms:
9-thianaphtho[2′,1′-3,4]fluorene; naphtho[2,1-*c*]-9-thiafluorene)

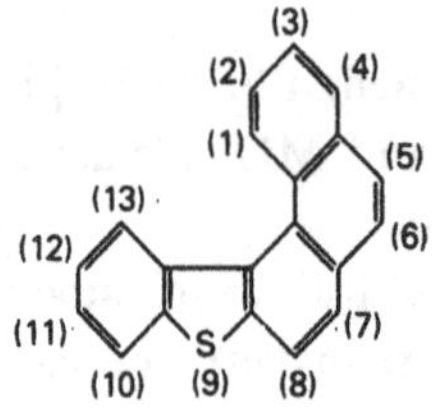

m.w.: 284 ($C_{20}H_{12}S$)

(151)

HPLC retention data for normal and reversed liquid chromatography have been published by Wise *et al.* (1983) and Wise and May (1983). The compound was synthesized starting with benzo[*b*]thiophene-2-aldehyde and 2-naphthyldiethylphosphonate by Pratap *et al.* (1982*b*):

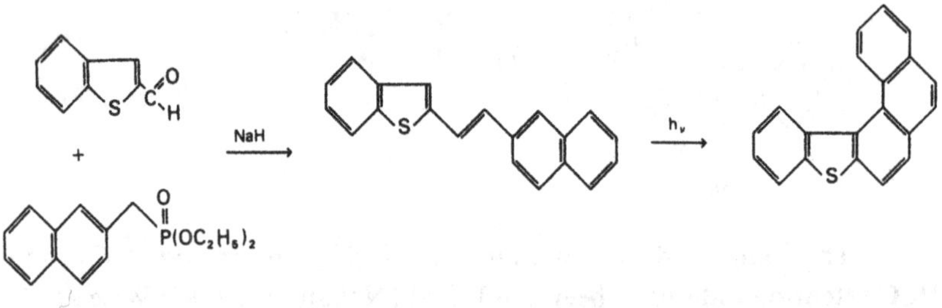

It may also be obtained in mixture with the [2,3-*d*]-isomer (as described there) from dibenzothiophene (Tedjamulia, 1983*c*).

Benzo[b]*phenanthro[9,10-d]thiophene* (synonyms: 1,2,3,4-dibenzo-9-thiafluorene; dibenzo[*a,c*]-9-thiafluorene)

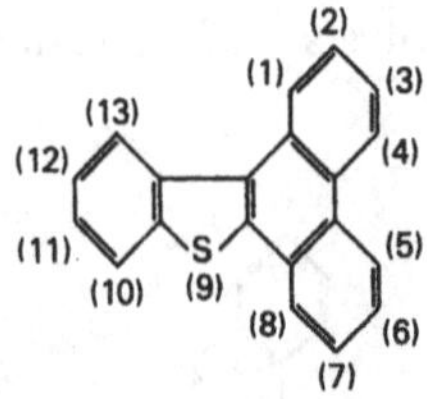

m.w.: 284 ($C_{20}H_{12}S$)
m.p.: 142°C

(152)

Benzo[*b*]phenanthro[9,10-*d*]thiophene occurs in coal oil. GC and HPLC retention data have been published (Nakamura, 1983; Wise *et al.*, 1983; Wise and May, 1983). The compound has been synthesized by condensation of 2-chlorocyclohexanone and phenanthrene-9-thiol and subsequent cyclization followed by dehydrogenation (Wilputte and Martin, 1956):

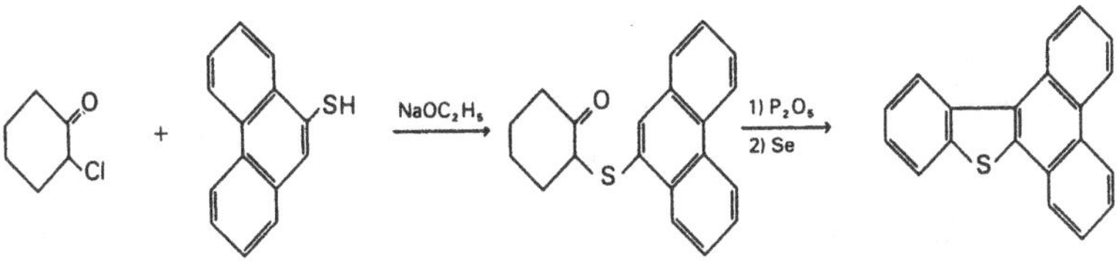

The system was also obtained by Gourier and Canonne (1973) who in a multistep synthesis prepared 1,3,6,8-tetramethylbenzo[*b*]phenanthro[9,10-*d*]thiophene (m.p.: 178°C) starting with dibenzothiophene. The latter was methylated and brominated with N-bromosuccinimide to 2,3-dibromomethyl-dibenzothiophene which upon reaction with propenyl-malonic ester and subsequent reduction, tosylation, reduction and BF₃-treatment resulted in the pentacyclic system 1,2,3,4,5,6,7,8-octahydro-1,3,6,8-tetramethylbenzo[*b*]phenanthro[9,10-*d*]thiophene which can be aromatized by Pd/C-treatment:

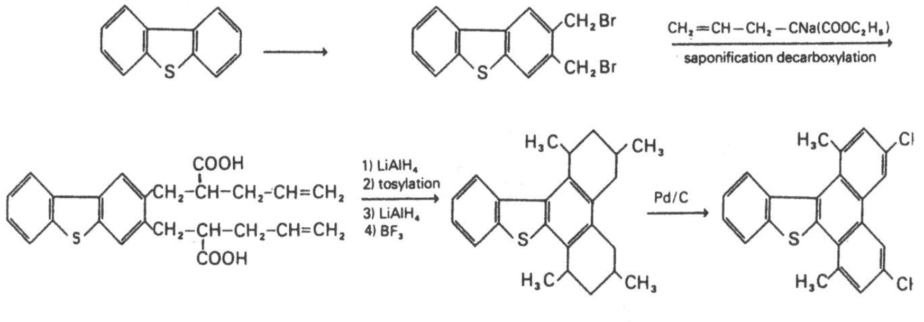

Buquet *et al.* (1981) prepared this thiaarene by irradiation of 2,3-diphenylbenzo[*b*]thiophene in the presence of iodine:

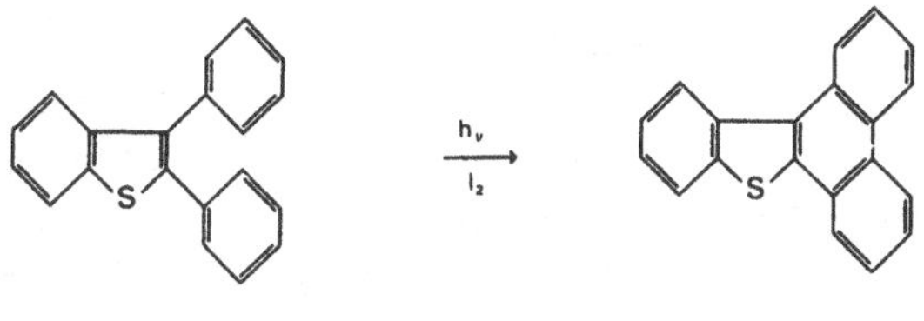

An interesting reaction of alkynes when treated with SbF_5 in benzene and liquid sulfur dioxide to obtain the sulfoxide of the above precursor of benzo[*b*]phenanthro[9,10-*d*]thiophene has been described by Fan *et al.* (1982).

Benzo[5,6]phenanthro[3,4-b]thiophene

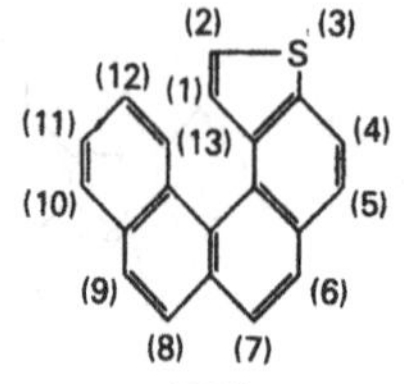

m.w.: 284 ($C_{20}H_{12}S$)
m.p.: 139°C

(*153*)

The formation of this system has been described by Dopper *et al.* (1975) through cyclization of 1-(2-thienyl)-2-(3-phenanthryl)ethene. The resulting benzo[5,6]phenanthro[3,4-*b*]thiophene can be further condensed by $AlCl_3$-treatment to benzo[8,9]pyreno[1,10-*bc*]thiophene:

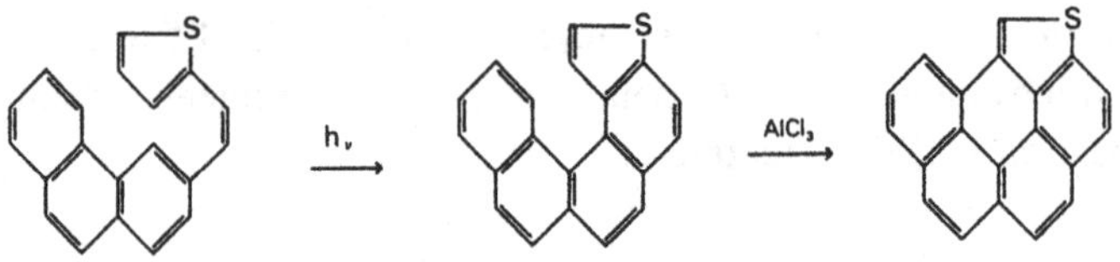

UV- and MS-spectral data have been provided by Dopper *et al.* (1975).

Benzo[2,3]phenanthro[4,5-bcd]thiophene (synonym: benz[*a*]anthraceno[11,12-*bcd*]thiophene)

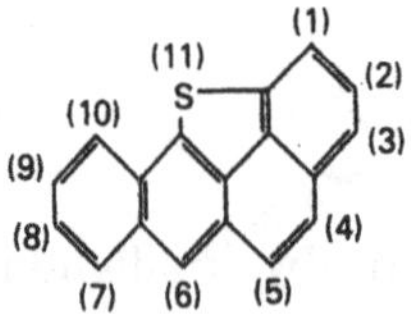

m.w.: 258 ($C_{18}H_{10}S$)
m.p.: 153°C

(*154*)

This thiaarene which is isoster to benzo[*a*]pyrene is a common attendant of the latter and, hence, occurs in various industrial products and in environmental matter. It has been detected in coal tar and pitch (Burchill *et al.*, 1982*a*; Nishioka *et al.*, 1986*b*), coal liquids and synfuels (Nakamura, 1983; Kong *et al.*, 1982, 1984; Wise *et al.*, 1983; Nishioka *et al.*, 1986*b*), carbon black (Silva *et al.*, 1982; Colmsjö *et al.*, 1982; Colmsjö and Östman, 1982), in commercial benzo[*a*]pyrene (Karcher *et al.*, 1979, 1981; Depaus, 1979), and in other tar related materials.

Thompson *et al.* (1981) prepared benzo[2,3]phenanthro[4,5-*bcd*]thiophene in a six-step synthesis starting from 3-acetyl-benzo[*b*]thiophene and diethylbenzylphosphonate (overall yield: 16%):

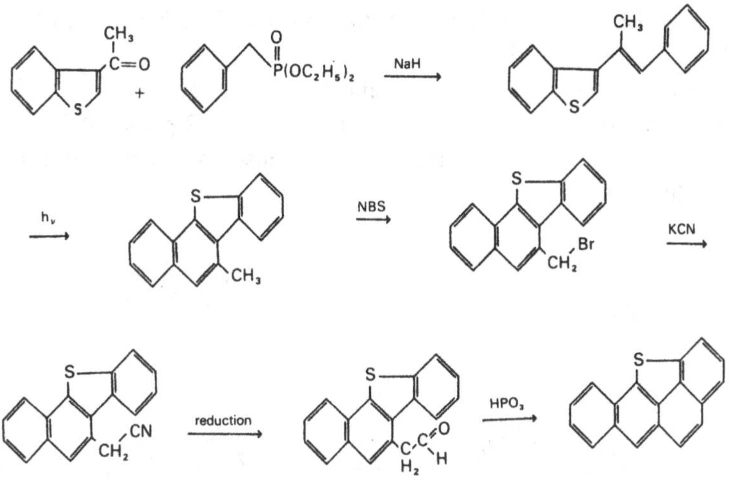

Sugiura *et al.* (1983) reported the synthesis of a series of monomethylbenzo[2,3]phenanthro[4,5-*bcd*]thiophenes (1-; 3-; 4-; 5-; 7-; 8-; 9- and 10-methyl derivative).

The UV- (Karcher *et al.*, 1979, 1981), fluorescence (Karcher *et al.*, 1979, 1981), mass- (Karcher *et al.*, 1979, 1981), low temperature fluorescence and phosphorescence- (Colmsjö *et al.*, 1982; Colmsjö and Östman, 1982) and NMR-spectra (Karcher *et al.*, 1981; Musmar *et al.*, 1984) have been recorded.

Benzo[2,3]phenanthro[4,5-*bcd*]thiophene was found to be a potent mutagen in the Ames test. On the basis of HMO-calculations Grünbauer and Wegener (1983) assumed identical metabolic activation routes for this thiaarene and its homocyclic parent compound benzo[*a*]pyrene.

*Chryseno[4,5-*bcd]*thiophene*

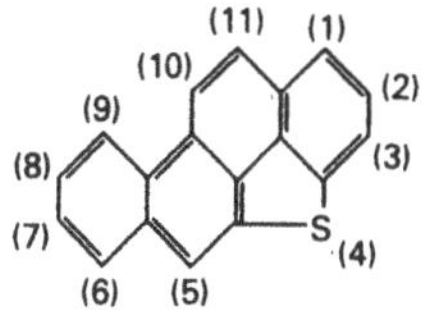

m.w.: 258 ($C_{18}H_{10}S$)
m.p.: 173°C

(*155*)

Chryseno[4,5-*bcd*]thiophene which is isoster to benzo[*a*]pyrene has been found in coal tar (Nishioka *et al.*, 1986*b*), in coal-derived products (Nakamura, 1983; Kong *et al.*, 1982, 1984; Karcher *et al.*, 1981; Wise *et al.*, 1983; Nishioka *et al.*, 1986*b*; Lee *et al.*, 1980), in shale oil (Kong *et al.*, 1984), carbon black (Colmsjö and Östman, 1982), as well as in commercial benzo[*a*]pyrene (Karcher *et al.*, 1979; Depaus, 1979). GC and HPLC retention data have been presented by Nakamura (1983) and by Wise *et al.* (1983).

A nine-step synthesis of chryseno[4,5-*bcd*]thiophene has been described by Thompson *et al.* (1981) starting with 2-phenyl-4,4-dimethyl-2-oxazoline which after lithiation was condensed with benzo[*b*]thiophene-2-aldehyde:

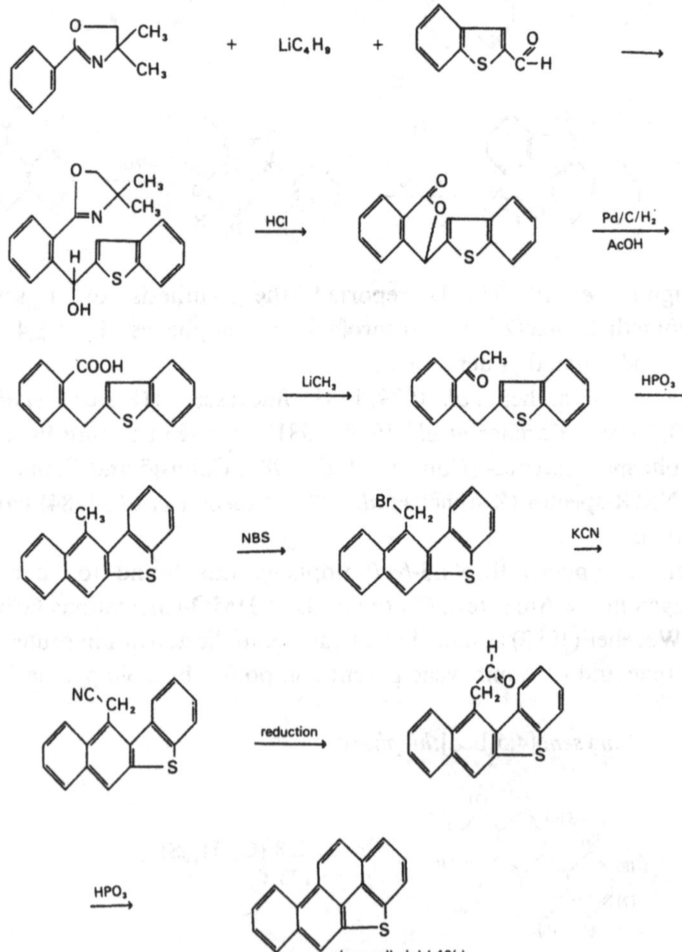

(overall yield 4%)

Colmsjö *et al.* (1985) reported the formation of the above thiaarene in mixture with chryseno[4,5-*bcd*: 10,11-*b'c'd'*]dithiophene by heating 4,5,10,11-tetrahydrochrysene (?) with sulfur in a sealed tube.

UV- (Karcher *et al.*, 1979, 1981), fluorescence- (Karcher *et al.*, 1979, 1981), low temperature fluorescence (Colmsjö *et al.*, 1982; Colmsjö and Östmann, 1982), NMR- (Karcher, 1979, 1981) and mass spectral data (Karcher *et al.*, 1979, 1981) have been published.

*Dinaphtho[1,2-*b: *1',2'*-d]thiophene* (synonyms: dibenzo[*a,g*]-9-thiafluorene; 1,2,5,6-dibenzo-9-thiafluorene)

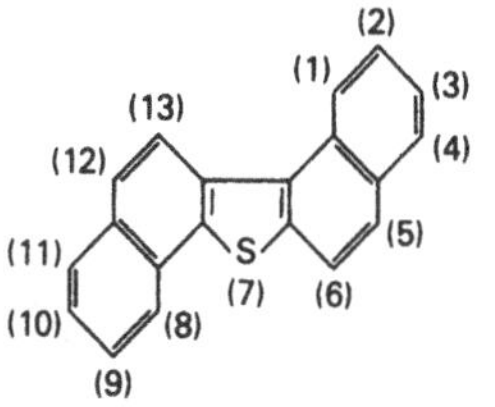

m.w.: 284 ($C_{20}H_{12}S$)
m.p.: 164°C

(*156*)

This compound being an isoster of benzo[*b*]chrysene was found in coal tar (Borwitzky and Schomburg, 1979), coal pitch (Shultz *et al.*, 1965) and accordingly in the working place atmosphere of coke-chemical production (Kumanova and Vasileva, 1983). HPLC retention data were determined by Wise *et al.* (1983) and Wise and May (1983).

The system was synthesized by Rabindran and Tilak (1953c) from naphthalene-1-thiol and 2-bromotetralone giving 2-(naphthyl-thio)tetralone which was cyclized with polyphosphoric acid to 5,6-dihydro-dinaphtho[1,2-*b*: 1',2'-*d*]thiophene which upon selenium dehydrogenation resulted in the above thiaarene:

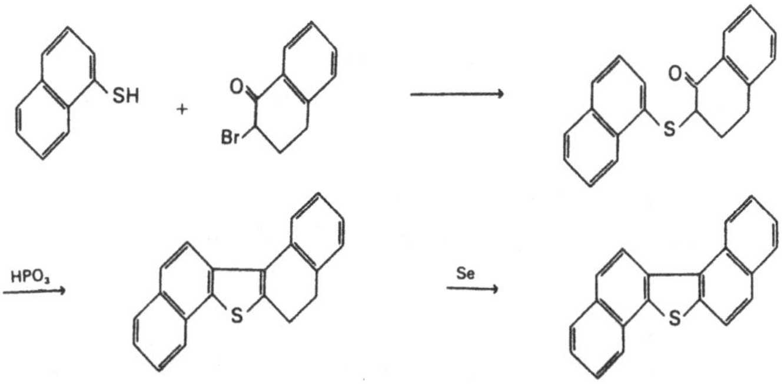

Blümer *et al.* (1977) described its formation from 1,2'-dinaphthylsulfide by photocyclization in cyclohexane under nitrogen in the presence of iodine:

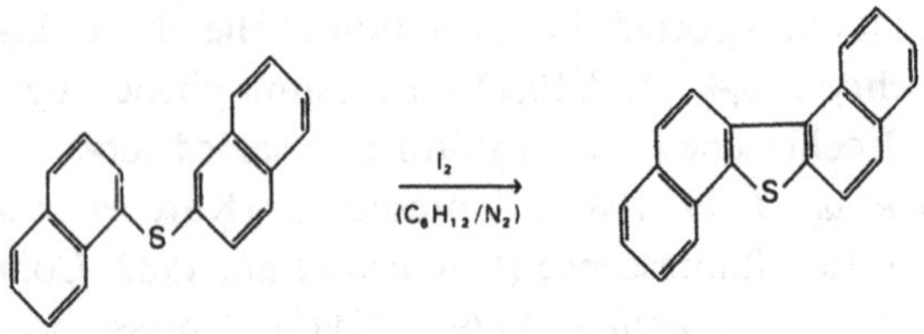

More recently, the compound has been prepared by Tedjamulia *et al.*
(1983*b*) from naphtho[1,2-*b*]thiophene-2-carboxylic ester in 4 steps with
an overall yield of 37%:

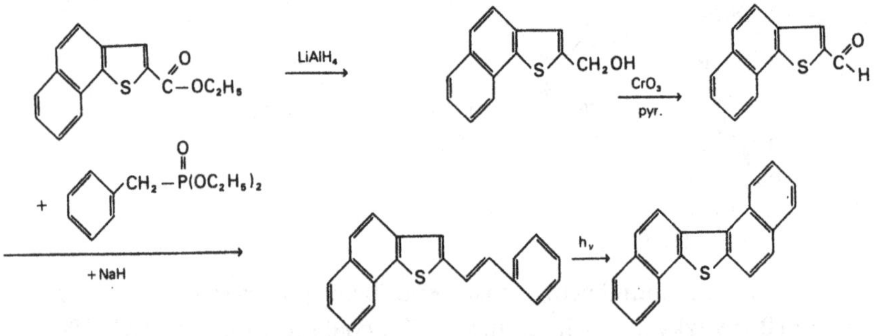

Blümer *et al.* (1977) described the AlCl₃-catalyzed rearrangement of
dinaphtho[1,2-*b*:1′,2′-*d*]thiophene to dinaphtho[1,2-*b*:2′,1′-*d*]thiophene:

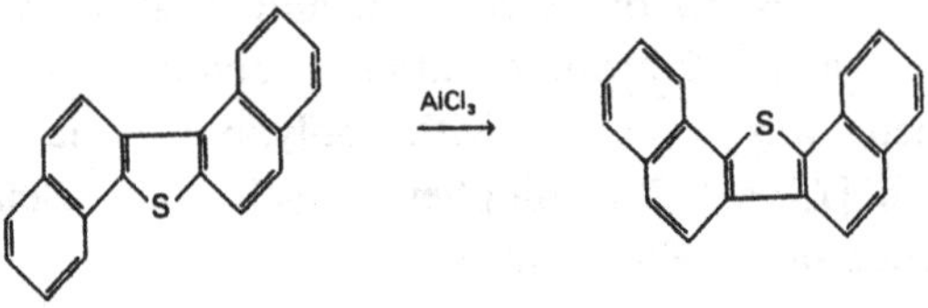

IR- (McDonald and Cook, 1967), mass- (Riepe and Zander, 1979), and
phosphorescence spectra (Zander, 1976) have been recorded.

*Dinaphtho[1,2-*b:*2′,1′-*d]thiophene* (synonyms: dibenzo[*a,i*]-9-
thiafluorene; 1,2,7,8-dibenzo-9-thiafluorene)

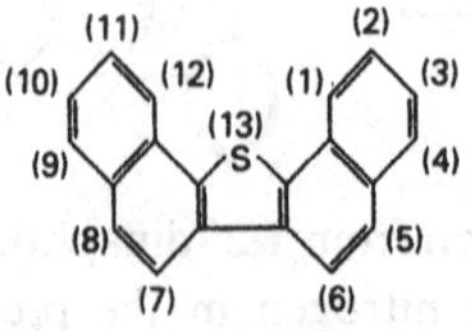

m.w.: 284 ($C_{20}H_{12}S$)
m.p.: 253°C (Wilputte and Martin, 1956)
         255–256°C (Armarego, 1960)

(157)

Dinaphtho[1,2-*b*:2′,1′-*d*]thiophene has been detected in coal products (Nakamura, 1983). GC- and HPLC-retention time studies have been carried out by Nakamura (1983), by Wise *et al.* (1983) and by Wise and May (1983). The compound has been synthesized by Wilputte and Martin (1956) by cyclodehydration of 1,1′-dinaphthyl sulfoxide:

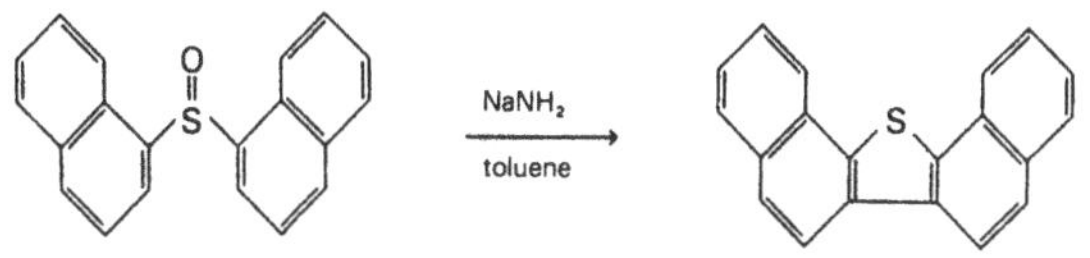

Armarego (1960) obtained it from 2-iodonaphthalene-1-sulfonate in the following way:

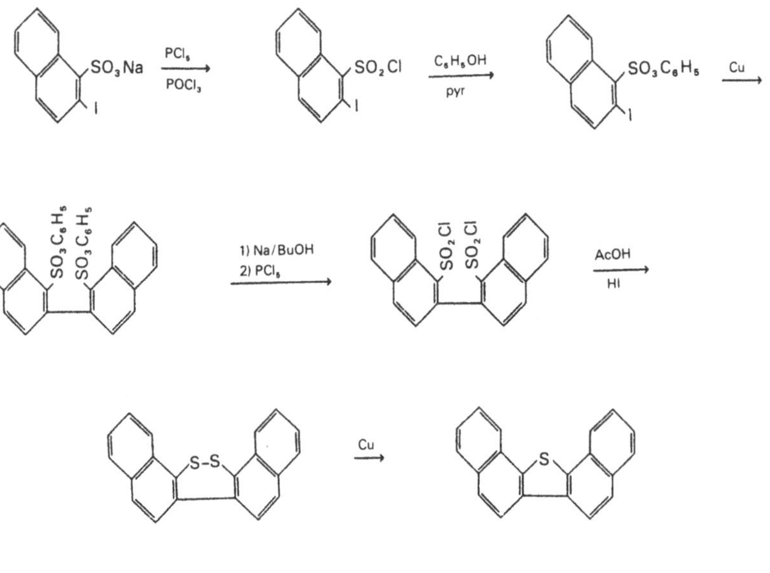

Tedjamulia *et al.* (1983*b*) described a synthesis from 1-naphthylamine which upon diazotization and treatment with potassium ethyl xanthate and subsequent reduction gave naphthalene-1-thiol. Reaction of the latter with α-bromoacetone and cyclization with polyphosphoric acid gives 3-methylnaphtho[1,2-*b*]thiophene which by SeO_2-oxidation resulted in the 3-aldehyde. This is condensed with diethylbenzylphosphonate to give 3-styrylnaphtho[1,2-*b*]thiophene which then is photocyclized to dinaphtho[1,2-*b*:2′,1′-*d*]thiophene (overall yield 23%):

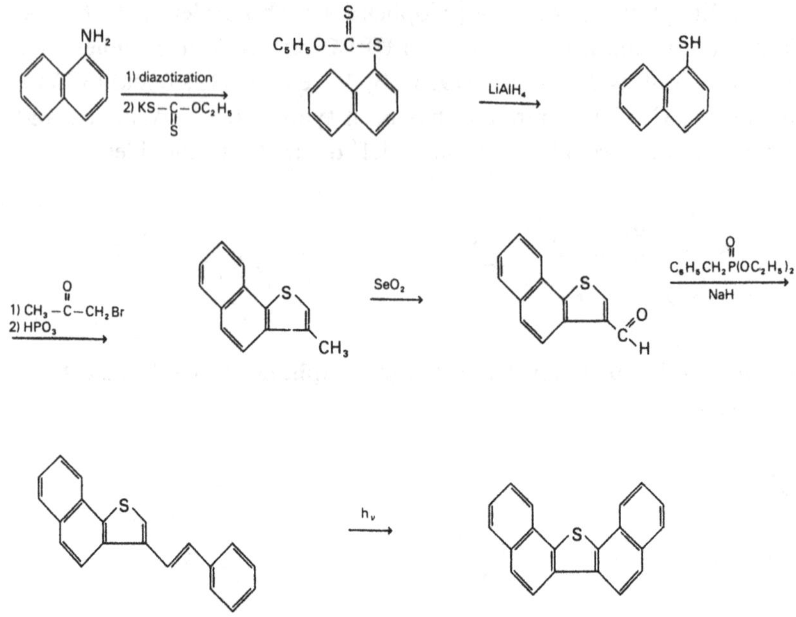

The mass spectroscopic behaviour of this thiaarene has been studied by Riepe and Zander (1979) and later by Glinzer *et al.* (1983*a*) who also recorded mass spectra of the sulfoxide and the sulfone (Glinzer *et al.*, 1983*b*). UV- (Armarego, 1960), IR- (McDonald and Cook, 1967) and phosphorescence spectra (Zander, 1976) have also been recorded.

Dinaphtho[1,2-b:2'3'd]thiophene (synonyms: dibenzo[*a,g*]-9-thiafluorene; 1,2,6,7-dibenzo-9-thiafluorene)

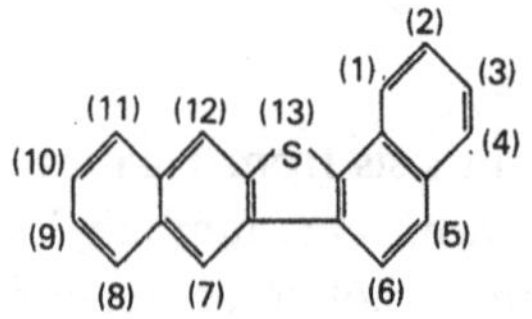

m.w.: 284 ($C_{20}H_{12}S$)
m.p.: 317°C

(*158*)

Its presence in coal tar (Nishioka *et al.*, 1986*b*) and in coal products (Nakamura, 1983; Nishioka *et al.*, 1986*b*) has been reported and GC- as well as HPLC-retention data have been published (Nakamura, 1983; Wise *et al.*, 1983). The compound can be obtained by 3 different routes. Wilputte and Martin (1956) synthesized it by condensation of naphthalene-1-thiol and 3-chloro-2-decalone which gives 3-(1-

naphthylthio)-2-tetralone. The latter then is cyclized by means of P_2O_5 and dehydrogenated to give the parent thiaarene:

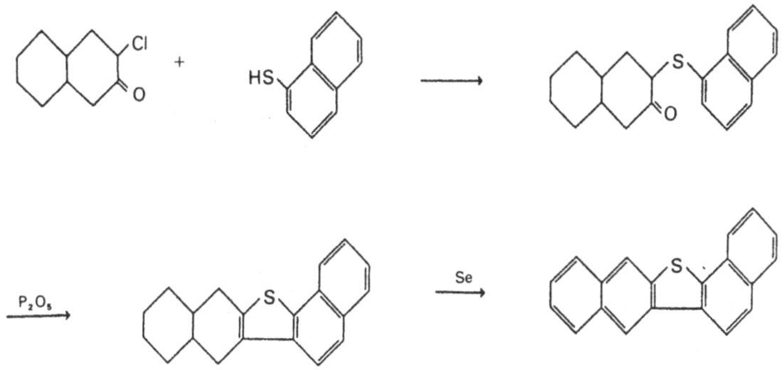

Armarego (1960) described a synthesis which starts from naphtho[1,2-*b*]thiophene and phthalic anhydride which under Friedel-Crafts conditions gives a keto acid. The latter is treated with polyphosphoric acid to give dinaphtho[1,2-*b*:2′,3′-*d*]thiophene-7,12-quinone which may be converted into the above thiaarene upon fusion with Zn-dust:

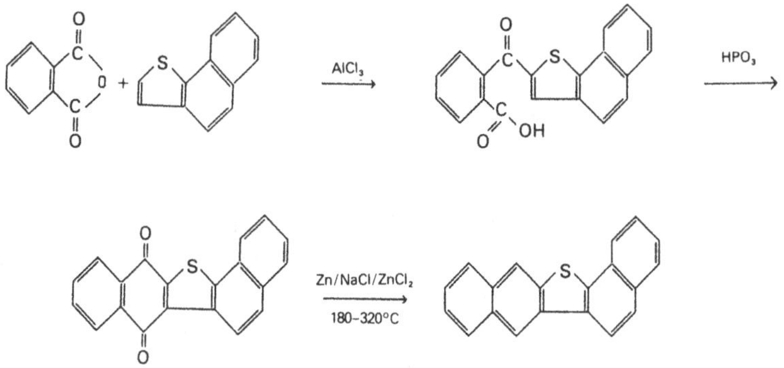

Tedjamulia used a very similar route also starting from naphtho[1,2-*b*]thiophene. The above keto acid, however, was first reduced and then the carboxyl group reduced to give the corresponding alcohol which was oxidized to the aldehyde by chromium trioxide. The latter was finally cyclized with polyphosphoric acid (Tedjamulia *et al.*, 1983*b*) (overall yield: 20%):

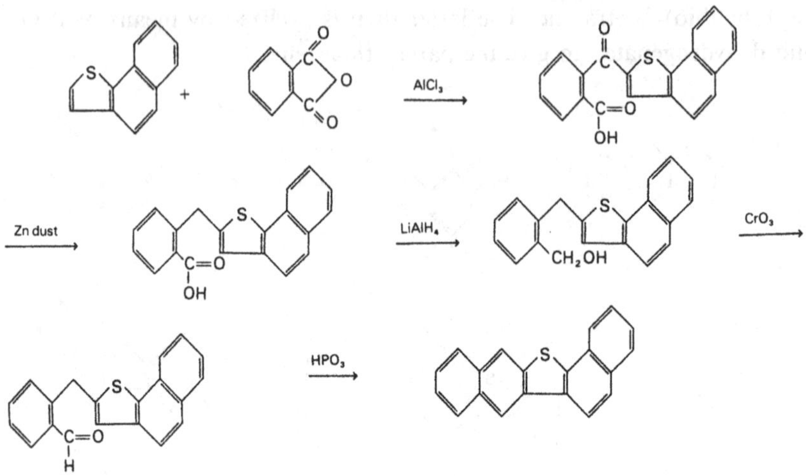

UV data have been presented by Armarego (1960).

Dinaphtho[2,1-b:1',2'-d]thiophene (synonyms: dinaphtho[2,1; 1',2']-thiophene; 3,4,5,6-dibenzo-9-thiafluorene; dibenzo[c,g]-9-thiafluorene)

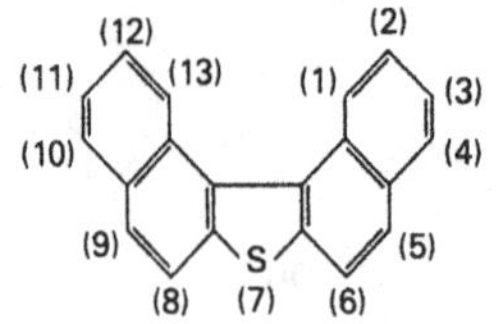

m.w.: 284 ($C_{20}H_{12}S$)
m.p.: 207°C (Rabindran and Tilak, 1953c)
208–209°C (Gogte *et al.*, 1960)

Dinaphtho[2,1-*b*:1',2'-*d*]thiophene has been found in coal extracts (Gundermann and Fuhrmann, 1978) and coal tar related materials (Karcher *et al.*, 1979, 1981). It has been synthesized by Rabindran and Tilak (1953c) by condensation of 2-bromotetralone with naphthalene-2-thiol giving 2-(2-naphthylthio)tetralone which on cyclization with polyphosphoric acid results in dihydrodinaphtho[2,1-*b*:1',2'-*d*]thiophene. The latter can be dehydrogenated with selenium to the parent thiaarene:

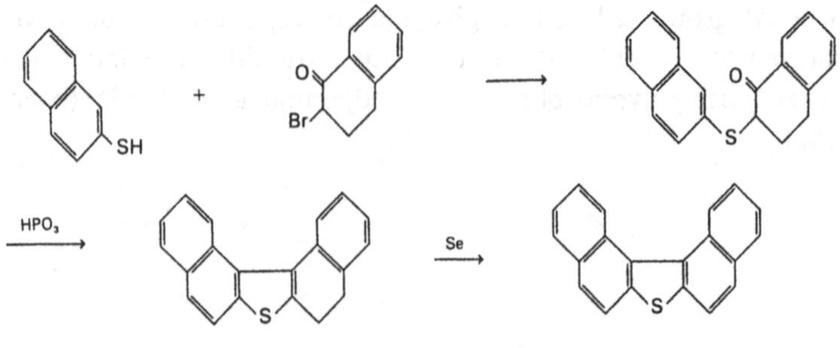

Gogte *et al.* (1960) obtained this thiaarene from β,β'-dinaphthylsulfone by lithiation and intramolecular thiannulation with anhydrous copper-2-chloride followed by LiAlH₄-reduction:

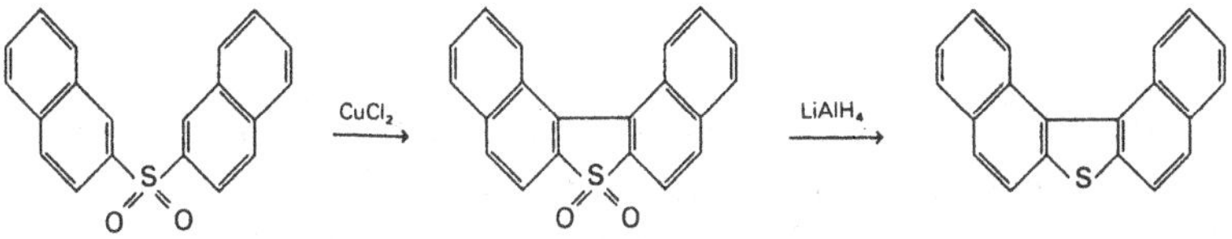

Blümer *et al.* (1977) described the formation of it from β,β'-dinaphthylsulfide by photocyclization in cyclohexane in the presence of iodine:

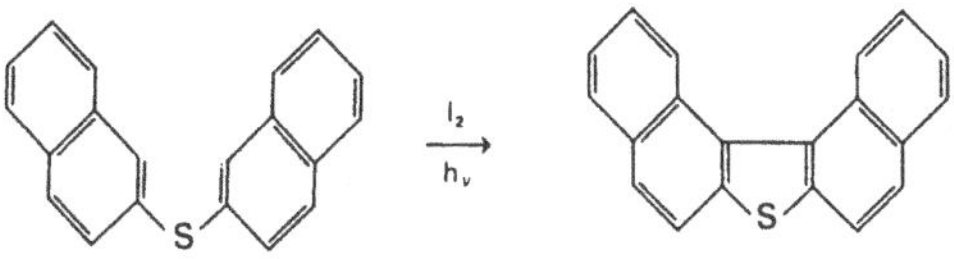

Similarly, it may be prepared by photocyclization of 1-phenyl-2-(2-naphtho[2,1-*b*]thienyl)ethene (Dopper, 1974):

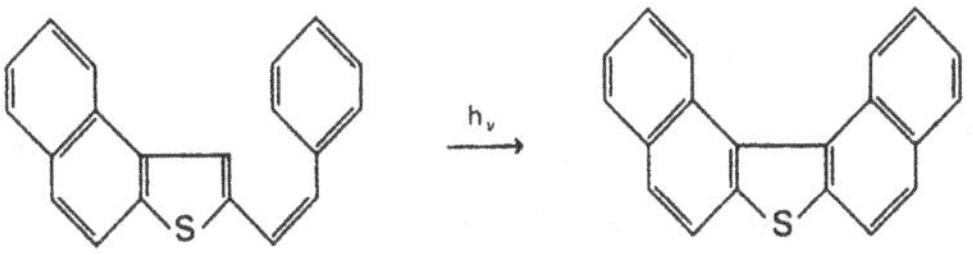

Its formation from dinaphtho[2,1-*b*:1',2'-*d*]di-1,2-thiin by heating with copper bronze has been described by Barber and Smiles (1928):

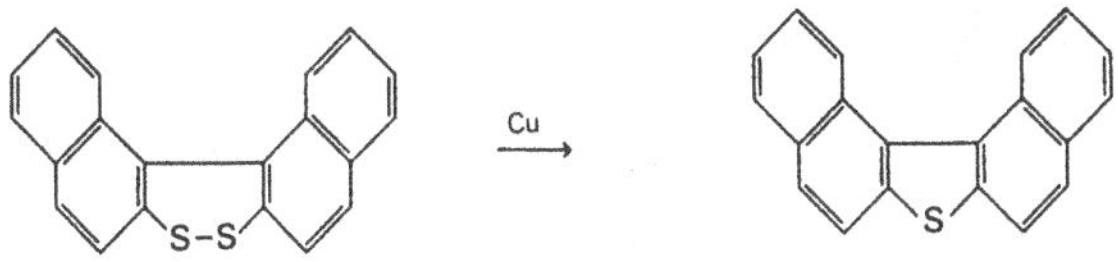

More recently Tedjamulia *et al.* (1983*b*) reported on a synthesis starting with 3-(1-naphthyl)-2-thiopropenoic acid. They obtained the thiaarene in a five step synthesis with an overall yield of 18%:

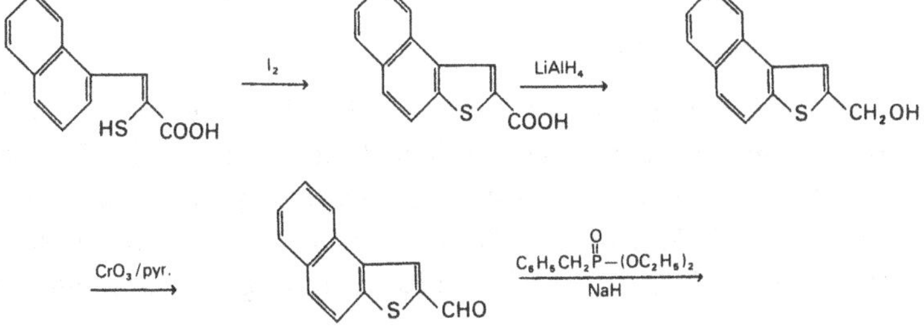

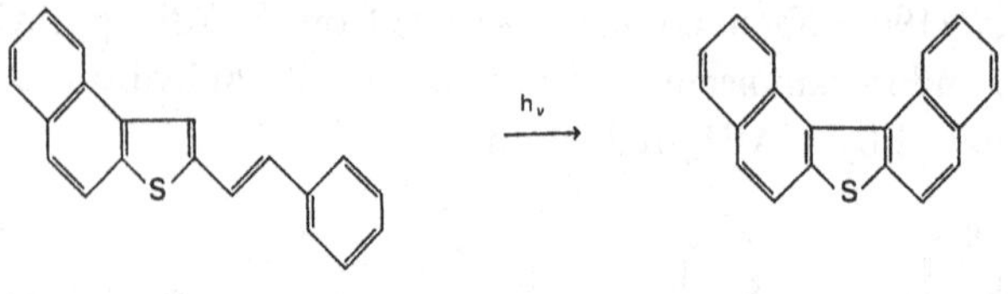

Dinaphtho[2,1-*b*:1',2'-*d*]thiophene can be desulfurized in tetralin at 360–380°C/85 bar by a molybdenum/cobalt catalyst yielding 1,1'-binaphthyl (Gundermann and Fuhrmann, 1978). It has also been reported by Blümer *et al.* (1977) that it rearranges in the presence of AlCl₃ to give both dinaphtho[1,2-*b*:2',1'-*d*]thiophene and perylo[1,12-*bcd*]thiophene:

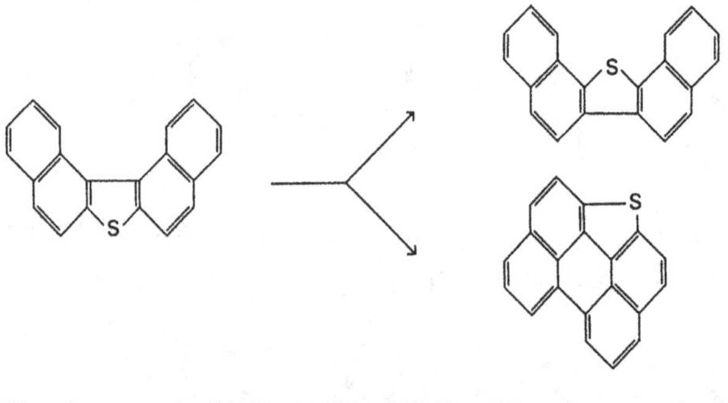

UV- (Karcher *et al.*, 1979, 1981), NMR- (Karcher *et al.*, 1979, 1981), fluorescence- (Karcher *et al.*, 1979, 1981), mass- (Riepe and Zander, 1979; Karcher *et al.*, 1979, 1981) and phosphorescence spectra (Zander, 1976) have been recorded.

Dinaphtho[2,1-*b*:1',2'-*d*]thiophene was found to be non-carcinogenic by Rabindran and Tilak (1953*c*).

*Dinaphtho[2,1-*b*:2',3'-d]thiophene* (synonyms: 2,3,5,6-dinaphtho 9-thiafluorene; dibenzo[*b,g*]-9-thiafluorene)

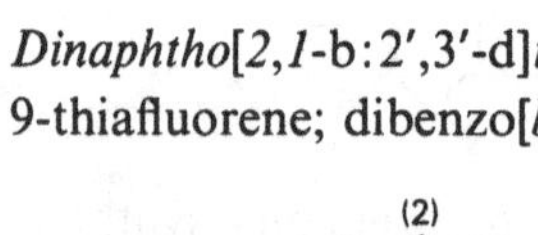

m.w.: 284 ($C_{20}H_{12}S$)
m.p.: 197°C

(160)

The compound was obtained by Wilputte and Martin (1956) through condensation of naphthalene-2-thiol and 3-chloro-2-decalone to give 3-(2-naphthylthio)-2-decalone which upon cyclization yields 8,8a,9,10,11,12,12a,13-octahydro-dinaphtho[2,1-*b*:2',3'-*d*]thiophene. The latter then is dehydrogenated with selenium to give the parent thiaarene:

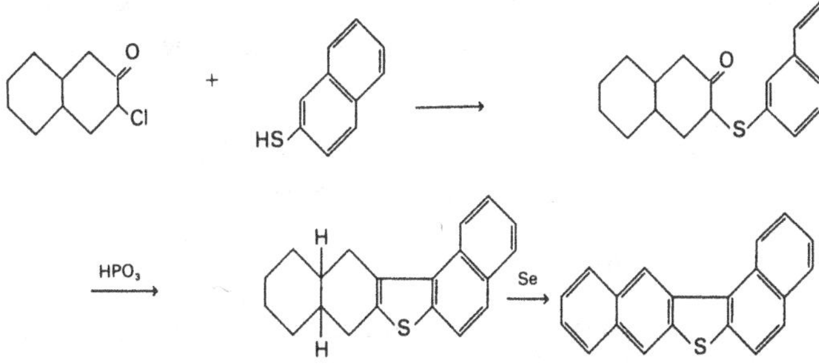

An alternative route has been described by Tedjamulia *et al.* (1983*b*). As starting material diethyl-2-thenylphosphonate and benzaldehyde were used leading to 2-styrylthiophene which upon photocyclization gives naphtho[2,1-*b*]thiophene. Friedel-Crafts reaction with phthalic anhydride results in a keto acid which is reduced with zinc dust to the corresponding carboxylic acid. After reduction to the alcohol followed by oxidation with chromium trioxide to the aldehyde, the latter was cyclized with polyphosphoric acid to give the above parent thiaarene in an overall yield of 14%:

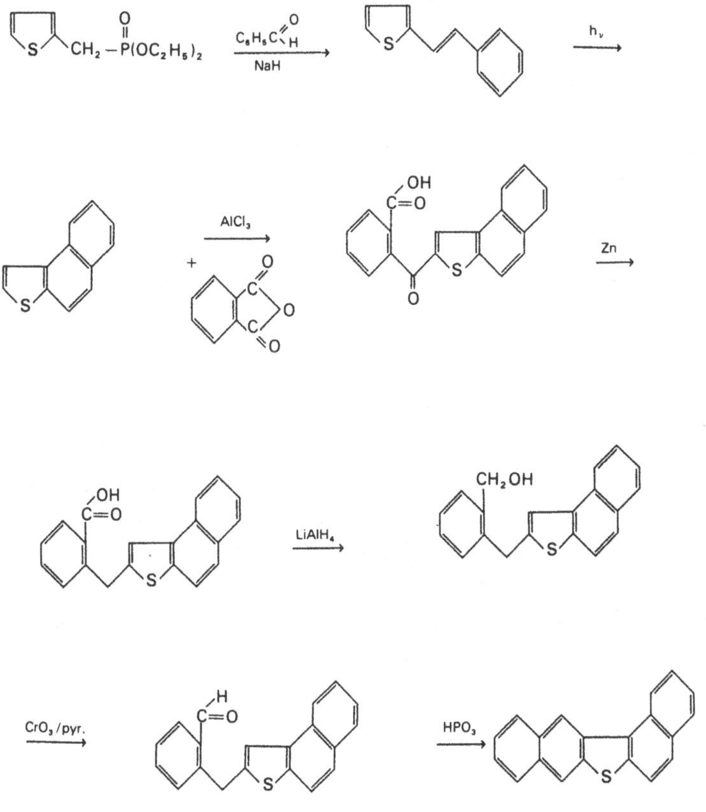

Dinaphtho[2,3-b:*2′,3′*-d]*thiophene* (synonym: dibenzo[*b,h*]-9-thiafluorene; 2,3,6,7-dinaphtho-9-thiafluorene)

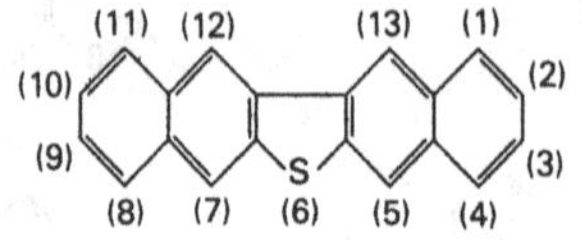

(11) (12)   (13) (1)
(10)   (2)
(9)   S   (3)
(8) (7) (6) (5) (4)

m.w.: 284 (C$_{20}$H$_{12}$S)
m.p.: 254°C

(161)

This compound was found in coal oil (Nakamura, 1983) and in commercial benzo[*a*]pyrene (Karcher *et al.*, 1979) which might have been prepared from a coal tar fraction. GC- and HPLC retention time data have been provided by Nakamura (1983) and Wise *et al.* (1983).

The compound can be obtained from the 5,7,12,13-diquinone by alkaline reduction with zinc (Wilputte and Martin, 1956):

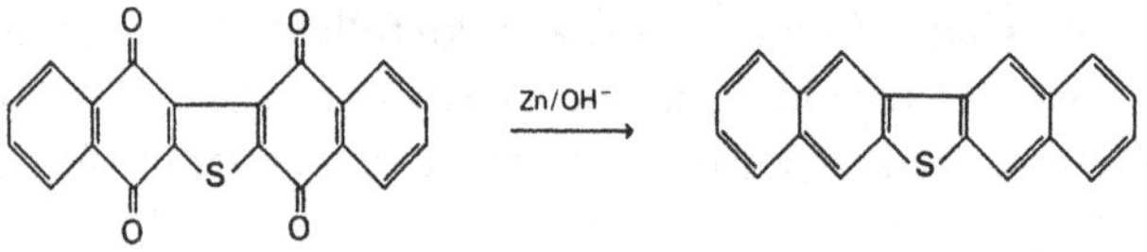

Zn/OH⁻ →

The above diquinone is obtainable from 2,3-dichloro-1,4-naphthoquinone through sulfurization with sodium sulfide giving a 1,4-dithiin product. This then can be partially desulfurized either by treatment with nitric acid (Brass and Köhler, 1922) or with hydroperoxide/acetic acid (Fickentscher *et al.*, 1969):

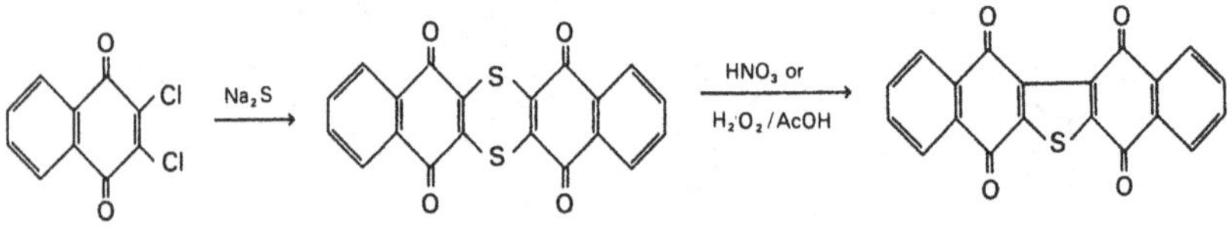

Na₂S →   HNO₃ or H₂O₂/AcOH →

Dinaphtho[2,3-*b*:2′,3′-*d*]thiophene probably is formed also by direct reaction between naphthalene and sulfur. A more specific synthesis has been described by Tedjamulia *et al.* (1983*b*) based on the reaction of naphtho[2,3-*b*]thiophene and phthalic anhydride under Friedel-Crafts condition. As in case of the [2,1-*b*:2′,3′-*d*]-isomer the resulting keto acid is reduced to the carboxylic acid which then is further reduced to the alcohol and finally oxidized to the corresponding aldehyde. The latter then is cyclized with polyphosphoric acid to the thiaarene:

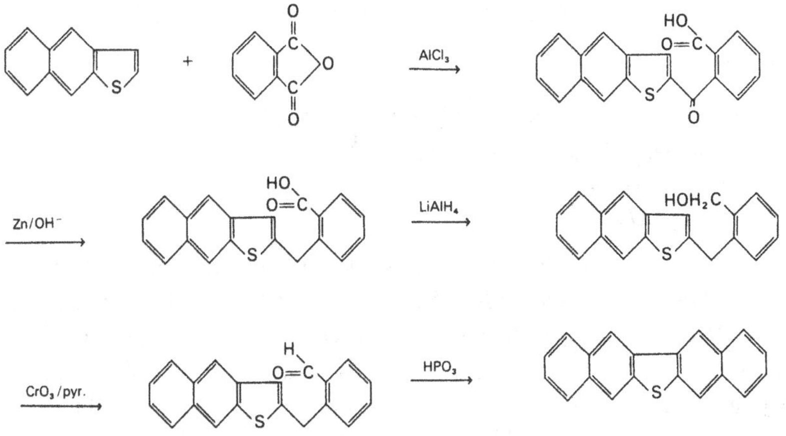

UV- (Karcher *et al.*, 1979), NMR- (Karcher *et al.*, 1979), IR- (Wilputte and Martin, 1956), and mass spectral data (Karcher *et al.*, 1979) have been presented. Molecular orbital studies on this compound have been carried out by Zahradnik and Parkanyi (1965).

Pyreno[1,2-b]thiophene (synonym: thieno[3,4-*b*]pyrene)

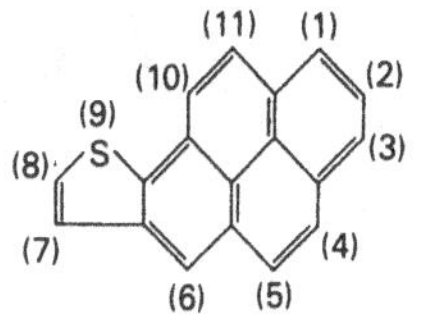

m.w.: 258 ($C_{18}H_{10}S$)
m.p.: 146°C

(*162*)

This thiaarene has been detected in coal liquids (Nakamura, 1983). GC- and HPLC retention times have been reported by Nakamura (1983), Wise *et al.* (1983) and by Wise and May (1983). Pandya and Tilak (1958, 1959*a*) have synthesized it by reaction of 2-oxoethyldisulfide dimethylacetale and 1-pyrenyllithium which can be obtained from 1-bromopyrene:

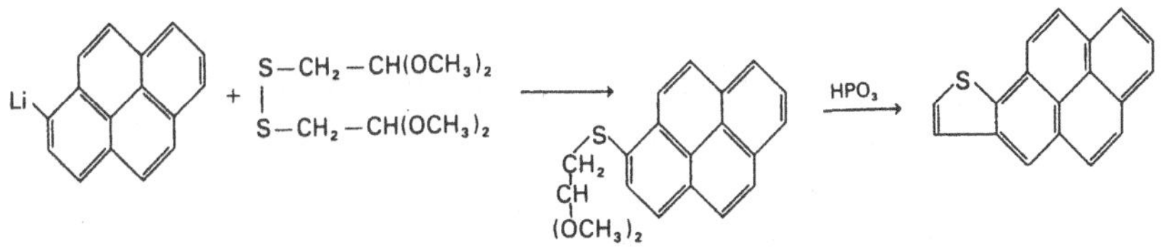

Pratap *et al.* (1981*b*) also have made use of this method. UV- (Pandya and Tilak, 1958) and fluorescence spectra (Colmsjö *et al.*, 1982) have been recorded. The compound was found to be non-carcinogenic after either subcutaneous or cutaneous application to mice (Pai and Ranadive, 1965).

Pyreno[2,1-b]thiophene (synonym:thieno[4,3-b]pyrene)

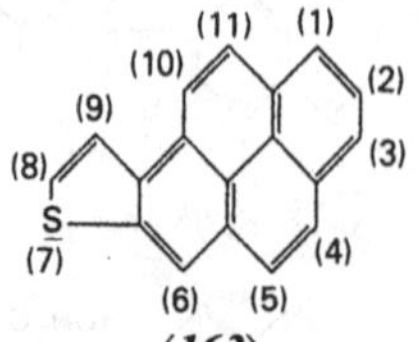

m.w.: 258 ($C_{19}H_{10}S$)
m.p.: 157°C

(*163*)

The compound was found in shale oil and coal liquids (Kong *et al.*, 1984; Nakamura, 1983). GC- (Nakamura, 1983) and HPLC- retention indices (Wise *et al.*, 1983) have been reported. It has been synthesized by Pratap *et al.* (1981*b*) in six steps with an overall yield of 1.5% from 1-acetyl-naphthalene and 2-thenylphosphonate giving 1-(2-thienyl)-2-(1-naphthyl)propene which can be photocyclized to 10-methylphenanthro[2,1-*b*]thiophene. The latter is brominated, bromine exchanged against a cyano group and the nitrile reduced with diisobutyl aluminiumhydride. The resulting aldehyde then is cyclized to pyreno[2,1-*b*]thiophene:

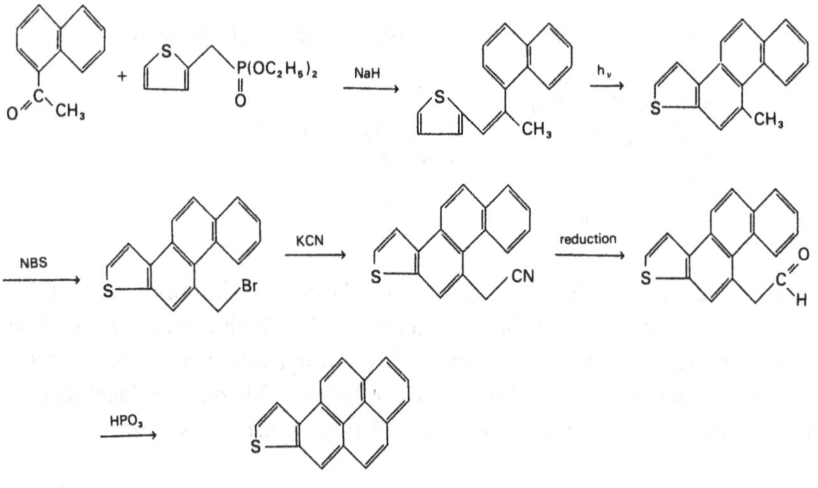

Pyreno[4,5-b]thiophene (synonym: thieno[4,5-b]pyrene)

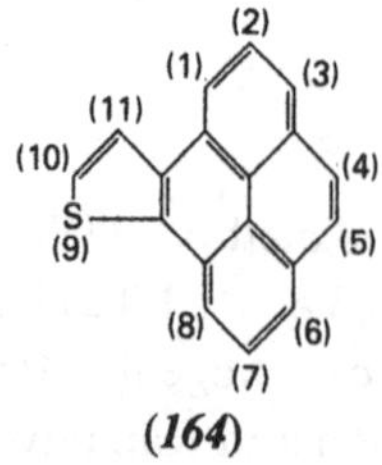

m.w.: 258 ($C_{18}H_{10}S$)
m.p.: 185°C

(*164*)

The compound occurs in coal liquids and GC- (Nakamura, 1983) as well as HPLC-retention indices (Wise *et al.*, 1983) have been recorded. This thiaarene which is isoster to benzo[*e*]pyrene has been prepared by Pratap *et al.* (1981*b*) from 1,2,3,6,7,8-hexahydropyrene which may be obtained from pyrene by reduction with sodium in pentanol. Bromination is then directed into the 4-position and the bromo-1,2,3,6,7,8-hexahydropyrene is aromatized with chloranil to 4-bromopyrene. This is lithiated with phenyllithium and reacts with 2-oxoethyldisulfide diethylacetal to 4-pyrenylthioethanal diethylacetal. Further treatment with polyphosphoric acid leads to pyreno[4,5-*b*]thiophene upon cyclization:

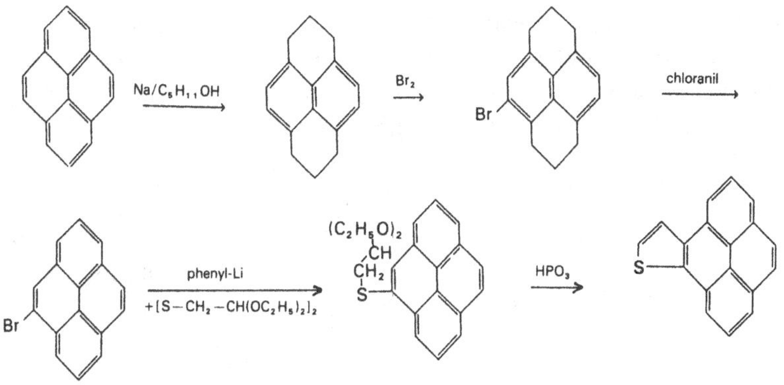

The formation of 2*H*- and 3*H*-pyreno[10,1-*bc*]thiophene from polycyclic aromatic thiones by cyclization has been reported by Lapouyade and De Mayo (1972) and by Cox *et al.* (1975).

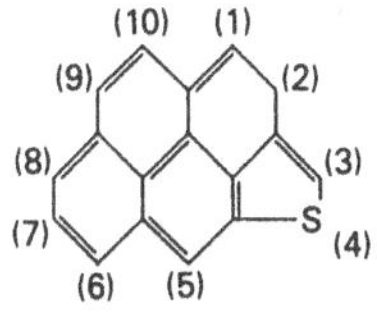

m.w.: 246 ($C_{17}H_{10}S$)

2*H*-pyreno[10,1-*bc*]thiophene
(*165*)

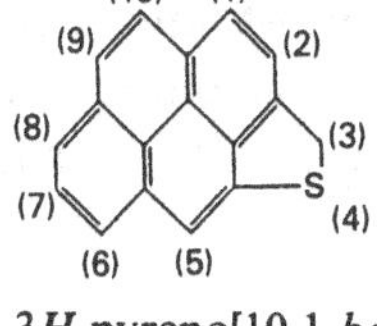

m.w.: 246 ($C_{17}H_{10}S$)

3*H*-pyreno[10,1-*bc*]thiophene
(*166*)

Triphenyleno[1,2-b]thiophene

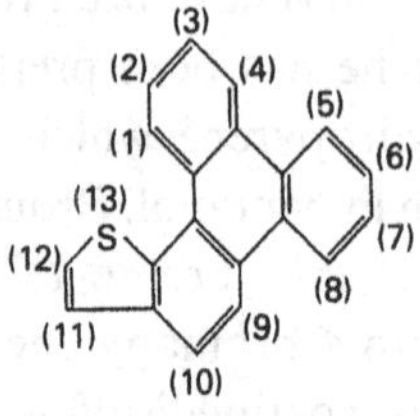

(*167*)

m.w.: 284 ($C_{20}H_{12}S$)

HPLC-retention time data of this compound have been provided by Wise *et al.* (1983) and by Wise and May (1983). It was synthesized by Pratap *et al.* (1981*a*) and Castle *et al.* (1983) in an overall yield of 14% from phenanthrene-9-aldehyde by Wadsworth-Emmons reaction with 3-thenylphosphonate giving 3-(9-phenanthrylethenyl)thiophene which can be photocyclized to triphenyleno[1,2-*b*]thiophene:

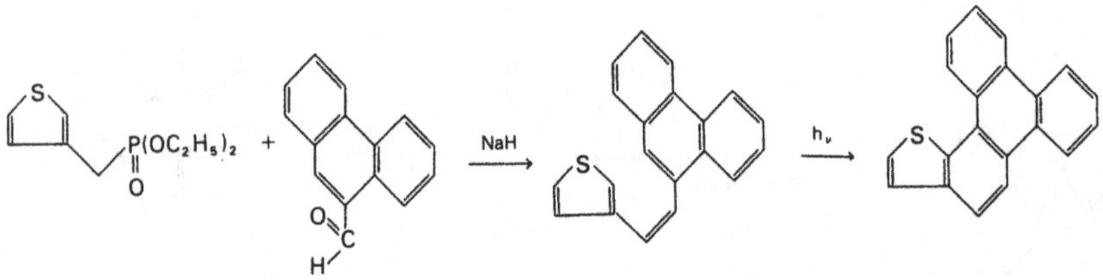

Triphenyleno[2,1-b]thiophene

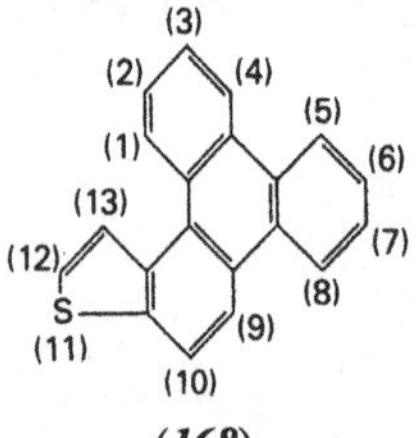

(*168*)

m.w.: 284 ($C_{20}H_{12}S$)

The compound was detected in coal liquids (Nakamura, 1983). GC- (Nakamura, 1983) and HPLC-retention indices have been published (Wise *et al.*, 1983; Wise and May, 1983). The compound was synthesized in analogy to the previous isomer by Wadsworth-Emmons reaction between phenanthrene-9-aldehyde and 2-thenylphosphonate with subsequent photocylization yielding 53% (Pratap *et al.*, 1981*a*; Castle *et al.*, 1983):

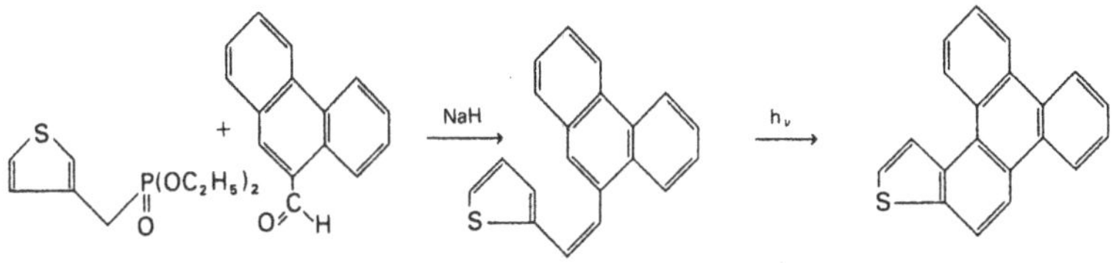

Triphenyleno[2,3-b]thiophene

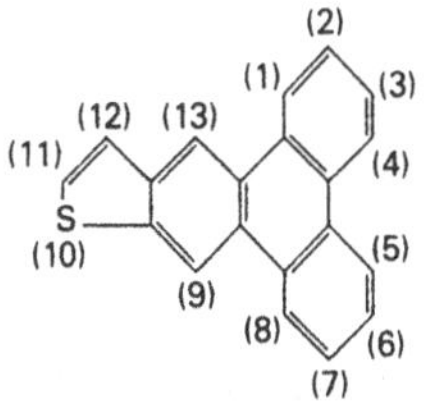

m.w.: 284 ($C_{20}H_{12}S$)
m.p.: 178°C

(*169*)

GC- (Nakamura, 1983) and HPLC-retention indices (Wise *et al.*, 1983; Wise and May, 1983) have been reported for this isomer. It was synthesized by Nicolaides (1976) by Wittig reaction starting with thiophene-2,3-dialdehyde via 9,13-dihydrotriphenyleno[2,3-*b*]thiophene which was subsequently dehydrogenated. The authors obtained also the 9,13-quinone upon oxidation with sodium bichromate in acetic acid:

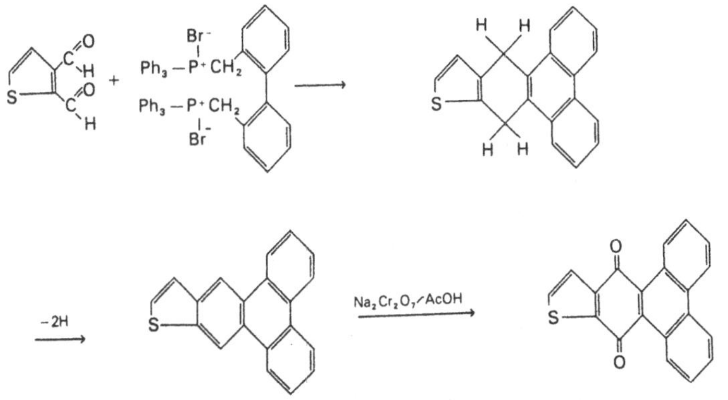

Triphenyleno(2,3-*b*)thiophene has been also synthesized by Pratap *et al.* (1981*a*) from 9-phenanthrenealdehyde and 2-(3-thienyl)-4,4-dimethyl-2-oxazoline-lithium in an overall yield of about 1%:

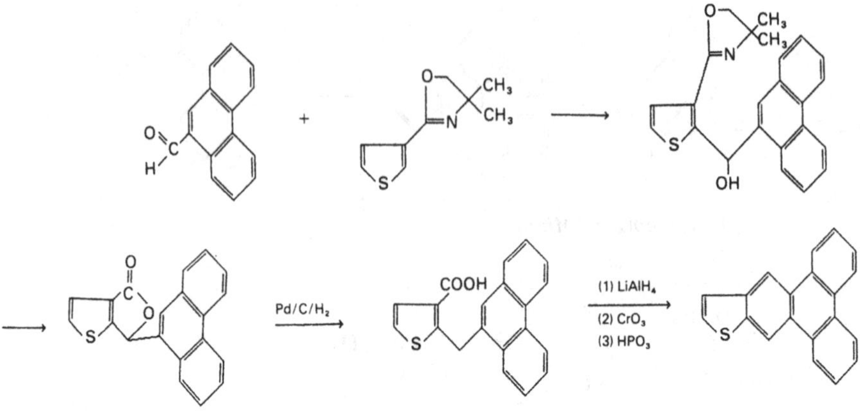

UV-, NMR-, IR- and mass spectra have been recorded (Nicolaides, 1976).

Triphenyleno[1,12-bcd]thiophene
(synonym: triphenyleno[4,5-*bcd*]thiophene)

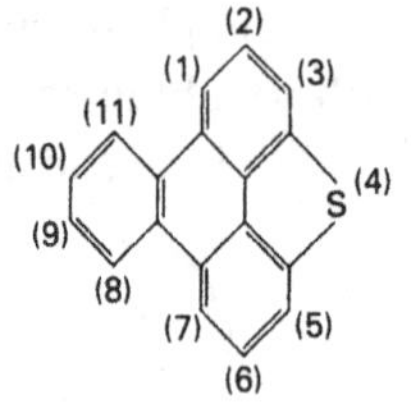

m.w.: 284 ($C_{20}H_{12}S$)
m.p.: 191°C

(170)

Triphenyleno[1,12-*bcd*]thiophene has been found in various environmental matrices such as carbon black (Fitch *et al.*, 1978; Fitch and Smith; Colmsjö and Östman, 1982), coal tar related products (Karcher *et al.*, 1981; Grimmer *et al.*, 1983a; Nishioka *et al.*, 1986b), coal liquids (Kong *et al.*, 1982; Nishioka *et al.*, 1986b), soil (Colmsjö and Östman, 1982), in crude oil (Grimmer *et al.*, 1983a), and in motor oils (Grimmer *et al.*, 1981a). Its GC- and HPLC-retention data have been indexed (Wise *et al.*, 1983; Wise and May, 1983). The compound can be obtained by sulfur insertion into triphenylene with H_2S and the catalytic action of a mixture of cobaltous, molybdic and aluminium oxide (Klemm and Lawrence, 1979):

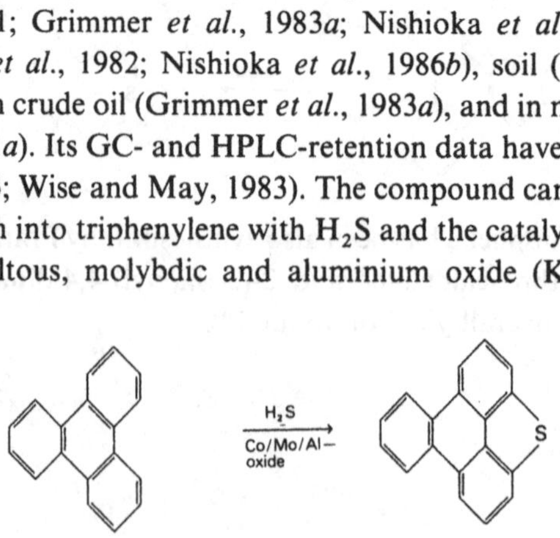

Colmsjö *et al.* (1985) obtained this thiaarene along with triphenyleno[1,12-*bcd*:4,5-*b'c'd'*]dithiophene by heating dodecahydro-triphenylene with sulfur in a sealed tube:

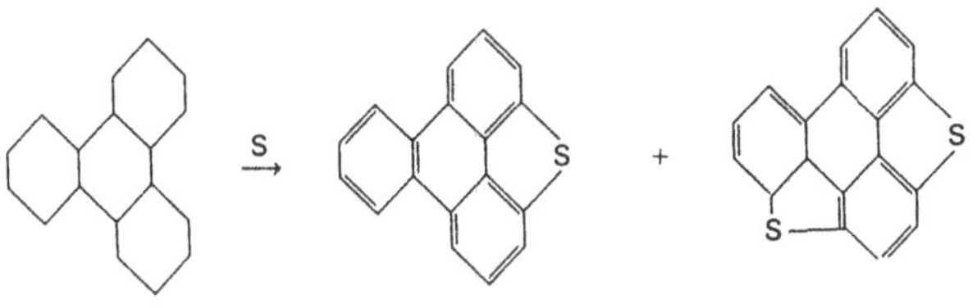

UV- (Klemm and Lawrence, 1979; Karcher *et al.*, 1981), fluorescence (Karcher *et al.*, 1981), mass (Klemm and Lawrence, 1979, Karcher *et al.*, 1981), NMR- (Klemm and Lawrence, 1979) and Shpol'skii spectra (Colmsjö and Östman, 1982; Colmsjö *et al.*, 1982) have been recorded. The adsorptivity on silica gel in comparison to PAH and other heteroatom-containing polycyclic aromatic compounds has been studied by Klemm *et al.* (1979*b*). Triphenyleno[1,12-*bcd*]thiophene has been tested for mutagenic activity in the AMES test, but was found to be negative in *S. typhimurium* TA 98 and TA 100 and in *E.coli* PKM 101 (Karcher *et al.*, 1981).

The synthesis of two further compounds belonging to this class of thiophenes, 4*H*-benzo[1,10]phenanthro[3,4-*c*]thiophene (MacDowell *et al.*, 1971) and 1*H*-chryseno[1,12-*bc*]thiophene (Cox *et al.*, 1975), has been described.

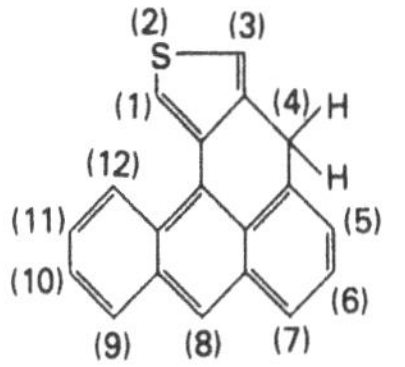

m.w.: 272 ($C_{19}H_{12}S$)

4*H*-benzo[1,10]phenanthro[3,4-*c*]thiophene
(*171*)

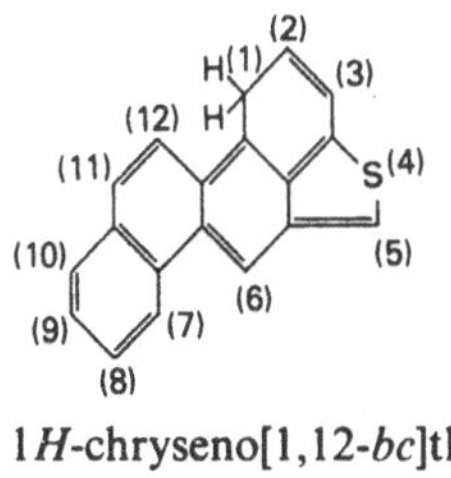

m.w.: 272 ($C_{19}H_{12}S$)

1*H*-chryseno[1,12-*bc*]thiophene
(*172*)

$C_4S–C_4S–C_6–C_6–C_6$

In this class of compounds anthradithiophenes, phenanthrodithi-ophenes, naphthobenzodithiophenes, naphthothienobenzothiophenes and benzobisbenzothiophenes are summarized.

Anthra[1,9-bc:5,10-b'c']dithiophene

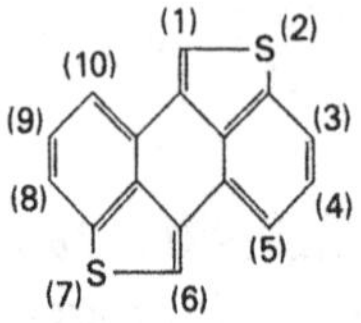

m.w.: 264 ($C_{16}H_8S_2$)
m.p.: 260°C

(*173*)

This thiaarene which is isoster to perylene has not been detected in environmental matter. It has been synthesized by Wudl *et al.* (1979) from 9,10-anthraquinone-1,5-dithiol by intramolecular thiannulation with monochloracetic acid:

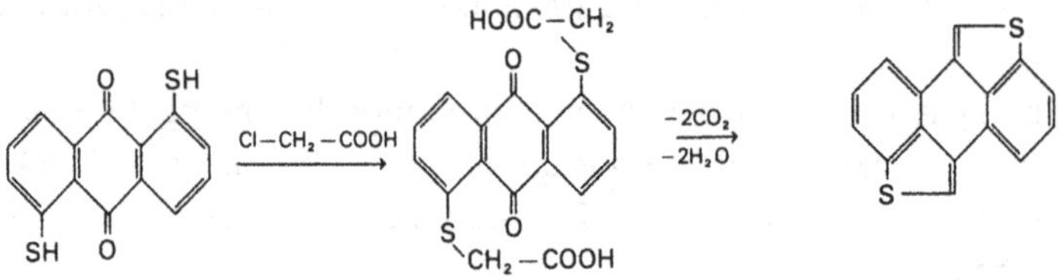

The authors recorded UV-, NMR-, fluorescence- and mass spectra; they also described that the compound readily forms an iodine complex with similar properties to the perylene-iodine solid.

Phenanthro[3,4-b:6,5-b']dithiophene

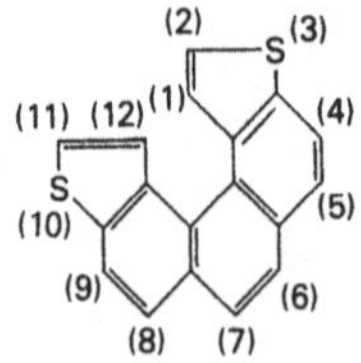

m.w.: 290 ($C_{18}H_{10}S_2$)

(*174*)

The synthesis of the thiaarene has not yet been described. However, its 6,7-dicarboxylic lactone may be obtained by the reaction of 4,4'-bis[6,7-dihydrobenzo[*b*]thiophene] with maleic anhydride:

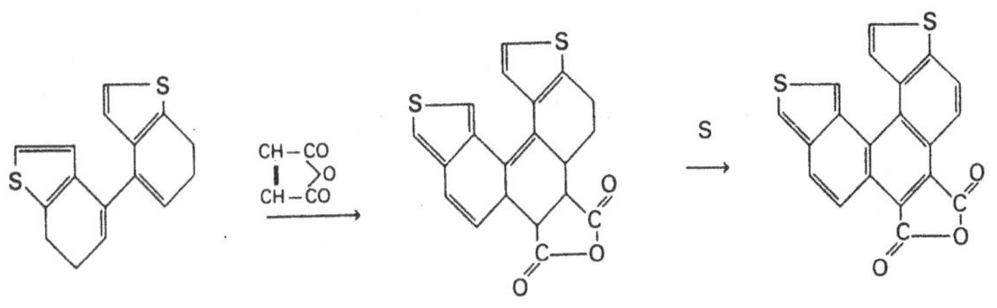

Naphtho[2,1-b]benzo[1,2-b:4,3-b']dithiophene

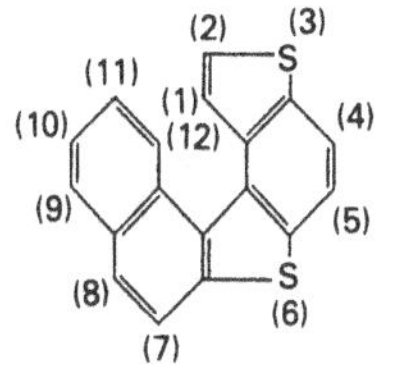

m.w.: 290 ($C_{18}H_{10}S_2$)
m.p.: 160°C

(175)

The compound has been synthesized by photocyclization of 2-(2-thienylethenyl)naphtho[2,1-*b*]thiophene by Dopper (1974) who also provided mass spectral data:

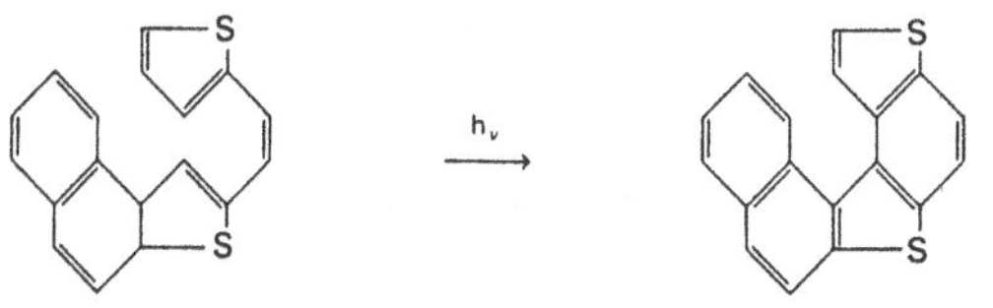

Benzo[1,2-b:3,4-b']bis[1]benzothiophene

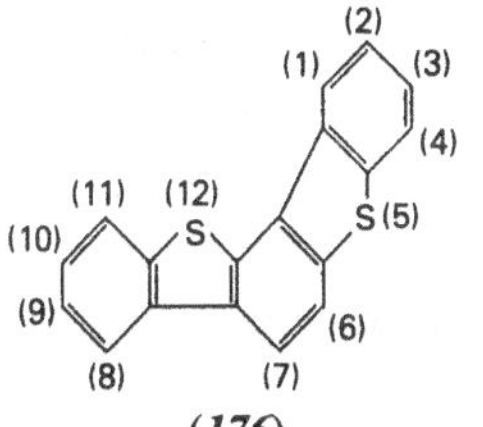

m.w.: 290 ($C_{18}H_{10}S_2$)
m.p.: 168°C

(176)

In mixture with other isomers the above system could be obtained by sulfur-bridging from *m*-terphenyl (Pandya and Tilak, 1959*b*):

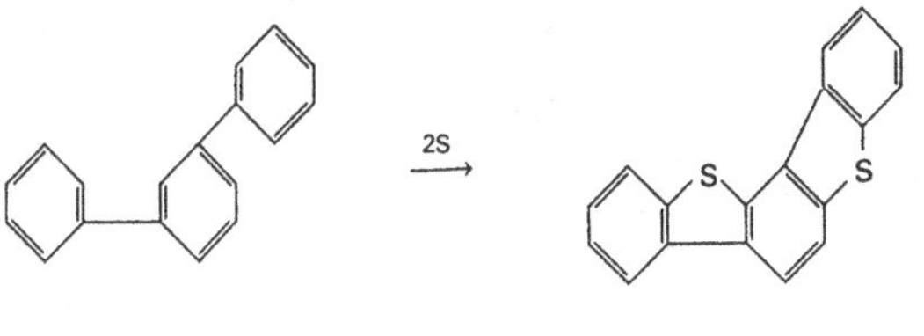

Rao and Tilak (1954) reported a synthesis starting with benzene-2,4-dithiol and 2-bromocyclohexanone. Subsequent dechlorination and dehydrogenation resulted in the above system in an overall yield of 26%:

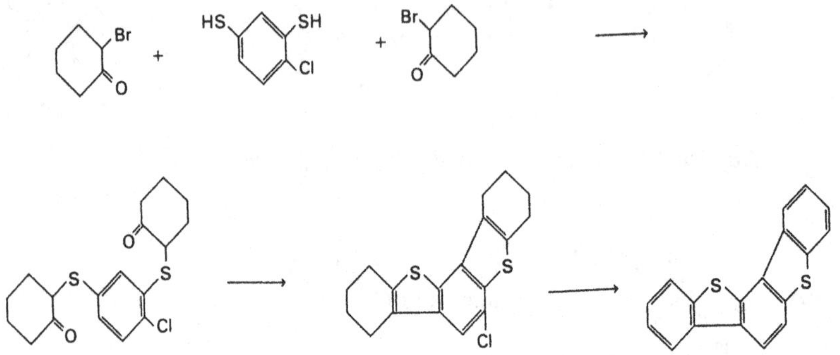

This thiaarene has also been obtained in good yield by treatment of 2,3'-bisbenzothiophene with maleic anhydride in the presence of chloranil and subsequent decarboxylation with soda lime at 400°C as described by Zander, 1977:

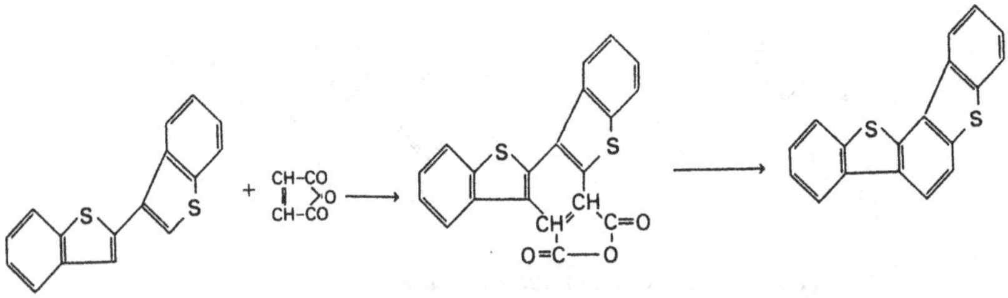

A multistep synthesis has been reported by Davies and Porter (1957c) and a more elegant synthesis has been provided by Kudo *et al.* (1984) using the Wadsworth-Emmons-reaction between 2-benzo[*b*]thiophenealdehyde and diethyl-3-benzo[*b*]thenylphosphonate giving 1-[2'-benzo[*b*]thienyl-2-(3'-benzo[*b*]thienyl)]ethene which can be photocyclized to the above thiaarene:

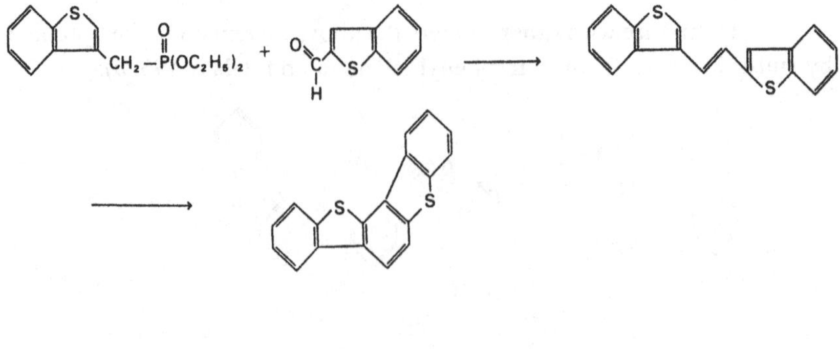

Mass spectral studies have been carried out with this compound by Collin (1963) and by Riepe and Zander (1979).

Benzo[1,2-b:3,4-e']bis[1]benzothiophene

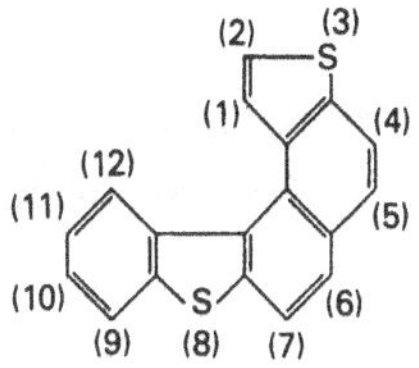

m.w.: 290 ($C_{18}H_{10}S_2$)

(*177*)

The compound was synthesized by Kudo *et al.* (1984) by Wadsworth-Emmons reaction of 2-dibenzothiophenealdehyde and diethyl 2-thenylphosphonate to give 2-(2-thienylethenyl)dibenzothiophene. The latter can be photocyclized to a mixture of the above system and benzo[1,2-*b*:5,4-*e'*]bis[1]benzothiophene which may be separated from each other by preparative HPLC (overall yield: 57%):

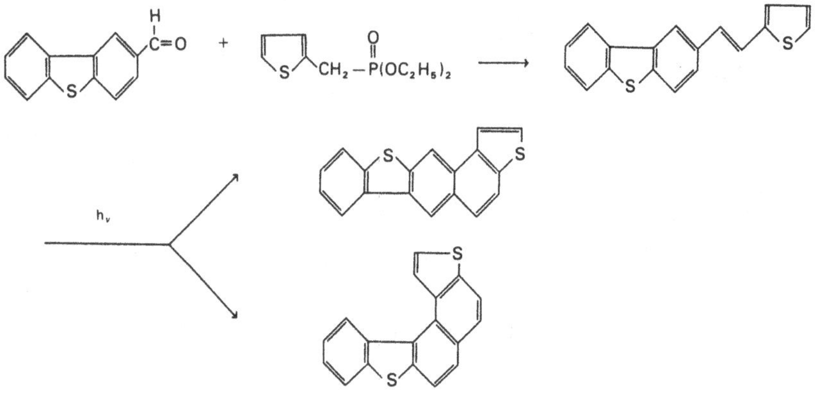

Benzo[1,2-b:4,3-b']bis[1]benzothiophene

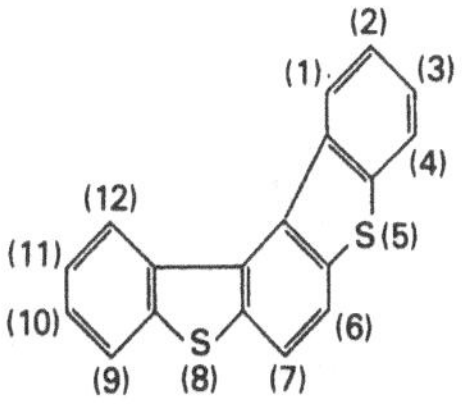

m.w.: 290 ($C_{18}H_{10}S_2$)
m.p.: 185°C

(*178*)

A first synthesis of this thiaarene was reported by Rao and Tilak (1958) who obtained it after condensation of 2-bromocyclohexanone with benzene-1,4-dithiol in aqueous NaOH. The resulting *p*-bis-[2-oxo-1-cyclohexylthio]benzene was treated with polyphosphoric acid to give a mixture of 1,2,3,4,7,8,9,10-octahydrobenzo[1,2-*b*:4,5-*b'*]bis[1]benzo-thiophene and its [1,2-*b*:4,3-*b'*]-isomer. After selenium dehydrogenation the mixture of the two isomeric thiaarenes was separated by fractional crystallization from benzene.

An isomer-free synthesis has been generated by Kudo *et al.* (1984) by Wadsworth-Emmons reaction in an overall yield of 69% according to the following scheme:

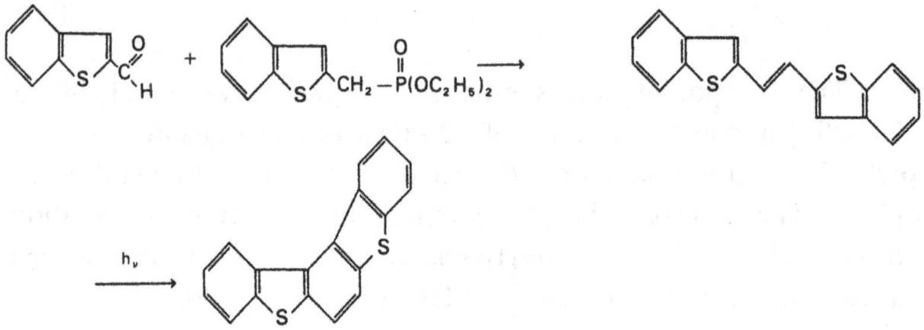

Groen *et al.* (1971) obtained this thiaarene by the following Wittig-reaction:

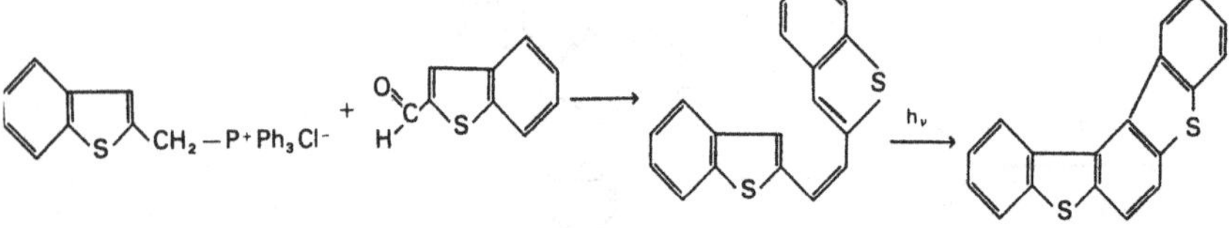

They also reported on the electron spectra of this compound (Groen and Wynberg (1971).

*Benzo[1,2-*b*:4,3-*g'*]bis[1]benzothiophene*

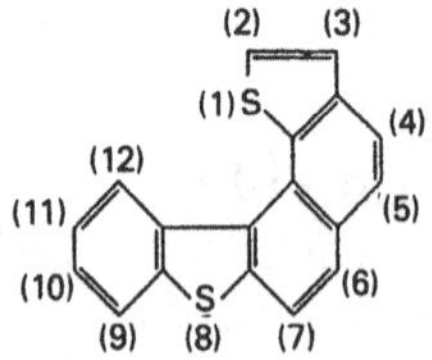

m.w.: 290 ($C_{18}H_{10}S_2$)

(*179*)

Kudo *et al.* (1984) obtained this compound in mixture with the [1,2-*b*:4,5-*g'*]-isomer by condensation of diethyl 3-thenylphosphonate with

2-dibenzothiophenealdehyde and subsequent photocyclization in overall yields of 34% and 13%, respectively:

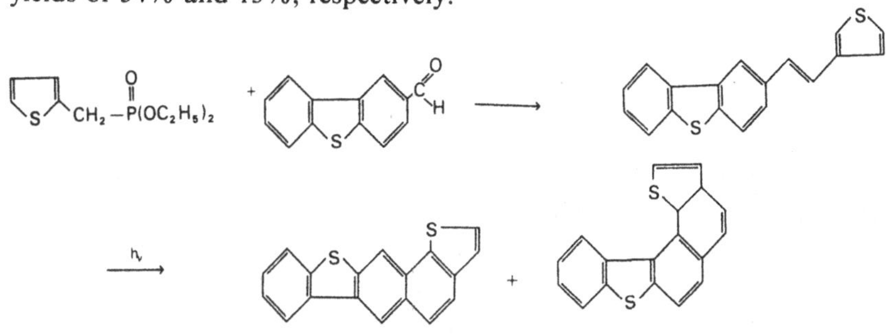

*Benzo[1,2-*b*:4,5-b']bis[1]benzothiophene*

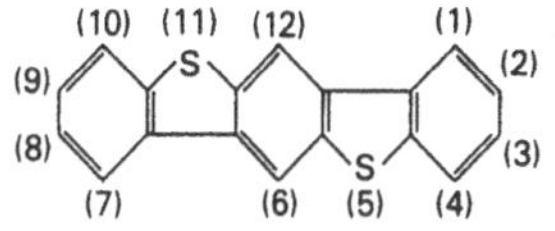

m.w.: 290°C ($C_{18}H_{10}S_2$)
m.p.: 315°C

(*180*)

This system seems to occur in petroleum. It has been synthesized by various routes and can also be obtained by sulfur insertion either into *m*-terphenyl (Pandya and Tilak, 1959*b*) forming a mixture with the [1,2-*b*:3,4-*b'*]- and the [1,2-*b*:5,4-*b'*]-isomer or into *p*-terphenyl formed in mixture with the [2,1-*b*:3,4-*b'*]-isomer (Rao and Tilak, 1958):

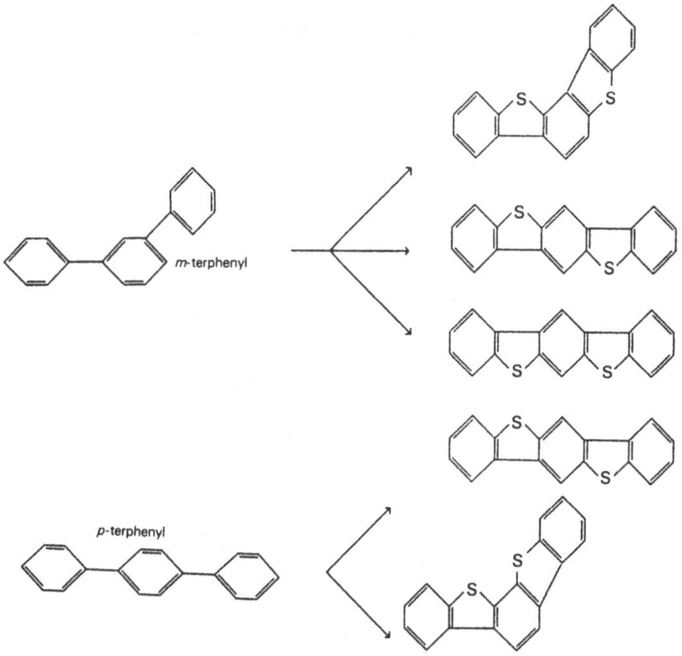

benzo[1,2-*b*:3,4-*b'*]-bis[1]-benzothiophene

benzo[1,2-*b*:4,5-*b'*]-bis[1]-benzothiophene

benzo[1,2-*b*:5,4-*b*]-bis[1]-benzothiophene

benzo[1,2-*b*:4,5-*b'*]-bis[1]-benzothiophene

benzo[2,1-*b*:3,4-*b'*]-bis[1]-benzothiophene

According to Ahmed *et al.* (1973) it can be synthesized from 2,3'-methylene-bis-(benzo[*b*]thiophene) by direct Bradsher reaction:

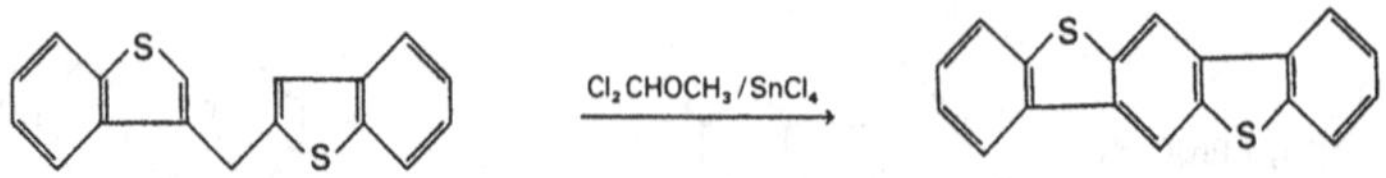

Collision-activated dissociation mass spectra have been studied by Hunt and Shabanowitz (1982).

The 6,12-dimethyl derivative being isosteric to 7,14-dimethyldibenz[*a,h*]anthracene has been studied for its carcinogenic potency in Swiss mice by skin painting and subcutaneous injection (Waravdekar and Ranadive, 1957; reviewed in Tilak, 1960). Its capacity of inducing malignant transformations in mouse, hamster and human fetal cells has been studied by Ranadive and Mashelkar (1972).

Benzo[1,2-b:5,4-b']bis[1]benzothiophene

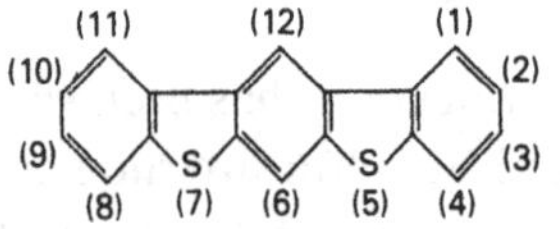

m.w.: 290 ($C_{18}H_{10}S_2$)
m.p.: 220°C

(181)

As mentioned under the preceding isomer, this thiaarene is formed by direct sulfur insertion into *m*-terphenyl (Pandya and Tilak, 1959*b*; Mayer *et al.*, 1931). The system is also formed in traces after heat polymerization of chloranil with sulfur (Rao and Tilak, 1958):

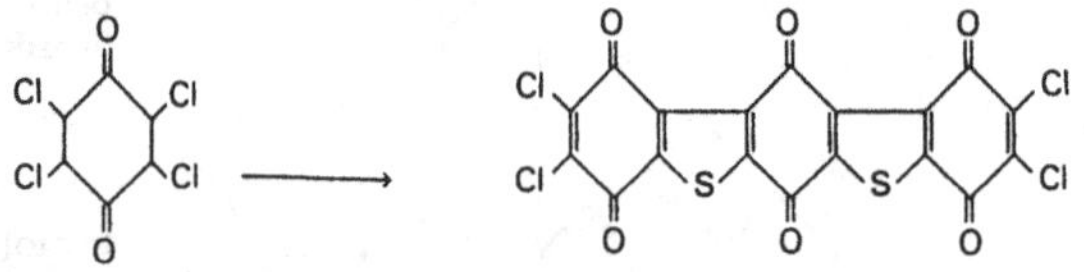

The 6,12-dimethyl derivative (m.p.: 189°C) has been prepared from *p*-xylene-1,3-dithiol and 2-bromocyclohexanone (Pillai *et al.*, 1963):

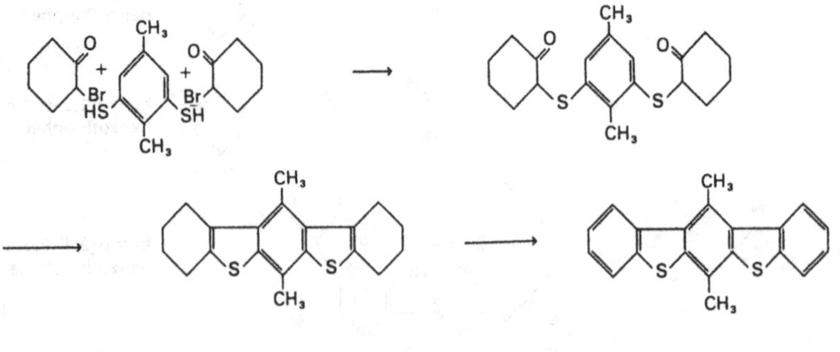

An elegant synthesis based on an intramolecular thiannulation has been described by Grandolino (1961) making use of the Pschorr cyclization of 1,5-diamino-2,4-di-(phenylsulfone) which leads to the disulfone of the above thiaarene. Further LiAlH$_4$-reduction gives the parent compound:

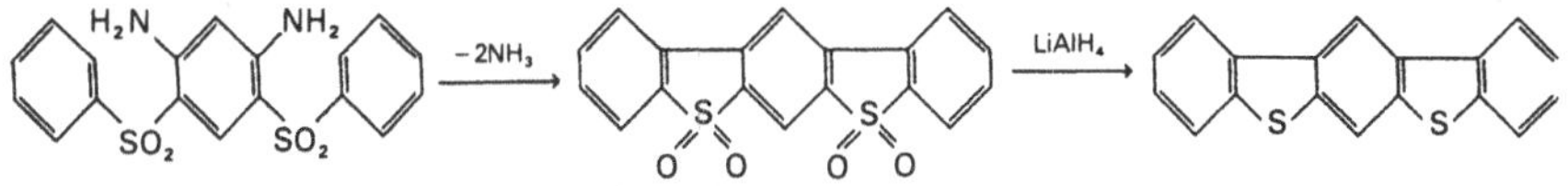

Similar to the preceding isomer benzo[1,2-*b*:5,4-*b*]bis[1]benzothiophene was obtained from 2,2'-methylene-bis(benzo[*b*]thiophene) by Bradsher reaction (Ahmed *et al.*, 1970, 1973):

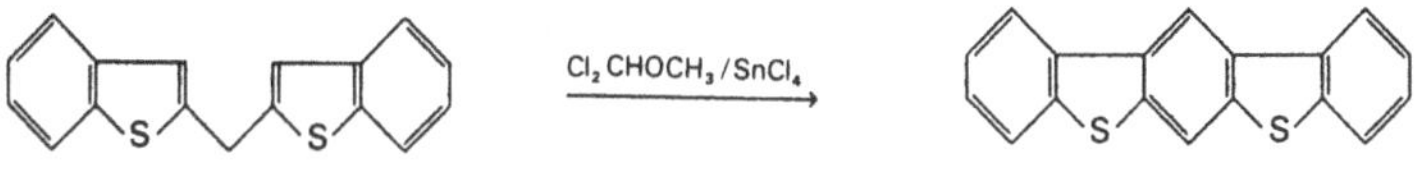

NMR- (Gogte, 1971) and mass spectra (Hunt and Shabanowitz, 1982) have been recorded.

The 6,12-dimethyl derivative being isosteric to 7,14-dimethyldibenz[*a,j*]anthracene has been tested for carcinogenicity (Waravdekar and Ranadive, 1957, reviewed in Tilak, 1960) and for micronuclei formation and lengthening of chromosomes on mouse skeletal fibroblasts cultivated *in vitro* (Ranadive *et al.*, 1963).

(182)

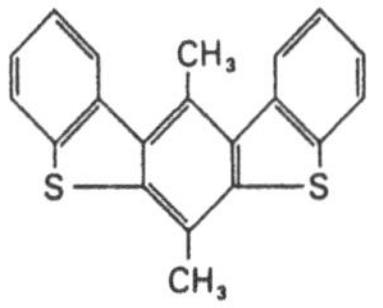

6,12-dimethylbenzo[1,2-*b*:5,4-*b*']
bis[1]benzothiophene

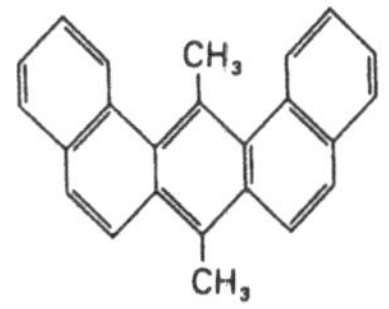

7,14-dimethyldibenz[*a,j*]anthracene

*Benzo[1,2-*b*:5,4-e']bis[1]benzothiophene*

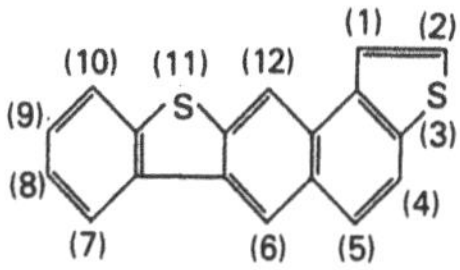

m.w.: 290 (C$_{18}$H$_{10}$S$_2$)

(183)

The compound has not been found in environmental matter. It has been synthesized in mixture with the [1,2-*b*:3,4-*e*']-isomer by reaction of 2-benzothiophenealdehyde and diethyl 2-thenylphosphonate resulting in 2-(2-thienylethenyl)dibenzothiophene which upon photocyclization gives a mixture of the above isomers which are separable by HPLC:

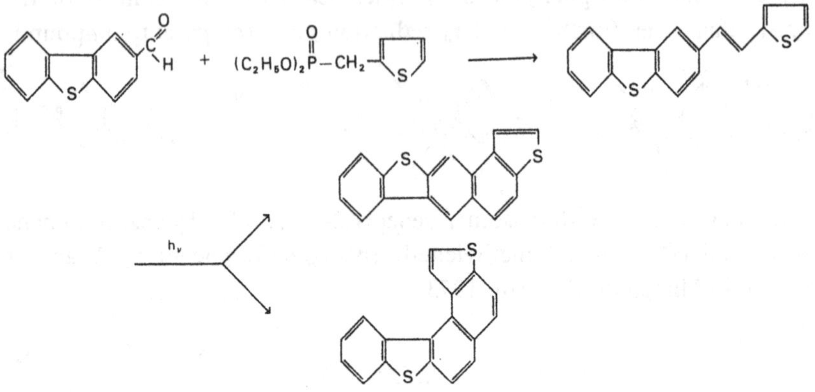

Benzo[2,1-b:3,4-b']bis[1]benzothiophene

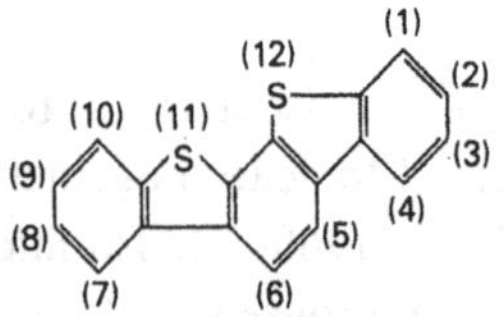

m.w.: 290 ($C_{18}H_{10}S_2$)
m.p.: 270°C

(184)

This compound is formed in low yield (3%) by direct sulfur insertion into *p*-terphenyl (Rao and Tilak, 1958):

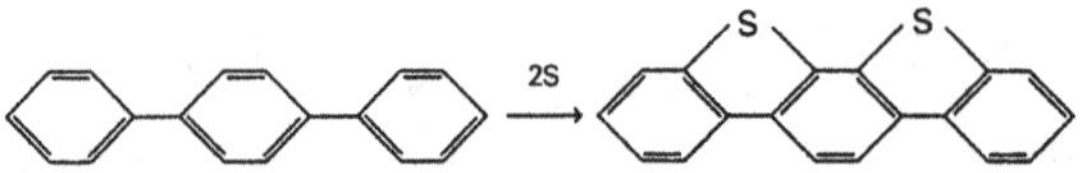

Zander (1977) obtained this thiaarene by treating 2,2'-bis-[benzothiophene] with maleic anhydride in the presence of chloranil. The resulting dicarboxylic anhydride then was hydrolyzed and decarboxylated with soda lime at 400°C:

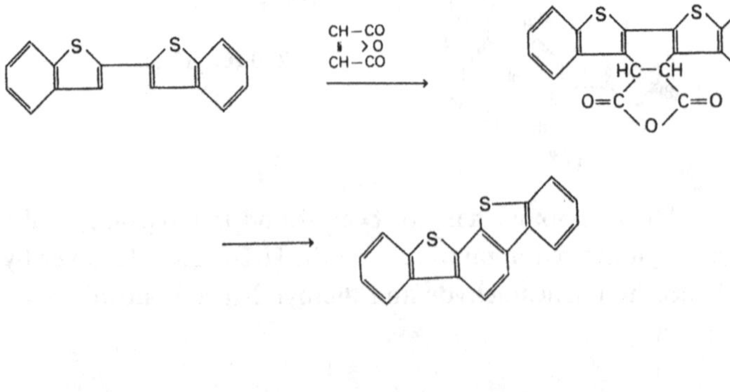

More recently Kudo *et al.* (1984) synthesized benzo[2,1-*b*:3,4-*b'*]bis[1]-benzothiophene in good yield (67%) by reaction of 2-benzo[*b*]thiophenealdehyde with 3-benzo[*b*]thenylphosphonate and subsequent photocyclization:

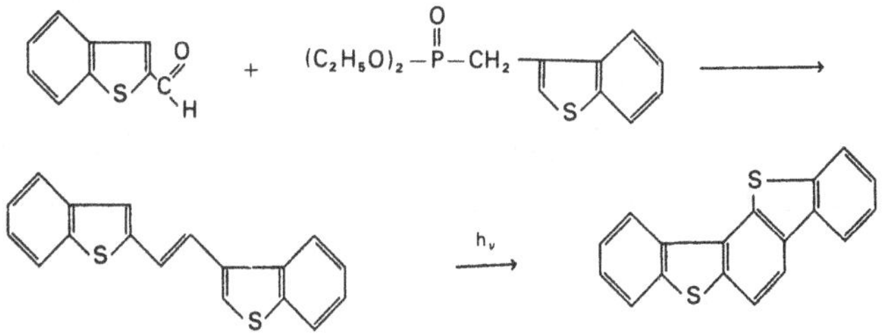

Electron impact (Riepe and Zander, 1979) and collision-activated dissociation mass spectra (Hunt and Shabanowitz, 1982) have been recorded.

Benzo[2,1-b:4,3-e']bis[1]benzothiophene

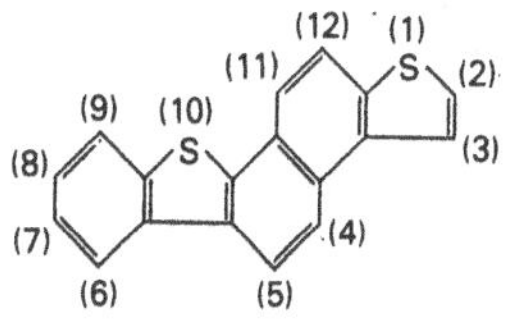

m.w.: 290 ($C_{18}H_{10}S_2$)

(185)

This compound was obtained in a 64% yield by condensation of 4-dibenzothiophenealdehyde with 2-thenylphosphonate followed by photocyclization of the intermediary 1-(4-dibenzothienyl)-2-(2-thienyl)ethene (Kudo *et al.*, 1984):

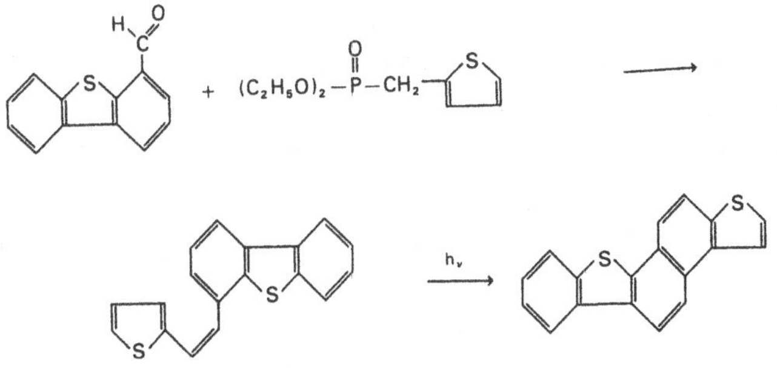

Benzo[2,1-b:3,4-g']bis[1]benzothiophene

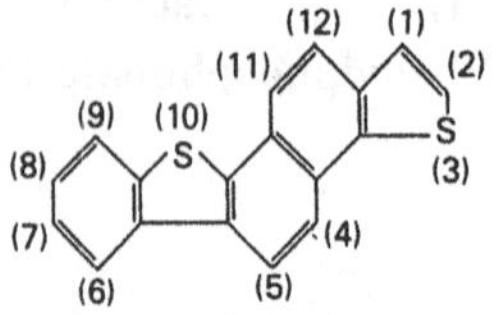

(186)

m.w.: 290 ($C_{18}H_{10}S_2$)

Similar to the preceding isomer this thiaarene has been synthesized in a 47% yield by Kudo *et al.* (1984) by condensing 4-dibenzothiophenealdehyde with 3-thenylphosphonate and subsequent photocyclization:

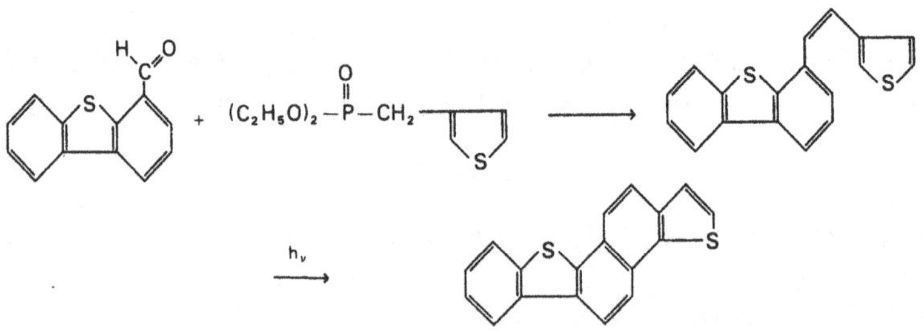

Naphtho[2',3':4,5]thieno[3,2-b][1]benzothiophene

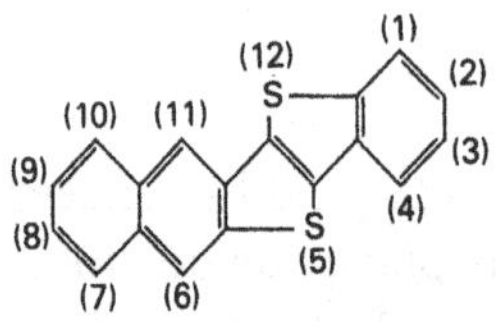

(187)

m.w.: 290 ($C_{18}H_{10}S_2$)
m.p.: 287°C

The compound was synthesized by Jacquignon *et al.* (1973) by Friedel-Crafts reaction of thieno[3,2-*b*][1]benzothiophene and 2-methylbenzoylchloride giving (methylbenzoyl)-thienobenzothiophene which cyclized upon pyrolysis. Similarly, the 8- and 10-methyl derivatives were obtained when 2,3- or 2,5-dimethylbenzoylchloride were employed (Jacquignon *et al.*, 1973):

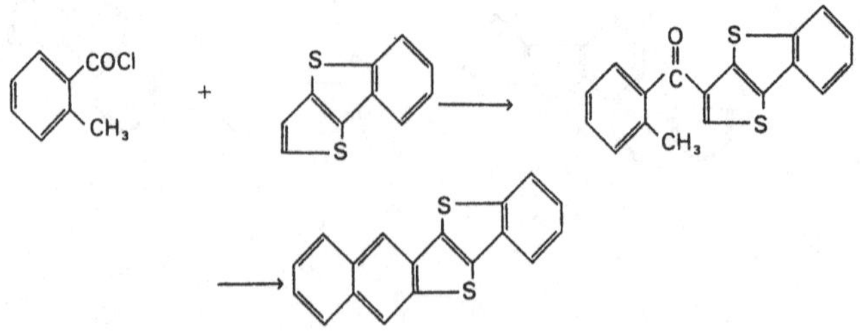

$C_5S-C_5S-C_6-C_6-C_6$ (*see under* $C_5S-C_5S-C_6-C_6$)
$C_5S-C_6-C_6-C_6-C_6$
Naphtho[1,2,3-kl]thioxanthene

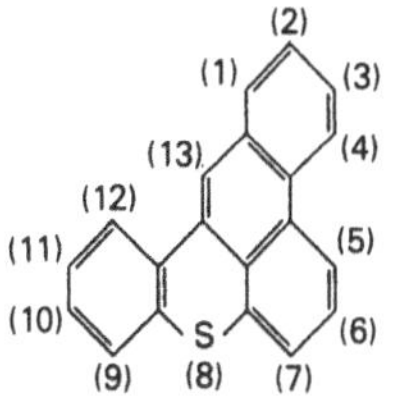

m.w.: 284 ($C_{20}H_{12}S$)

(**188**)

This system has been prepared by dehydrocyclization of benzyl-idenethioxanthene with UV-light in acetone or benzene under nitrogen (Schoenberg and Sidky, 1974):

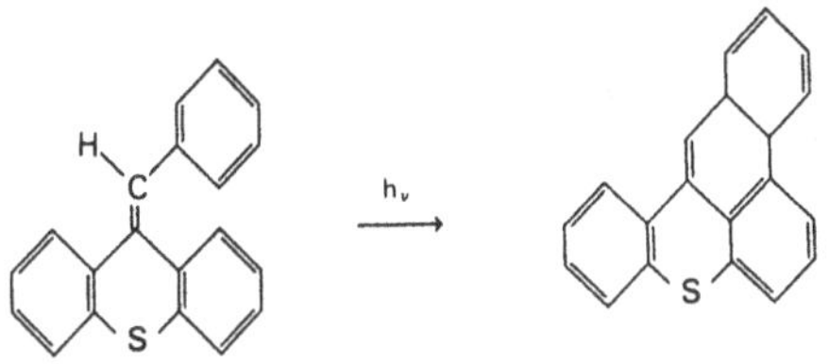

Pyreno[3,4-bc]thiopyran

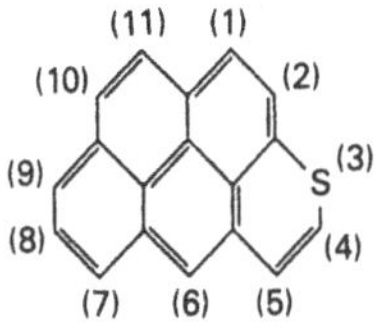

m.w.: 258 ($C_{18}H_{10}S$)

(**189**)

The 5-keto-4,5-dihydropyreno[3,4-*bc*]thiopyran was synthesized from pyrene by Shevchuk and Paramonov (1976):

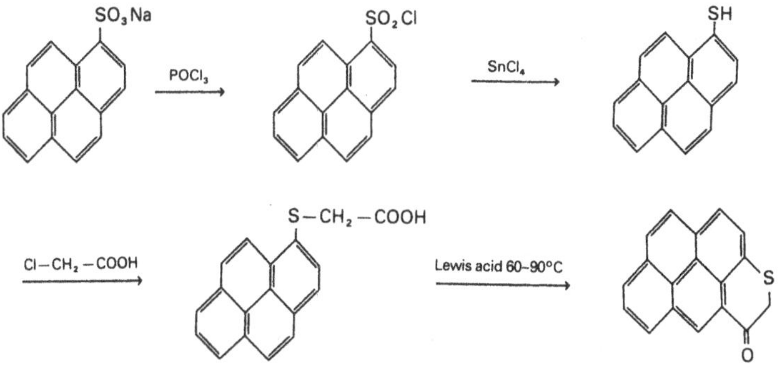

The same authors (Paramonov *et al.*, 1978) observed the formation of the following dimer after air oxidation of the above keto compound (46% yield):

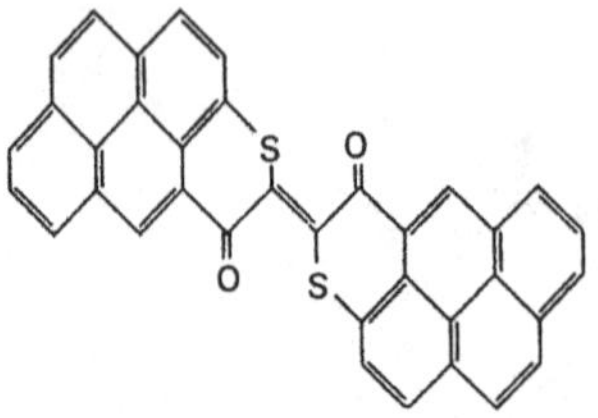

Derivatives of 1*H*-dibenzo[*c,h*]thioxanthene and 14*H*-dibenzo[*a,j*]-thioxanthene have been prepared (Lawrence, 1971; Fedotova *et al.*, 1977).

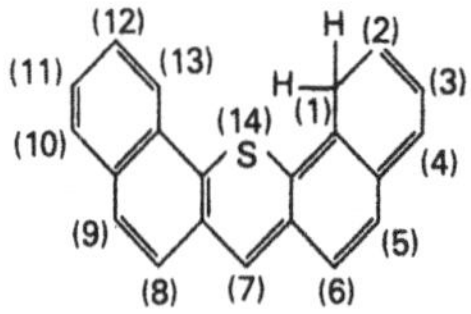

m.w.: 298 (C$_{21}$H$_{14}$S)

1*H*-dibenzo[*c,h*]thioxanthene
(**190**)

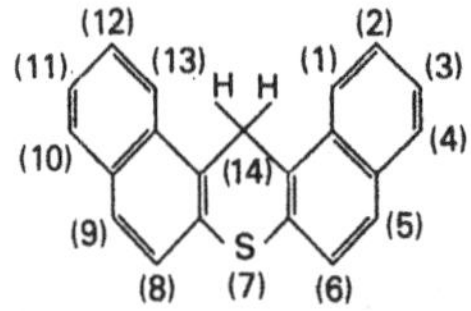

m.w.: 298 (C$_{21}$H$_{14}$S)

14*H*-dibenzo[*a,j*]thioxanthene
(**191**)

2.5   Hexacyclic compounds
$C_4S-C_5-C_6-C_6-C_6-C_6$

The following systems from this class of compounds have been described and synthesized; they are, however, of no environmental relevance, as far as known today.

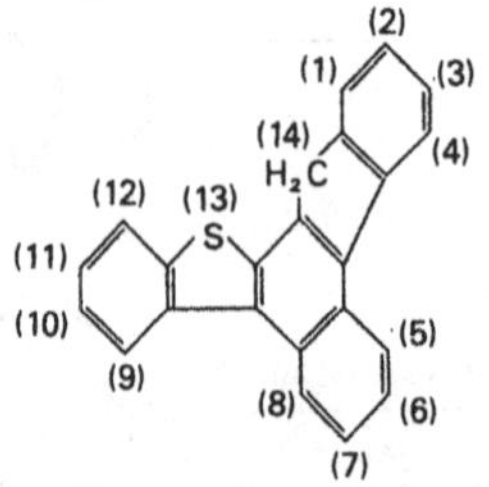

m.w.: 322 (C$_{23}$H$_{14}$S)

14*H*-benzo[*b*]benzo[3,4]fluoreno[2,1-*d*]thiophene
(**192**)

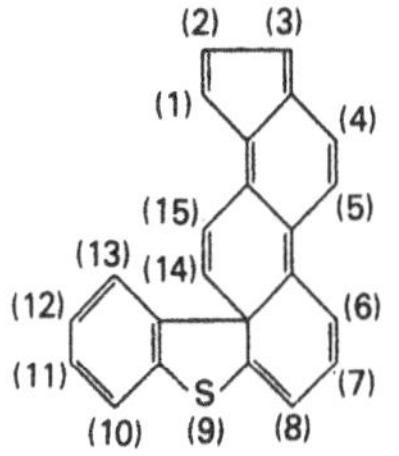

benzo[*b*]cyclopenta[7,8]phenanthro[10a,1-*d*]thiophene
(193)

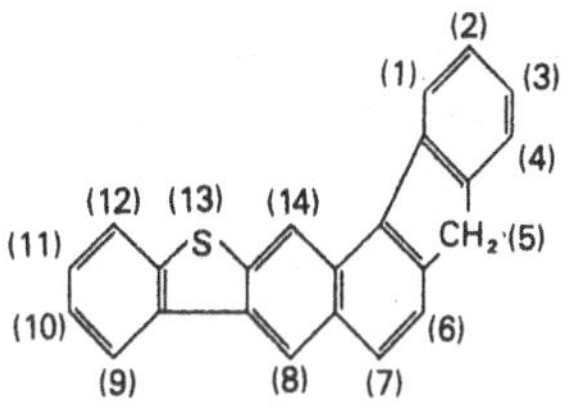

m.w.: 322 ($C_{23}H_{14}S$)

5*H*-fluoreno[3,4-*b*]dibenzothiophene
(194)

m.w.: 322 ($C_{23}H_{14}S$)

C_4S–C_6–C_6–C_6–C_6–C_6

The main structures found in this class are benzopyrenothiophenes, benzochrysenothiophenes, benzotriphenylenothiophenes, perylothiophenes, and naphthophenanthrothiophenes. Several of these systems have been detected in environmental matter as a result of their occurrence in coal tar.

Benzo[8,9]pyreno[1,10-bc]thiophene

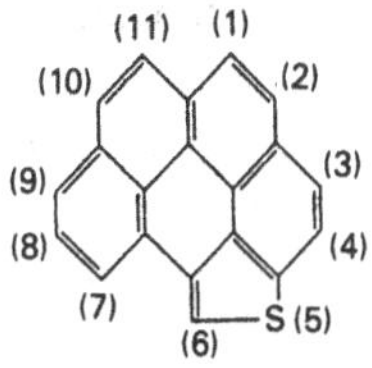

m.w.: 282 ($C_{20}H_{10}S$)

(195)

Dopper *et al.* (1975) obtained this system by AlCl$_3$-catalyzed dehydrogenation from the hetero[5]helicene benzo[5,6]phenanthro[3,4-*b*]thiophene:

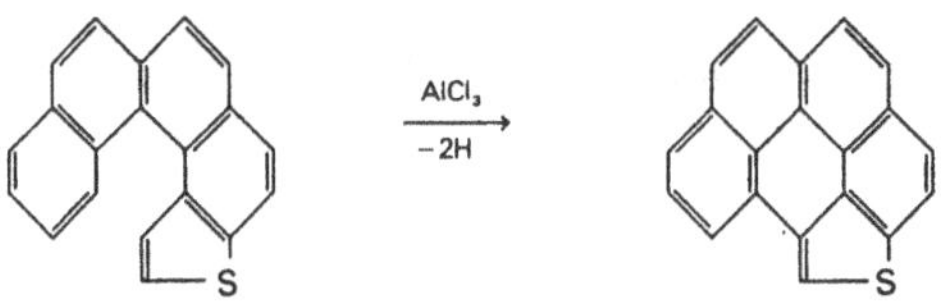

Mass- and UV-data have been presented also by Dopper *et al.* (1975).

Benzo[10,11]chryseno[4,5-bcd]thiophene (synonym:
10,11-epithiobenzo[a]pyrene)

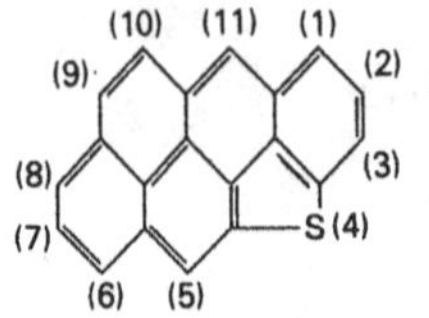

(10) (11) (1)
(9)
(8)
(7)
(6) (5)
(2)
(3)
S (4)

m.w.: 282 ($C_{20}H_{10}S$)

(196)

This thiaarene being isosteric to the carcinogen anthanthrene has
been found in carbon black and soil (Colmsjö and Östman, 1982; Colmsjö
et al., 1982). It is possibly formed from benzo[a]pyrene by sulfur insertion
during the coalification process. Low temperature fluorescence and
phosphorescence spectra have been recorded by Colmsjö and Östman
(1982) and by Colmsjö *et al.* (1982).

Benzo[4,5]triphenyleno[1,12-bcd]thiophene
(synonym: 1,12-epithiobenzo[e]pyrene)

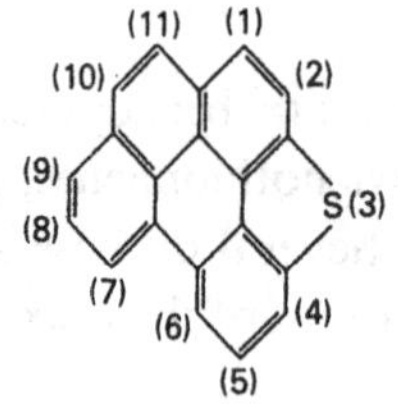

(11) (1)
(10)
(9)
(8)
(7)
(6)
(5)
(4)
(2)
S (3)

m.w.: 282 ($C_{20}H_{10}S$)

(197)

This compound which is isosteric to benzo[*ghi*]perylene has also
been found in carbon black and in soil (Colmsjö and Östman, 1982;
Colmsjö *et al.*, 1982) and benzo[e]pyrene might be its geochemical
precusor. Colmsjö *et al.* (1982) have recorded its Shpol'skii spectra. They
obtained   the   compound   by   heating   1,2,3,6,7,8,9,10,11,12-
decahydrobenzo[e]pyrene with sulfur in a sealed tube (Colmsjö *et al.*,
1985).

Perylo[1,12-bcd]thiophene (synonym: 1,12-epithioperylene)

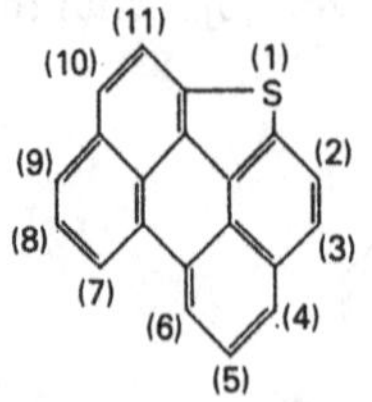

(11)
(10)
(9)
(8)
(7)
(6)
(5)
(1)
S
(2)
(3)
(4)

m.w.: 282 ($C_{20}H_{10}S$)

(198)

Perylo[1,12-*bcd*]thiophene, another benzo[*ghi*]perylene isoster, has been detected in coal products (Nishioka *et al.*, 1986*b*) and in a vacuum distillate fraction from coal tar (200–600°C) by Borwitzky *et al.* (1977) and by other investigators (Burchill *et al.*, 1982*a*). It has also been detected as an impurity of commercial benzo[*ghi*]perylene (Karcher *et al.*, 1979) and in carbon black (Colmsjö *et al.*, 1982; Lee and Hites, 1976; Colmsjö and Östman, 1982). Colmsjö *et al.* (1985) prepared perylo[1,12-*bcd*]thiophene by heating 1,2,3,10,11,12-hexahydroperylene with sulfur in a sealed tube. It has also been obtained by Rogovik and coworkers (Rogovik, 1970, 1974; El'tsov *et al.*, 1982) from the sulfone of perylene-3,4,9,10-tetracarboxylic acid by boiling with sulfur in KOH and subsequent heating of the thiaarene acid with copper in quinoline. The latter is readily converted into its sulfone by H_2O_2-treatment:

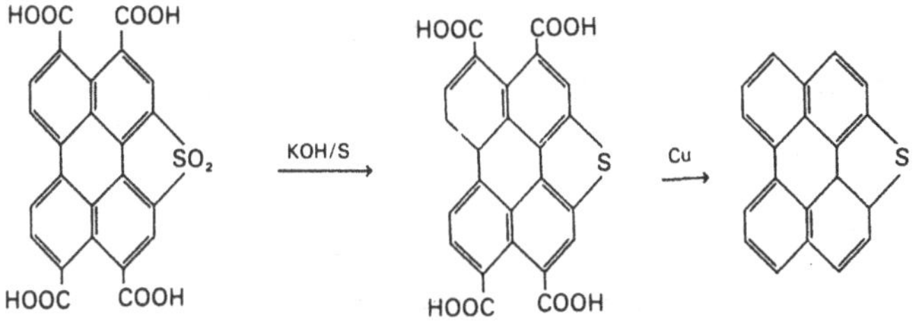

HOOC   COOH SO_2 $\xrightarrow{\text{KOH/S}}$ HOOC   COOH S HOOC   COOH $\xrightarrow{\text{Cu}}$ S

HOOC   COOH   HOOC   COOH

Mass- (Karcher *et al.*, 1979) and Shpol'skii fluorescence spectra (Colmsjö *et al.*, 1982) have been recorded.

Naphtho[2,1-b]phenanthro[1,2-d]thiophene (synonyms: 5,6-benzonaphtho[1′,2′,3,4]-9-thiafluorene; 9-thia-5,6-benzonaphtho[1′,2′,3,4]fluorene)

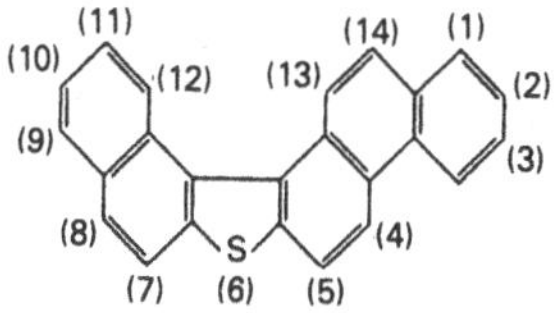

(11) (10) (12) (14) (13) (1) (2) (9) (3) (8) S (4) (7) (6) (5)

m.w.: 334 ($C_{24}H_{14}S$)

(*199*)

The compound has been synthesized by Davies and Porter (1956) by heating naphtho[2,1-*b*]thiophene-sulfone in xylene. The resulting 6a,13c-dihydronaphtho[2,1-*b*]phenanthro[1,2-*d*]thiophene-7,7-dioxide can be converted into the parent thiaarene by dehydrogenation and subsequent reduction of the sulfone formed:

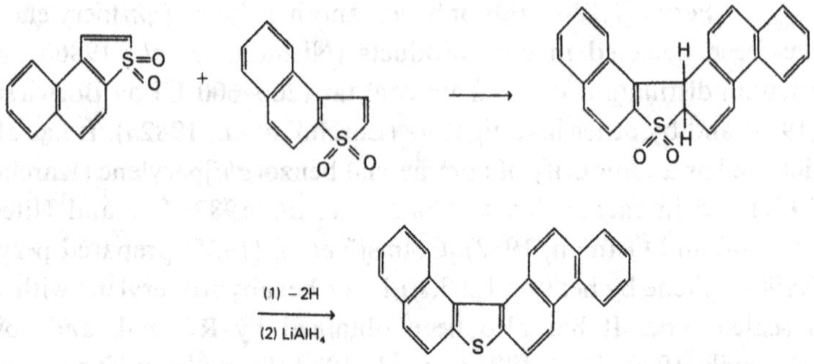

It was also obtained by the above authors from 1-vinylnaphthalene and naphtho[2,1-*b*]thiophene-sulfone in a similar way (Davies and Porter, 1957*a*).

*Naphtho[2,1-*b*]phenanthro[9,10-*d*]thiophene*
(synonym: 1,2,3,4,5,6-tribenzo-9-thiafluorene)

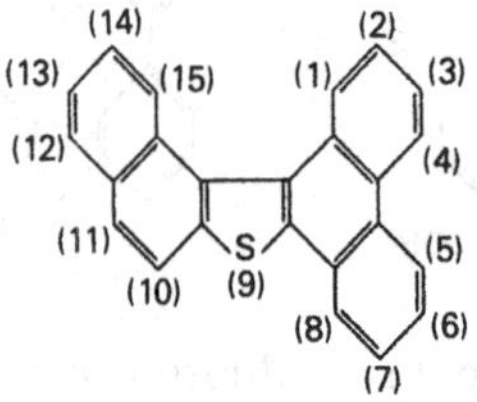

m.w.: 334 ($C_{24}H_{14}S$)
m.p.: 196°C

(*200*)

The above system was obtained by Wilputte and Martin (1956) by condensation of phenanthrene-9-thiol and 2-chlorotetralone which upon loss of water gives the 9-10-dihydro derivative. After dehydrogenation the latter yields naphtho[2,1-*b*]phenanthro[9,10-*d*]thiophene:

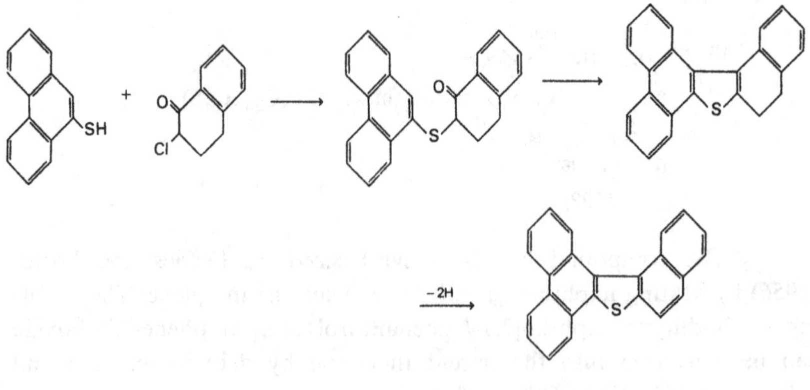

Naphtho[2,3-b]phenanthro[9,10-d]thiophene
(synonym: 1,2,3,4,6,7-tribenzo-9-thiafluorene)

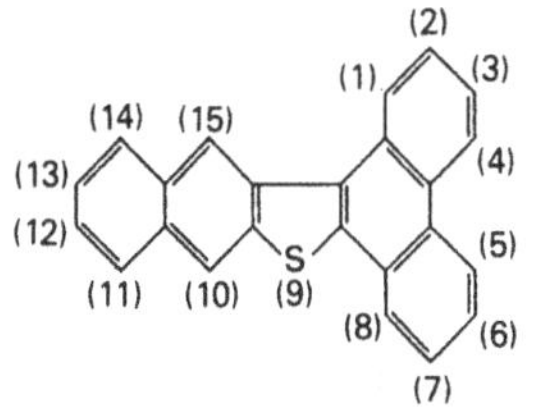

m.w.: 334 ($C_{24}H_{14}S$)
m.p.: 243°C

(201)

Wilputte and Martin (1956) have synthesized this system by condensation of phenanthrene-9-thiol and 3-chloro-2-decalone via 10,11,12-13,14,15-hexahydro-naphtho[2,3-*b*]phenanthro[9,10-*d*]thiophene, which upon dehydrogenation gives the parent thiaarene:

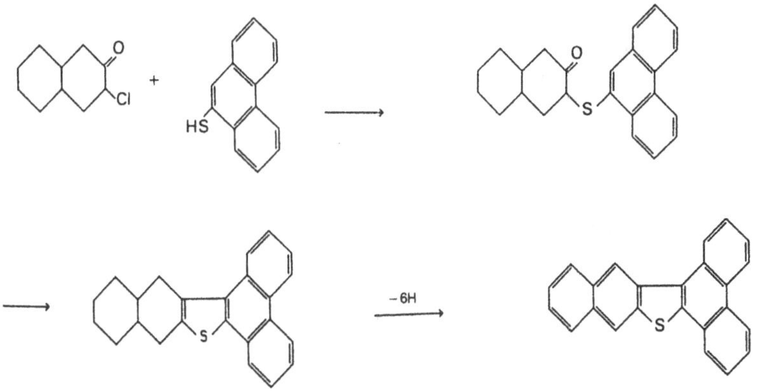

Naphtho[2',3':9,10]phenanthro[4,5-bcd]thiophene

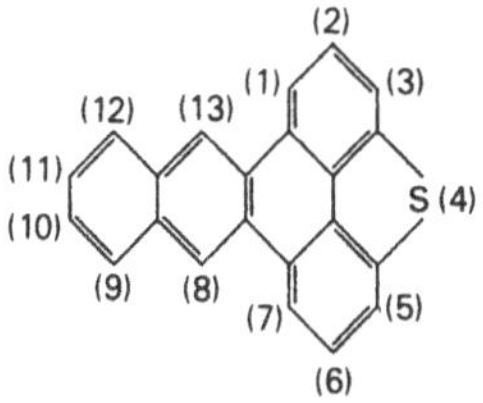

m.w.: 334 ($C_{24}H_{14}S$)

(202)

This compound has been tentatively identified in synfuel (Kong *et al.*, 1984).

The syntheses of some heterotriptycenes such as 6,11(1',2')-benzenobenzo[*b*]naphtho[2,3-*d*]thiophene (Reinecke and Ballard, 1979),

4,11(1′,2′)-benzenoanthra[2,3-*b*]- and -[2,3-*c*]thiophene (Wynberg *et al.*, 1970; DeWit and Wynberg, 1973; McKinnon and Wong, 1971) and 7,11(1′,2′)benzenophenanthro[2,3-*c*]thiophene (McKinnon and Wong, 1971) have been described.

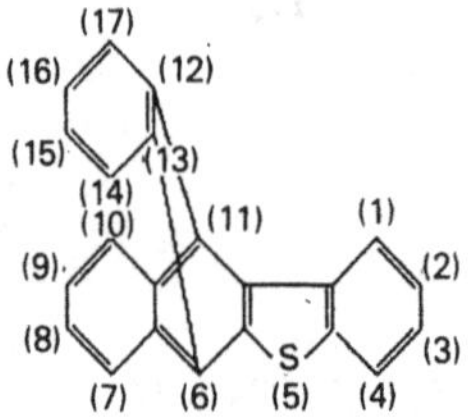

m.w.: 308 ($C_{22}H_{12}S$)

6,11(1′,2′)benzenobenzo[*b*]naphtho[2,3-*d*]thiophene
(**203**)

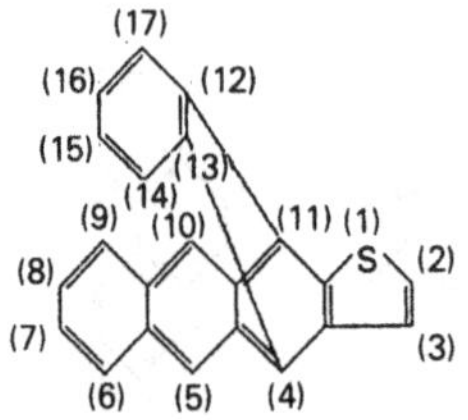

m.w.: 308 ($C_{22}H_{12}S$)

4,11(1′,2′)benzenoanthra[2,3-*b*]thiophene
(**204**)

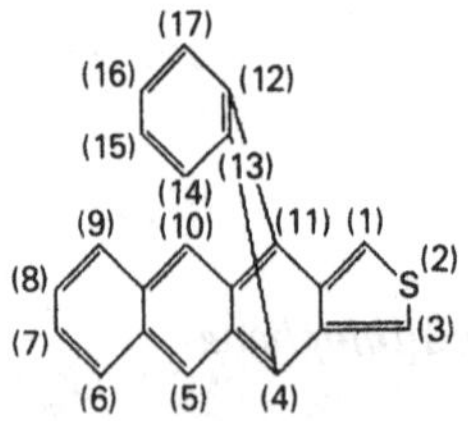

m.w.: 308 ($C_{22}H_{12}S$)

4,11(1′,2′)benzenoanthra[2,3-*c*]thiophene
(**205**)

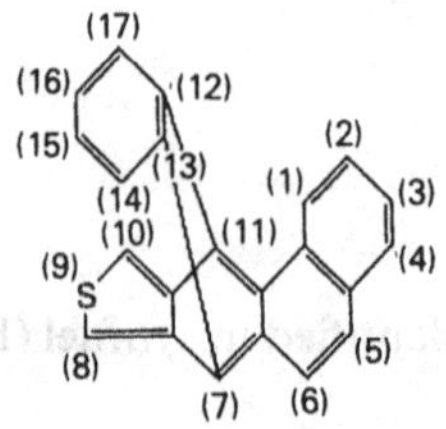

m.w.: 308 ($C_{22}H_{12}S$)

7,11(1′,2′)benzenophenanthro[2,3-*c*]thiophene
(**206**)

$C_5S-C_6-C_6-C_6-C_6-C_6$

14H-Anthra[2,1,9-mna]thioxanthene

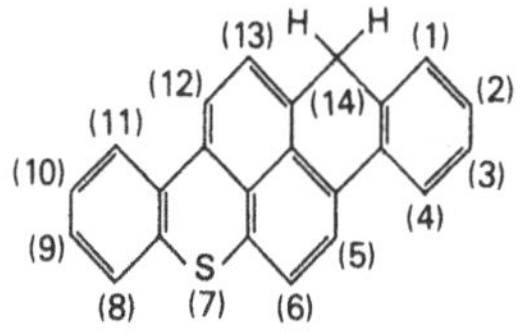

(207)

m.w.: 322 ($C_{23}H_{14}S$)

The 14-oxo-compound and derivatives of it are used as dye materials and have been prepared in a one-step reaction by diazotization of 3-(2-aminophenylthio)-benzanthrone and subsequent cyclization by heating in the presence of copper sulfate at 110–115°C for 3 h (Farbwerke Hoechst AG, 1967; Spietschka and Landler, 1971, 1972).

$C_4S-C_4S-C_6-C_6-C_6-C_6$

Benzonaphthobenzodithiophenes and naphtho-bis-benzo-thiophenes belong to these six-rings containing thiaarene systems.

Benzo[d]naphtho[1,2-d']benzo[1,2-b:4,3-b']dithiophene

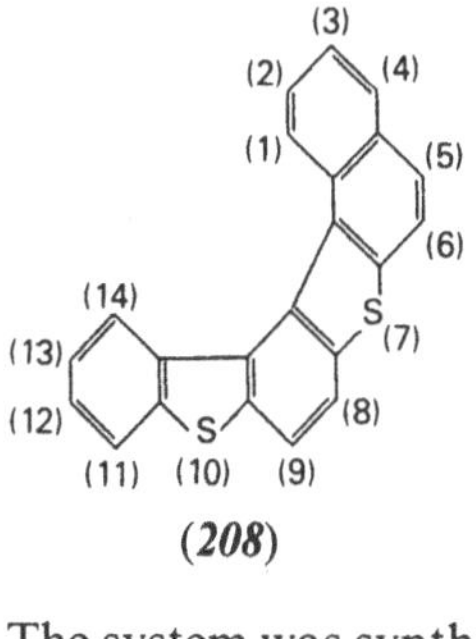

(208)

m.w.: 308 ($C_{22}H_{12}S_2$)

The system was synthesized by photolysis of 1-benzo[*b*]thien-2-yl-2-naphtho[2,1-*b*]thien-2-yl-ethene (Wynberg and Groen, 1968; Wynberg *et al.*, 1970). The same authors obtained optically active crystals of this compound by slow crystallization from benzene. The optically pure forms racemize in chloroform solution (Wynberg and Groen, 1969). The molecular structure of this system and of its 1-tert-butyl derivative have been studied by Groen and Wynberg (1971), Stulen and Visser (1969) and by Wijmenga *et al.* (1978).

Numan and Wynberg (1975) synthesized methano-bridged hetero-helicenes from the 14-methyl- or 14-ethyl derivative of the above system by treatment with N-bromosuccinimide in tetrachloromethane containing traces of azoisobutyronitrile at 160°C.

UV-, NMR- and mass spectra as well as ORD- and CD-spectra have been recorded (Wynberg *et al.*, 1970; Groen and Wynberg, 1971).

Naphtho[1,2-b:4,3-b']bis[1]benzothiophene
(synonyms: naphtho[1,2-*b*:4,3-*b'*]dibenzothiophene;
naphtho[1,2-*b*:4,3-*b'*]dithionaphthene

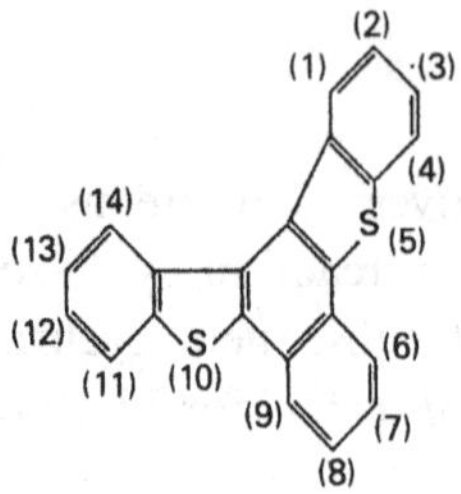

m.w.: 308 (C$_{22}$H$_{12}$S$_2$)
m.p.: 215°C

(209)

Desai and Tilak (1961) synthesized this compound by condensation of naphthalene-1,4-dithiol with 2-bromocyclohexanone and subsequent ring-closure of the intermediary product. The resulting 1,2,3,4,11,12,13,14-octahydronaphtho[1,2-*b*:4,3-*b'*]bis[1]benzothiophene leads to the above thiaarene upon selenium dehydrogenation:

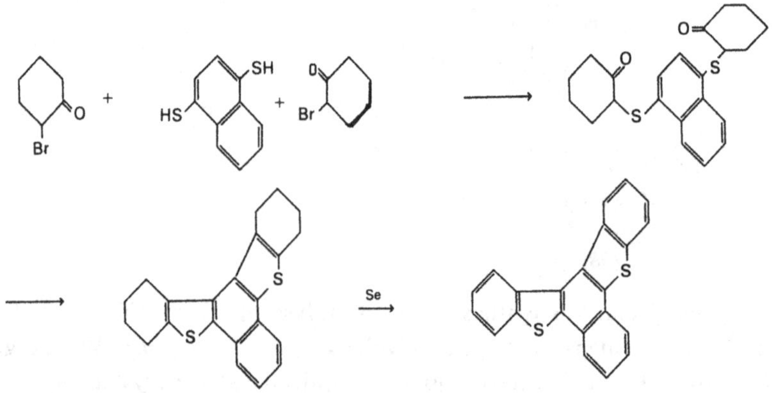

Naphtho[1,2-b:5,6-b']bis[1]benzothiophene
(synonyms: naphtho[1,2-*b*:5.6-*b'*]dibenzothiophene;
naphtho[1,2-*b*:5,6-*b'*]dithionaphthene)

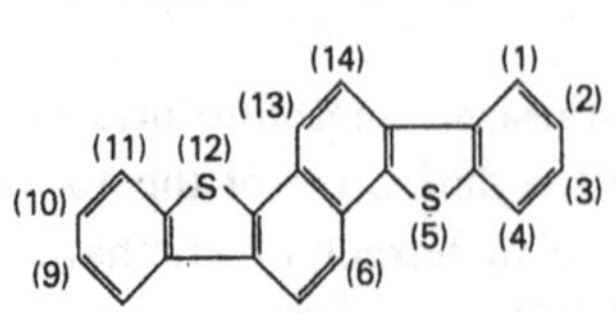

m.w.: 308 (C$_{22}$H$_{12}$S$_2$)
m.p.: >360°C

(210)

In analogy to the preceding system Desai and Tilak (1961) synthesized this thiaarene by condensation of naphthalene-1,5-dithiol and 2-bromocyclohexanone to 1,5-bis(2-oxocyclohexylthio)naphthalene. Cyclization and subsequent selenium dehydrogenation of the 1,2,3,4,8,9,10,11-octahydro compound yielded the parent thiaarene:

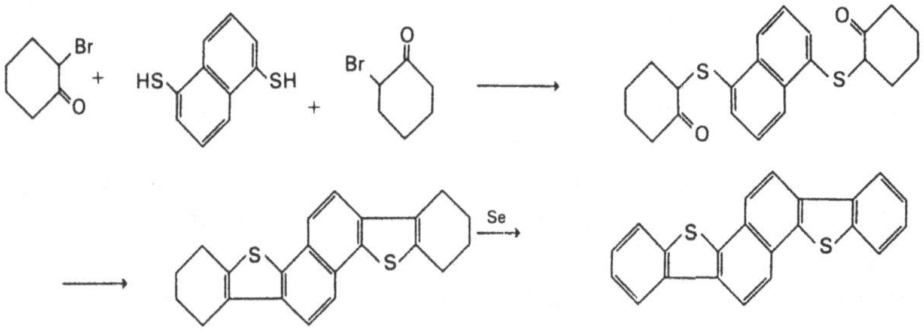

Naphtho[1,2-b:6,5-b']bis[1]benzothiophene
(synonyms: naphtho[1,2-*b*:6,5-*b'*]dibenzothiophene;
naphtho[1,2-*b*:6,5-*b'*]dithionaphthene)

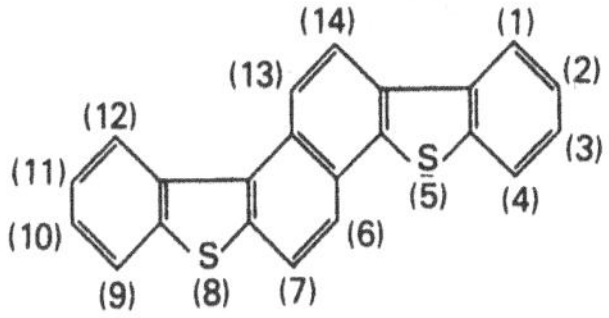

m.w.: 308 ($C_{22}H_{12}S_2$)

(211)

The synthesis of the above thiaarene has been described by Tedjamulia *et al*, (1984) who obtained it by condensation of dibenzothiophene-4-aldehyde and 2-benzo[*b*]thenylphosphonate and subsequent photocylization in 61% yield:

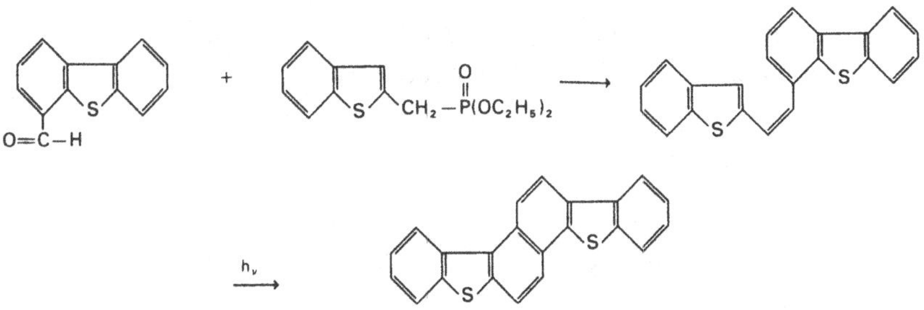

*Naphtho[1,2-*b:*7,6-*b'*]bis[1]benzothiophene*
(synonyms: naphtho[1,2-*b*:7,6-*b'*]dibenzothiophene;
naphtho[1,2-*b*:7,6-*b'*]dithionaphthene)

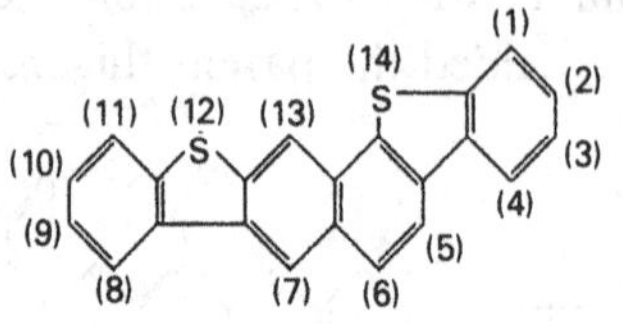

(212)

m.w.: 308 (C$_{22}$H$_{12}$S$_2$)

Similar to the preceding system this thiaarene was prepared by Tedjamulia *et al.* (1984) in a 19% yield by condensation of dibenzothiophene-2-aldehyde and 3-benzo[*b*]thenylphosphonate. Photocyclization of the resulting 1-(3-benzo[*b*]thienyl)-2-(2-dibenzothienyl)ethene unfortunately gives a mixture of naphtho[1,2-*b*:7,6-*b'*]- and -[1,2-*b*:7,8-*b'*]-bis[1]-benzothiophene which, however, can be separated by preparative HPLC:

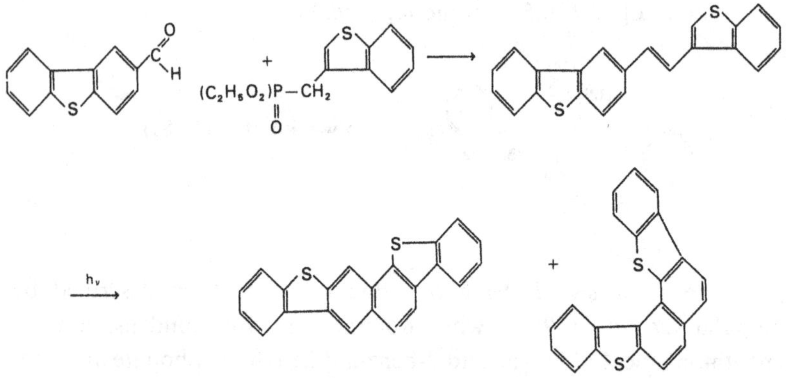

*Naphtho[1,2-*b:*7,8-*b'*]bis[1]benzothiophene*
(synonyms: naphtho[1,2-*b*:7,8-*b'*]dibenzothiophene;
naphtho[1,2-*b*:7,8-*b'*]dithionaphthene)

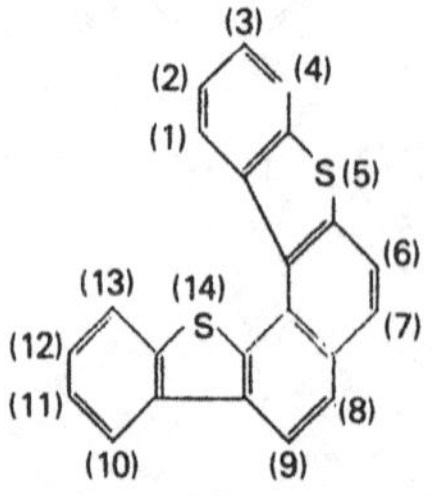

(213)

m.w.: 308 (C$_{22}$H$_{12}$S$_2$)

The compound has been obtained in a 34% yield from dibenzothiophene-2-aldehyde and 3-benzo[*b*]thenylphosphonate as described under the preceding thiaarene (Tedjamulia *et al.*, 1984).

Naphtho[2,1-b:6,5-b']bis[1]benzothiophene
(synonyms: naphtho[2,1-*b*:6,5-*b*']dibenzothiophene;
naphtho[2,1-*b*:6,5-*b*']dithionaphthene)

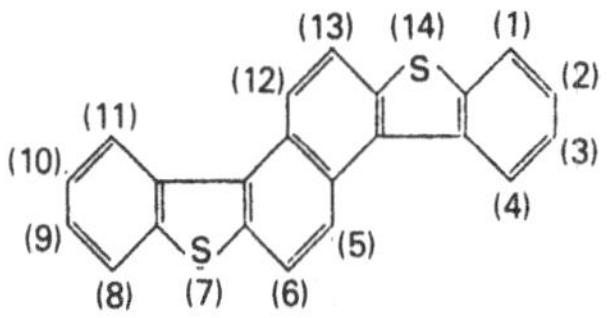

m.w.: 308 ($C_{22}H_{12}S_2$)

(214)

Tedjamulia *et al.* (1984) have prepared this thiaarene from dibenzothiophene-1-aldehyde and 2-benzothenylphosphonate to give 1-(2-benzo[*b*]thienyl)-2-(1-dibenzothienyl)ethene which can be photocyclized to naphtho[2,1-*b*:6,5-*b*']bis[1]benzothiophene:

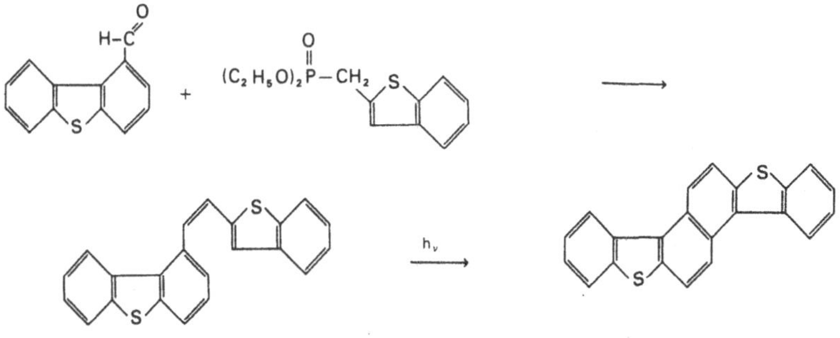

Naphtho[2,1-b:7,6-b']bis[1]benzothiophene
(synonyms: naphtho[2,1-*b*:7,6-*b*']dibenzothiophene;
naphtho[2,1-*b*:7,6-*b*']dithionaphthene)

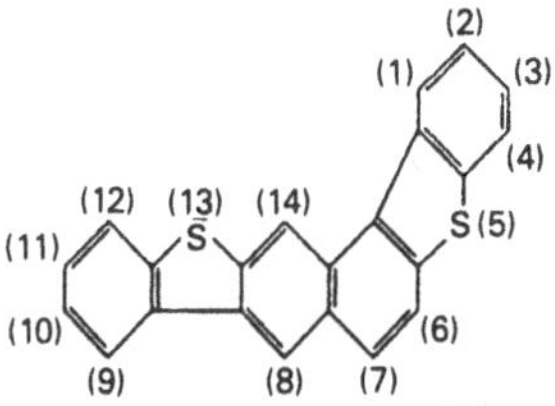

m.w.: 308 ($C_{22}H_{12}S_2$)

(215)

Tedjamulia *et al.* (1984) have synthesized the above system in an overall yield of 11% by condensing dibenzothiophene-2-aldehyde and 2-

benzo[*b*]thenylphosphonate. Subsequent photocyclization results in the formation of the separable isomers, naphtho[2,1-*b*:7,6-*b'*]- and -[2,1-*b*:7,8-*b'*]bis[1]benzothiophene:

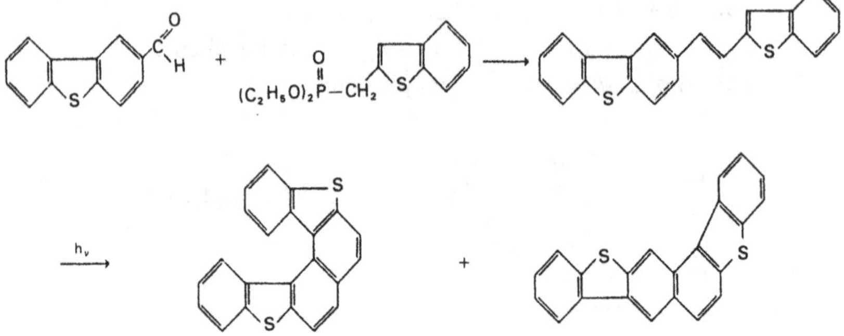

Naphtho[2,1-b:7,8-b']bis[1]benzothiophene
(synonyms: naphtho[2,1-*b*:7,8-*b'*]dibenzothiophene;
naphtho[2,1-*b*:7,8-*b'*]dithionaphthene)

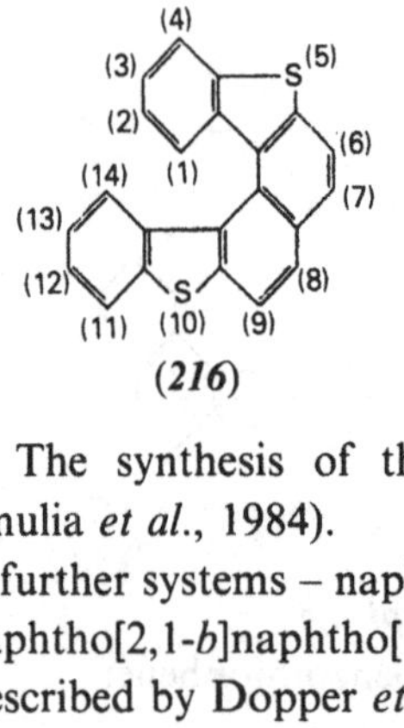

m.w.: 308 ($C_{22}H_{12}S_2$)

(*216*)

The synthesis of this compound has been described above (Tedjamulia *et al.*, 1984).

Two further systems – naphtho[1,2-*e*:8,7-*e'*]bis[1]benzothiophene (*217*) and naphtho[2,1-*b*]naphtho[1',2':4,5]thieno[3,2-*d*]thiophene (*218*) have been described by Dopper *et al.* (1973, 1975):

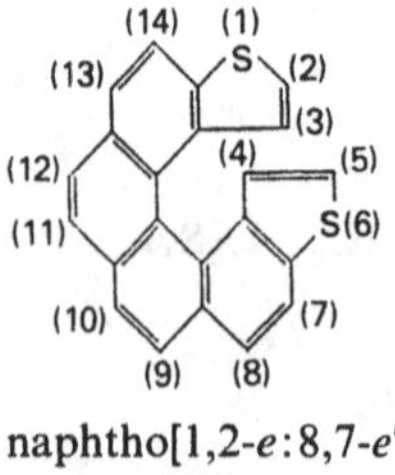

m.w.: 308 ($C_{22}H_{12}S_2$)

naphtho[1,2-*e*:8,7-*e'*]bis[1]benzothiophene
(*217*)

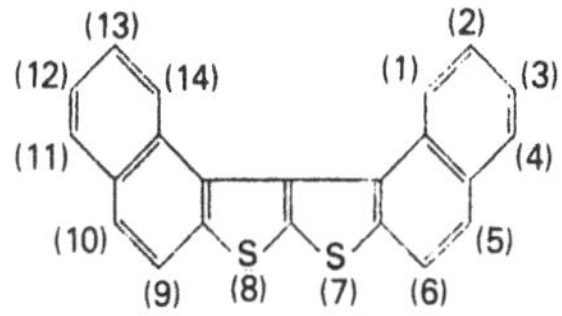

(13)   (2)
(12) (14)   (1) (3)
(11)   (4)   m.w.: 308 ($C_{22}H_{12}S_2$)
(10) S S (5)
(9) (8) (7) (6)

naphtho[2,1-*b*]naphtho[1',2':4,5]thieno[3,2-*d*]thiophene
(218)

2.6   Heptacyclic compounds

$C_4S-C_5-C_5-C_6-C_6-C_6-C_6$

*Diacenaphtho[1,2-*b*:1',2'-d]thiophene* (synonyms:
dinaphthylenethiophene; di-peri-naphthylenethiophene)

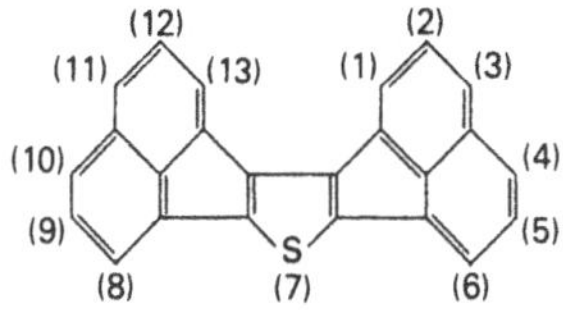

(12)   (2)
(11) (13)   (1) (3)
(10)   (4)   m.w.: 332 ($C_{24}H_{12}S$)
(9)   S (5)
(8)   (7)   (6)

(219)

The system has been found in airborne particulates (Sun, 1983). The incorporation of sulfur into tars from this thiaarene has been studied by Greinke and Lewis (1979*a,b*). Its stability against hydrogenation in comparison to other thiophene systems has been investigated by Landa and Mrnkova (1966). It sensitizes the oxygen transfer in the formation of sulfones from sulfoxides as reported by Schenck and Krauch (1963).

Fluorescence- (Sawicki *et al.*, 1964) and mass spectra (Riepe and Zander, 1979; Glinzer *et al.*, 1983*a*) as well as the molecular refraction (Schuyer *et al.*, 1983) have been recorded and semi-empirical molecular calculations have been carried out by Fabian *et al.* (1968).

$C_4S-C_5-C_6-C_6-C_6-C_6-C_6$

Two systems belonging to this class have been synthesized:

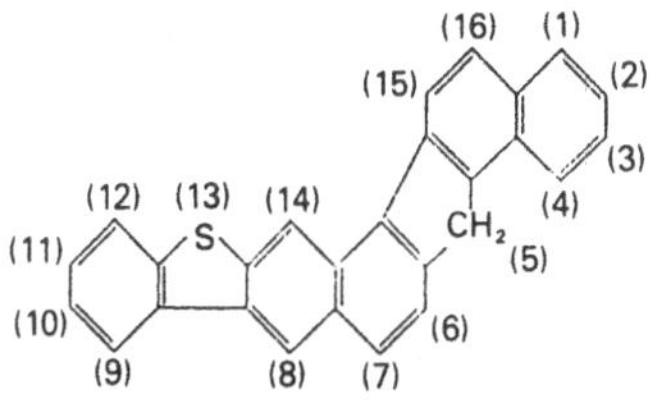

(16) (1)
(15) (2)
      (3)
(12) (13) (14)   (4)   m.w.: 372 ($C_{27}H_{16}S$)
(11)   S CH_2 (5)
(10)   (6)
(9) (8) (7)

5*H*-benzo[7,8]fluoreno[3,4-*b*]dibenzothiophene (Saint-Ruf *et al.*, 1959)
(220)

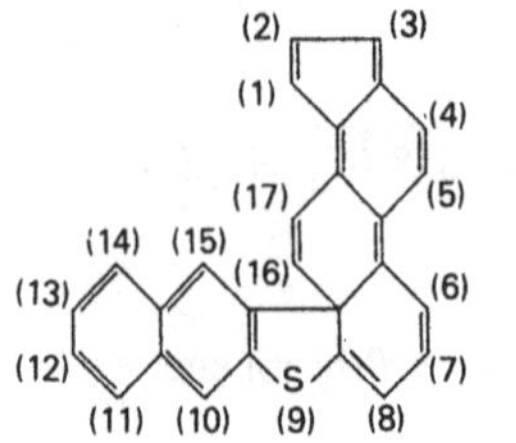

m.w.: 374 ($C_{27}H_{18}S$)

cyclopenta [7,8]phenanthro[1,10a-*b*]naphtho[2,3-*d*]thiophene (Schultz *et al.*, 1978)

(221)

$C_4S-C_6-C_6-C_6-C_6-C_6-C_6$
*Diphenanthro[9,10-*b:9',10'*-d]thiophene*
(synonym: 1,2,3,4,5,6,7,8-tetrabenzo-9-thiafluorene)

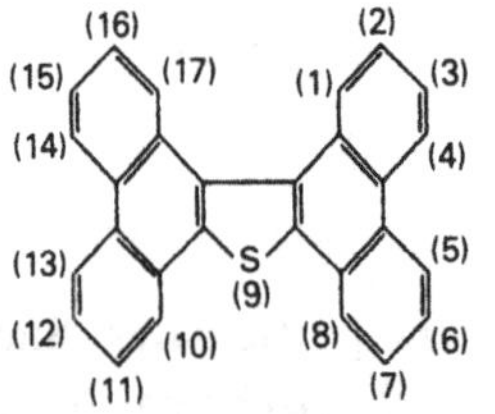

m.w.: 384 ($C_{28}H_{16}S$)
m.p.: 259–260°C

(222)

Although not definitely identified in environmental matter, the system has been synthesized by cyclodehydration of 9,9'-diphenan-thrylsulfoxide by Wilputte and Martin (1965):

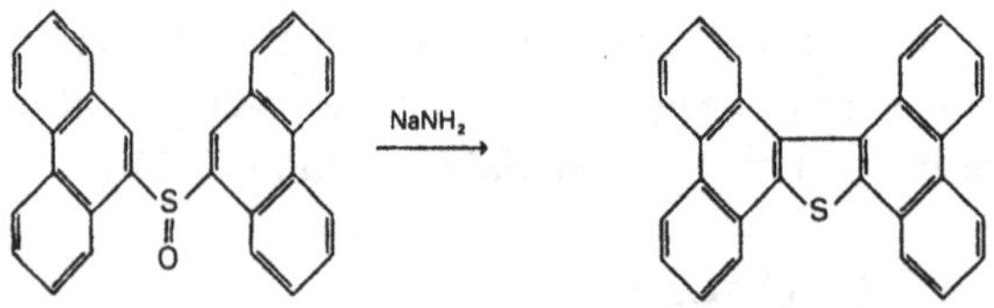

Zander and Franke (1973) obtained it by direct sulfur linking of two phenanthrene molecules via tetrabenzothianthrene which was desul-furized with copper at 439°C:

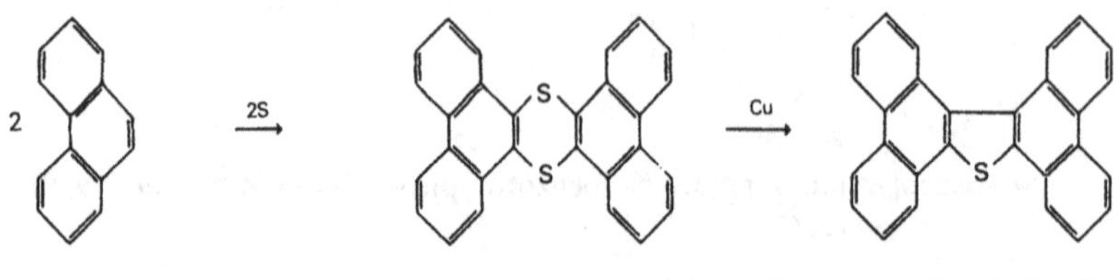

Mass spectral data have been provided by Glinzer *et al.* (1983a,b).

*Benzo[6,7]perylo[1,12-*bcd]*thiophene*
(synonym: 7,8-epithiobenzo[*ghi*]perylene)

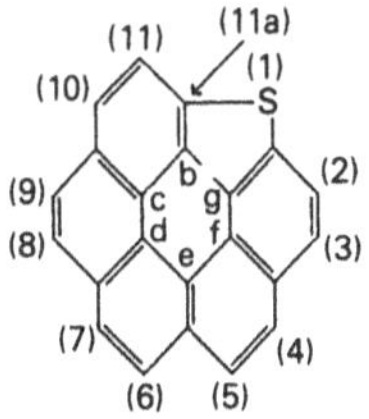

m.w.: 306 ($C_{22}H_{10}S$)

(*223*)

Benzo[6,7]perylo[1,12-*bcd*]thiophene has been detected in carbon black (Alsberg *et al.*, 1982; Lee and Hites, 1976; Colmsjö and Östman, 1982) and in other carbonaceous materials (Stenberg and Alsberg, 1981). The synthesis of this system can be achieved by irradiation of (2,2'),(3,3')-biphenylo-*p*-cyclophane-1,9-diene (Lawson *et al.*, 1973; DuVernet *et al.*, 1978) or by Diels-Alder reaction of dehydro[5]heterohelicene with maleic anhydride, followed by decarboxylation of the intermediary dicarboxylic anhydride with soda lime and subsequent dehydrogenation (Dopper and Wynberg, 1975):

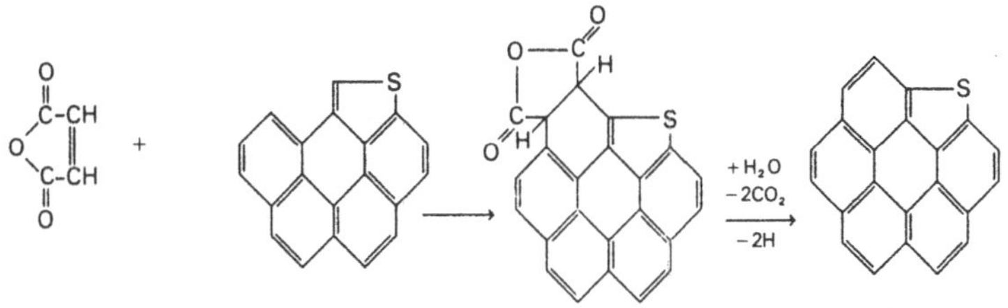

$+H_2O$
$-2CO_2$
$-2H$

NMR- (DuVernet *et al.*, 1978), and low temperature fluorescence and phosphorescence spectra (Colmsjö *et al.*, 1982; Colmsjö and Östman, 1982) have been recorded.

The synthesis of two other thiaarenes from this class have been reported – benzo[*b*]benzo[10,11]chryseno[6,5-*d*]thiophene (Vingiello and Henson, 1966) and 6,13(1',2')benzanthra[2,3-*b*]benzo[*d*]thiophene (Davies and Porter, 1957*a*).

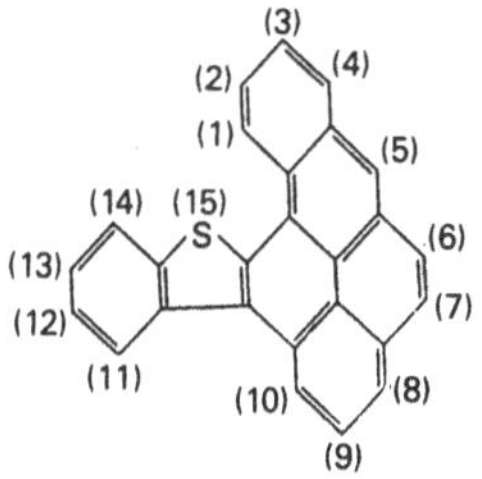

m.w.: 358 ($C_{26}H_{14}S$)

benzo[*b*]benzo[10,11]chryseno[6,5-*d*]thiophene
(*224*)

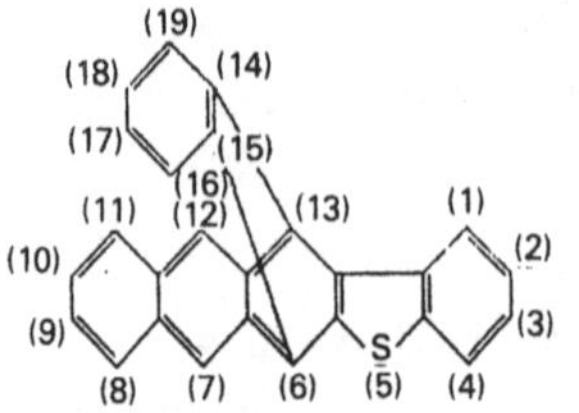

6,13(1',2')benzanthra[2,3-*b*]benzo[*d*]thiophene
(**225**)

m.w.: 358 (C$_{26}$H$_{14}$S)

$C_4S-C_4S-C_6-C_6-C_6-C_6-C_6$
Dinaphtho[1,2-d:1',2'-d']benzo[1,2-b:4,3-b']dithiophene

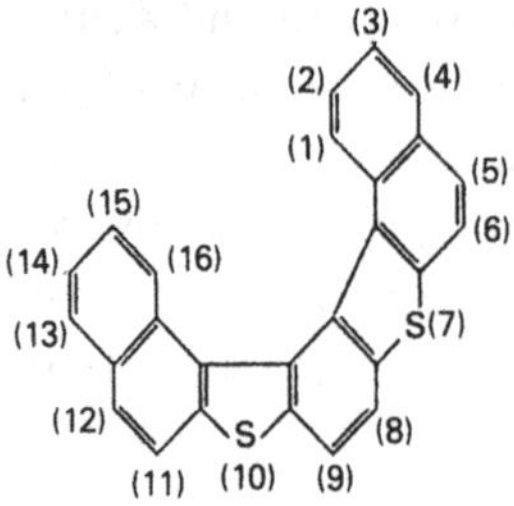

m.w.: 390 (C$_{26}$H$_{14}$S$_2$)

(**226**)

The compound was obtained by photolysis of 1,2-di(2-naphtho-[2,1-*b*]thien-2-yl)ethene in benzene in the presence of iodine (Wynberg *et al.*, 1971):

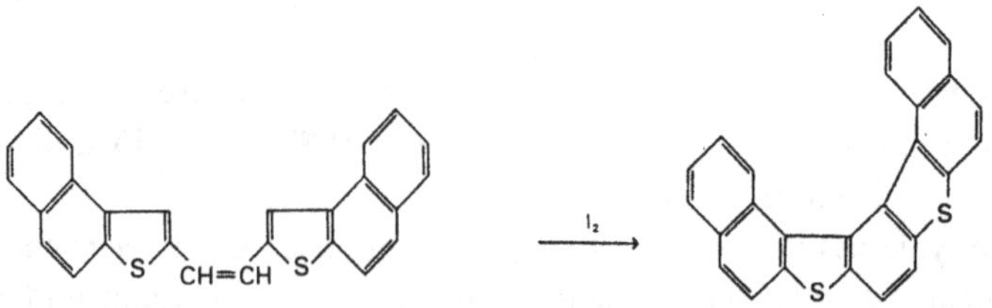

Electronic spectra, ORD- and CD-spectra have been recorded by Groen and Wynberg (1971) and its HPLC behaviour has been studied by Numan *et al.* (1976) and by Mikes and Boshart (1978).

$C_5S-C_6-C_6-C_6-C_6-C_6-C_6$

16H-Benzo[4,5]phenaleno[1,2,3-kl]thioxanthene (synonyms:
13*H*-dibenzo[*f,j*]1-4-thiaperylene; 16*H*-7-thiabenzo[*a,o*]perylene)

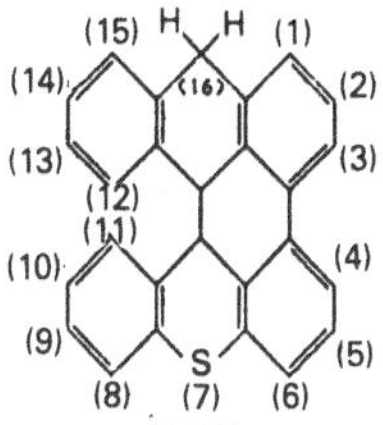

m.w.: 372 ($C_{27}H_{16}S$)

(*227*)

The formation of the 16-oxo derivative from 10,9'-anthrony-lidenethioxanthene by photodehydrogenation has been described by Ismail and El-shafei (1957):

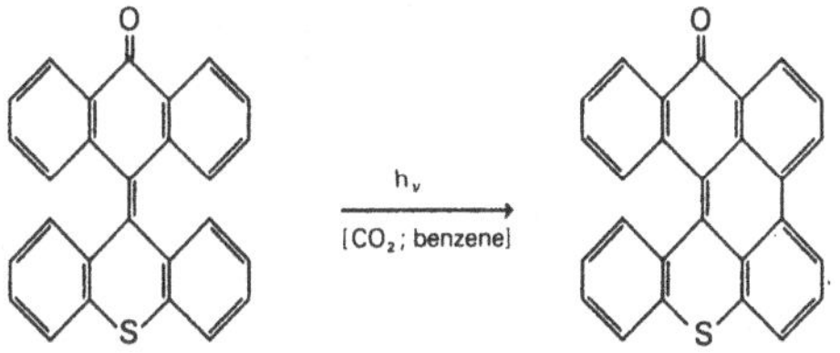

2.7   Higher-condensed systems
$C_4S-C_5-C_5-C_6-C_6-C_6-C_6-C_6$

Indeno[1',7':6,7,8]fluoreno[3,4-b]dibenzothiophene

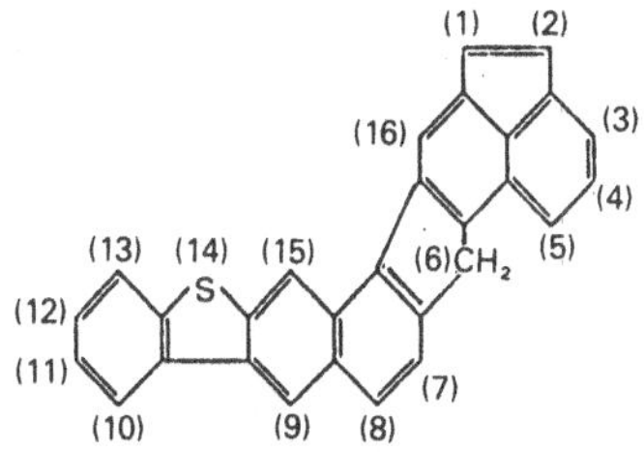

m.w.: 396 ($C_{29}H_{16}S$)

(*228*)

The synthesis of a 2,6-dihydro derivative of this system has been described by Saint-Ruf *et al.* (1959).

$C_4S-C_5-C_6-C_6-C_6-C_6-C_6-C_6$

*8H-Pyreno[1′,2′:6,7]indeno[1,2-*b*][*1*]benzothiophene*
(synonym: pyreno[1′,2′:6,7]indeno[1,2-*b*]thianaphthene)

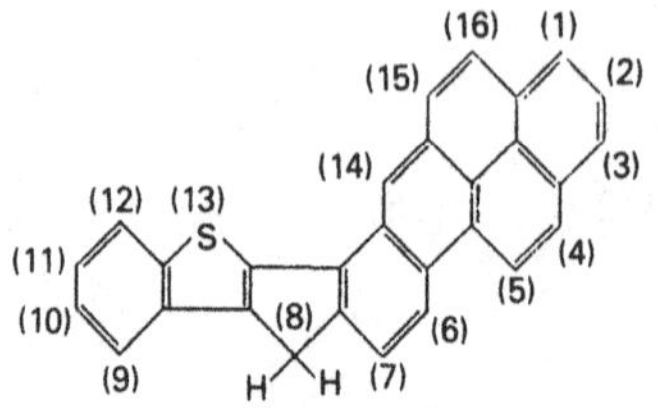

m.w.: 398 ($C_{29}H_{18}S$)
m.p.: 276°C

(229)

The synthesis of this system has been reported by Saint-Ruf (1959).

$C_4S-C_5-C_5-C_6-C_6-C_6-C_6-C_6-C_6-C_6$

Biscyclopenta[7,8]phenanthro[2,3-b:3′,2′-d]thiophene

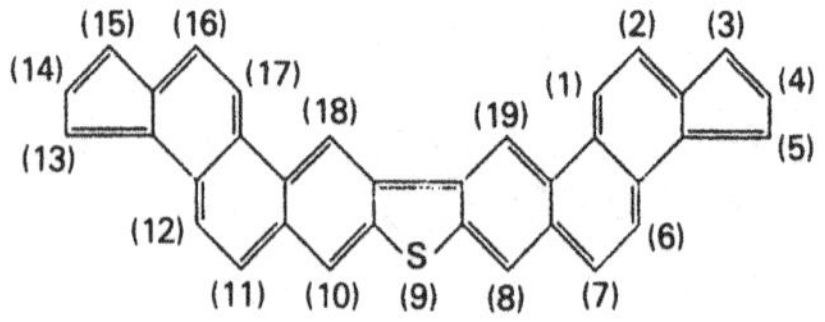

m.w.: 458 ($C_{34}H_{18}S$)

(230)

This system has been described by Jones *et al.* (1970).

$C_4S-C_6-C_6-C_6-C_6-C_6-C_6-C_6$

Dibenzo- and naphthoperylo[1,12-*bcd*]thiophenes are found in this class of compounds.

*Dibenzo[2,3:10,11]perylo[1,12-*bcd*]thiophene*

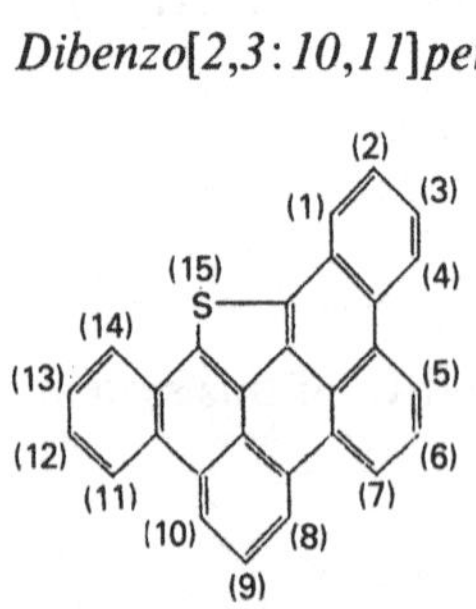

m.w.: 382 ($C_{28}H_{14}S$)
m.p.: 378–380°C

(231)

Zander and Franke (1973) obtained the above thiaarene by heating dibenzoperylene with sulfur at 320°C:

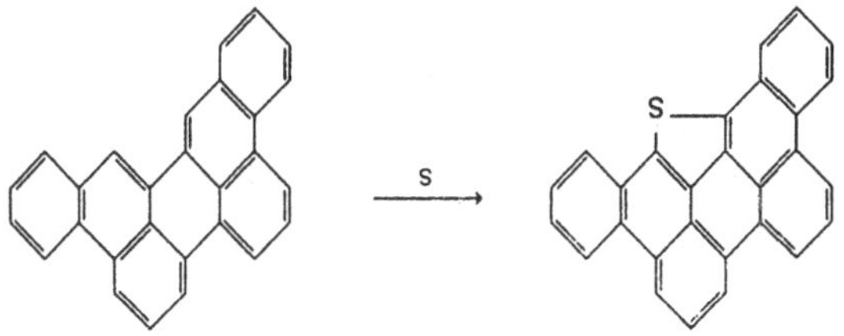

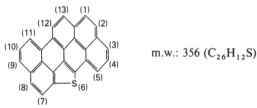

It is also formed by $AlCl_3$-treatment of tetraphenylthiophene (Stein-kopf, 1935; Badger *et al.*, 1957). The Raney-Ni-induced desulfurization of this thiaarene has been studied by Badger *et al.* (1957).

Dibenzo[4,5:6,7]perylo[1,12-bcd]thiophene

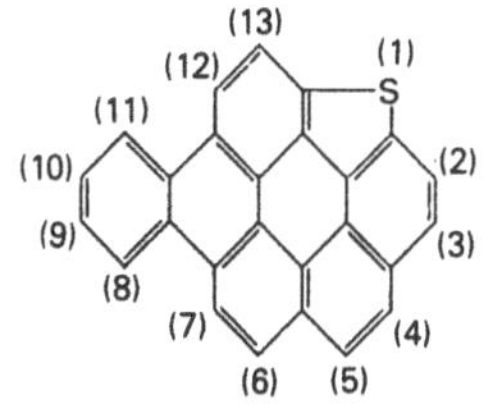

m.w.: 356 ($C_{26}H_{12}S$)

(232)

Peaden *et al.* (1980) have tentatively identified this compound in carbon black extracts after reversed-phase HPLC separation by mass spectrometry and spectrofluorimetry. According to these authors the following two naphthoperylo[1,12-*bcd*]thiophenes also seem to be present in carbon black:

m.w.: 356 ($C_{26}H_{12}S$)

naphtho[8′,1′,2′:2,3,4]perylo[1,12-*bcd*]thiophene
(233)

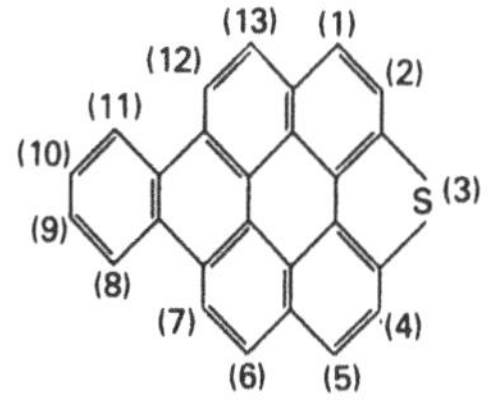

m.w.: 356 ($C_{26}H_{12}S$)

naphtho[1′,2′,3′,4′:6,7]perylo[1,12-*bcd*]thiophene
(234)

$C_4S-C_6-C_6-C_6-C_6-C_6-C_6-C_6-C_6$

Two structures of this class have been tentatively identified in high-molecular weight polyaromatic thiophene fractions of carbon black extracts after HPLC-separation – coroneno[3,2,1-*bcd*][1]benzothiophene (**235**) and phenanthro[5′,4′,3′,2′:4,5,6,7]perylo[1,12-*bcd*]thiophene (**236**) (Peaden *et al.*, 1980).

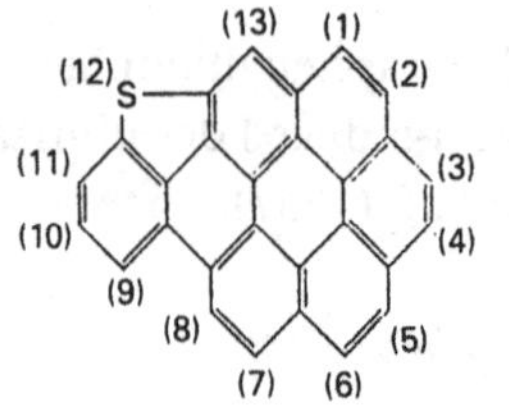

m.w.: 380 ($C_{28}H_{12}S$)

coroneno[3,2,1-*bcd*][1]benzothiophene
(**235**)

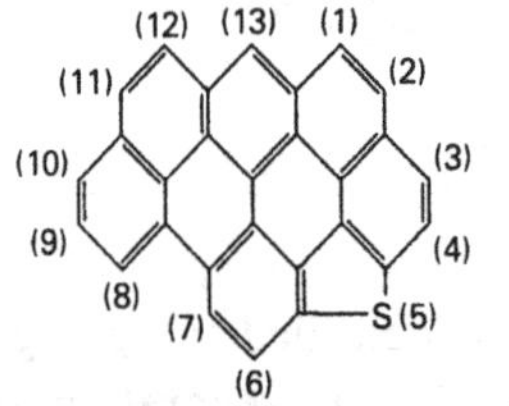

m.w.: 380 ($C_{28}H_{12}S$)

phenanthro[5′,4′,3′,2′:4,5,6,7]perylo[1,12-*bcd*]thiophene
(**236**)

3

References

Adlard, E. R. (1972). A review for the methods of the identification of persistent hydrocarbon pollutants on seas and beaches. *J. Inst. Petrol.*, **58**, 63–74.

Adlard, E. R., Creaser, L. F. and Matthews, P. H. D. (1972). Identification of hydrocarbon pollutants on seas and beaches by gas chromatography, *Anal. Chem.*, **44**, 64–73.

Aggarwal, N. and MacDowell, D. W. H. (1979). Benzo[1,2-*b*:4,5-*b'*]dithiophene. *Org. Prep. Proceed. Int.*, **11**, 247–9.

Ahmed, M., Ashby, J. and Meth-Cohn, O. (1970). Direct Bradsher reaction: Synthesis of benzodithiophenes and related systems. *J. Chem. Soc.*, **D1970**, 1094–5.

Ahmed, M., Ashby, J., Ayad, M. and Meth-Cohn, O. (1973). Direct Bradsher reaction: Synthesis of thiophene analogs of linear polycyclic hydrocarbons. *J. Chem. Soc., Perkin Trans.*, **1**, 1099–103.

Aitken, J., Heeps, T. and Steedman, W. (1968). Organic sulfur in coal: model compound studies. II. The pyrolysis of thianthrene and dibenzothiophene. *Fuel*, **47**, 353–7.

Akhobadze, R. N., Teplitskaya, T. A. and Utkina, L. F. (1975a). Spectroscopy of naphthobenzothiophenes at 77K. *Tezisy Dokl.-Vses. Soveshch. Lyumin.* 22nd, 58.

Akhobadze, R. N., Teplitskaya, T. A. and Utkina, L. F. (1975b). Spectroscopy of naphthobenzothiophenes at 77K. *Izv. Akad. Nauk SSSR, Ser. Fiz.*, **39**, 2390–4.

Akhobadze, R. N., Utkina, L. F. and Teplitskaya, T. A. (1975c). Quasilinear fluorescence and absorption spectra of benzo[*b*]naphtho[2,3-*d*]thiophene, 7-methyl-benzo[*b*]naphtho[2,3-*d*]thiophene and 9,10-dihydro-7-methylbenzo[*b*]naphtho[2,3-*d*]-thiophene. *Soobshch. Akad. Nauk Gruz. SSR*, **77**, 369–72.

Akhobadze, R. N., Utkina, L. F. and Teplitskaya, T. A. (1975d). Quasilinear phosphorescence spectra of benzo[*b*]naphtho[2,3-*d*]thiophene and 7-methylbenzo-[*b*]naphtho[2,3-*d*]thiophene. *Soobshch. Akad. Nauk Gruz. SSR.*, **78**, 365–8.

Akhobadze, R. N., Teplitskaya, T. A., Utkina, L. F. and Melikadze, L. D. (1976). Qualitative analysis of organic sulfur compounds in complex mixtures by luminescence and luminescence excitation spectra. *Soobshch. Akad. Nauk Gruz. SSR*, **84**, 109–12.

Akhobadze, R. N., Melikadze, L. D., Teplitskaya, A. T. and Utkina, L. F. (1977). Possibility of identifying thiophene derivatives in spectra. *Zh. Prike. Spektrosk.*, **27**, 263–7.

Alsberg, T., Rannug, U., Stenberg, U. and Sundvall, A. (1982). Evaluation of extraction methods for carbon black: POM analysis and mutagenicity assay. In: *Polynuclear Aromatic Hydrocarbons: Phys. Biol. Chem.* (M. Cooke, A. J. Dennis and G. L. Fisher, eds.), pp. 73–82. Columbus/Ohio. Battelle Press.

Albers, G. (1980). Untersuchung hochsiedender Erdölanteile mit Hilfe der

Massenspektrometrie. EKEP-Synopse 8044. *Erdöl und Kohle-Erdgas-Petrolchem.*, **33**, 484.

Andersson, J. T. (1987*a*). Separations on a mercuri-acetate-substituted phenyl-silica phase in normal-phase liquid chromatography. *Fresenius Z. Anal. Chem.*, **326**, 425–33.

Andersson, G. (1987*b*). Ligand-exchange chromatography of polycyclic sulfur heterocycles on silica gel modified with silver nitrate or palladium chloride. *Fresenius Z. Anal. Chem.*, **327**, 38.

Andersson, J. T. (1987*c*). Retention properties of a palladium chloride/silica sorbent for the liquid chromatographic separation of polycyclic aromatic sulfur heterocycles. *Anal. Chem.*, **59**, 2207–9.

Andersson, J. T. (1987*d*). Isomer distribution of alkylated benzothiophenes and dibenzothiophenes in petroleum products. 11th Int. Symp. on Polynuclear Aromatic Hydrocarbons. Sept. 1987. Gaithersburg/Wash. USA (in press).

Anisimow, A. V., Aukharieve, R. G., Federov, N. V. and Viktorova, E. A. (1983). Reactions of 1-naphthalenethiol with bifunctional compounds in the synthesis of sulfur-containing heteroatomic compounds. *Vestn. Mosk. Univ., Ser. 2 Khim.*, **24**, 584–8.

Armarego, W. L. F. (1960). Synthesis of two dinaphthothiophenes. *J. Chem. Soc.*, 433–6.

Armstrong, K. J., Martin-Smith, M., Brown, N. M. D., Brophy, G. C. and Sternhell, S. (1969). Benzo[*b*]thiophene derivates. Part IX. Nitration of benzo[*b*]thiophene and the isomeric nitrobenzo[*b*]thiophenes. *J. Chem. Soc. C.*, 1766–80.

Arsic, S., Butkovic, V., Humski, K., Kasinc, L. and Marcec, R. (1983). Determination of aromatic compounds in lubricating base oils. *Nafta (Zagreb)*, **34**, 701–7.

Ashby, J. and Cook, C. C. (1974). Recent advances in the chemistry of dibenzothiophenes. *Adv. Heterocycl. Chemistry*, **16**, 181–288.

Ashby, J., Ayad, M. and Meth-Cohn, O. (1974). Direct bradsher reaction. III. New method for the benzologation of heterocycles. *J. Chem. Soc., Perkin Trans.*, **1**, 1744–7.

Bachman, W. E. and Wilds, A. L. (1940). The synthesis of cis and trans 17-equilenone. *J. Am. Chem. Soc.*, **62**, 2084–8.

Badger, G. M. and Christie, B. J. (1956*a*). Polynuclear heterocyclic systems. Part X. The Elbs reaction with heterocyclic ketones. *J. Chem. Soc.*, 3435–7.

Badger, G. M. and Christie, B. J. (1956*b*). Absorption spectra of compounds containing 5-membered rings. *J. Chem. Soc.*, 3438–42.

Badger, G. M. and Christie, B. J. (1958). Polynuclear heterocyclic systems. XII. Further examples of the Elbs reaction with heterocyclic ketones. *J. Chem. Soc.*, 913–15.

Badger, G. M., Christie, B. J., Pryke, J. M. and Sasse, W. H. F. (1957). Synthetic applications of activated metal catalysis. V. Desulfurization of flavophene and of tetraphenylthiophene. *J. Chem. Soc.*, 4417–19.

Baig, A. R., Cowper, C. J. and Gibbons, P. A. (1982). Application of a flame photometric detector to the gas chromatographic measurement of sulfur compounds in hydrocarbon fractions. *Chromatographia*, **16**, 297–300.

Bailey, R. J., Card, P. and Shechter, H. (1983). Chemistry of 8-substituted 1-naphthylmethylenes and 2-substituted benzylidenes. *J. Chem. Soc.*, **105**, 6096–103.

Bailey, W. J. and Cummings, E. W. (1954). Cyclic dienes. III. The synthesis of thiophene-1,1-dioxide. *J. Am. Chem. Soc.*, **76**, 1932–6.

Banfield, J. E., Davies, W., Gamble, N. W. and Middleton, S. (1956*a*). Derivates of thianaphthene. II. Thianaphthene derivatives formed by cyclization of acetonyl aryl sulfides and aryl phenacyl sulfides. *J. Chem. Soc.*, 4791–9.

Banfield, J. E., Davies, W., Ennis, B. C., Middleton, S. and Porter, Q. N. (1956*b*). The synthesis of thiaarene derivatives. I. The cyclization of (arylthio)acetaldehyde diethylacetals. *J. Chem. Soc.*, 2603–8.

Barber, H. J. and Smiles, S. (1928). Cyclic disulphides derived from diphenyl. *J. Chem. Soc.*, 1141–9.

Bartle, K. D. (1973). Correlation of molecular orbital indexes of reactivity and proton chemical shifts. Acenaphtho[1,2-*b*] and [1,2-*c*]thiophenes. *Org. Magn. Resonance*, **5**, 95–7.

Bartle, K. D., Jones, D. W. and Matthews, R. S. (1971*a*). High-resolution proton magnetic resonance spectra of polynuclear heterocycles. II. Benzo[*b*]thiophene and dibenzothiophene. *Tetrahedron*, **27**, 5177–89.

Bartle, K. D., Jones, D. W., Matthews, R. S., Birch, A. and Cromble, D. A. (1971). High-resolution proton magnetic resonance spectra of polynuclear heterocycles. III. Electronic spectra and high-resolution proton magnetic resonance of acenaphtho[1,2-*b*]thiophene and acenaphtho[1,2-*c*]thiophene. *J. Chem. Soc. B*, 2092–6.

Bartle, K. D., Lee, M. L. and Wise, S. A. (1981). Modern analytical methods for environmental polycyclic aromatic compounds. *Repr. Chem. Soc. Rev.*, **10**, 113–58.

Barton, T. J., Nelson, A. J. and Clardy, J. (1972). Novel two-step synthesis of 10*H*-benzo[*b*]indeno[2,1-*d*]thiophene. Heterocyclopentadienes. III. *J. Org. Chem.*, **36**, 3995–8.

Barudi, A. L., Zheltov, A. Y. and Stepanov, B. I. (1980*a*). Synthesis of difficulty accessible 2,7-disubstituted 4b,9b-dihydrodibenzothieno[3,2-*b*]benzothiophenes. *Zh. Org. Khim.*, **16**, 2448–9.

Barudi, A. L., Kudryavtsev, A. B., Zheltov, A. Y. and Stepanov, B. I. (1980*b*). Nitration of benzothieno[3,2-*b*]benzothiophene. *Zh. Org. Khim.* **16**, 438–43.

Bates, T. S. and Carpenter, T. (1979*a*). Determination of organosulfur compounds extracted from marine sediments. *Anal. Chem.* **51**, 551–4.

Bates, T. S. and Carpenter, R. (1979*b*). Organosulfur compounds in sediments of the Puget Sound basin. *Geochim. Cosmochim. Acta*, **43**, 1209–21.

Baumann, P. C., Smith, W. D. and Ribick, M. (1982). Hepatic tumor rates and polynuclear aromatic hydrocarbon levels in two populations of brown bullhead (*Ictalurus nebulosus*). In '*Polynuclear Aromatic Hydrocarbons: Chem. Biol. Chem.*' (M. Cooke, A. J. Dennis and G. L. Fisher, eds.), pp. 93–102. Columbus/Ohio, Battelle Press.

Beck, J. and Stoebet, M. B. (1982). Polycyclic aromatic hydrocarbons in Danish leafy crops. Part I. PAH in kale and beets related to point sources of PAH. *Rep. Nord. PAH. Proj.*, **15**, 3–22.

Behringer, H. and Meinetsberger, E. (1981). 1,1',2,2'-Tetrathiafulbalenes. II. Thieno[3,2-*b*]thiophenes from 1,2-dithiol compounds; 3*H*-1,2-dithiol-3-ylidenes(1,2-dithiol-3-carbenes) as supposed intermediates. *Liebigs Ann. Chem.*, **10**, 1729–50.

Bergamasco, T. and Porter, Q. N. (1977). Vinylindenes and some heteroanalogs in the Diels-Alder reaction. III. Benzoquinone, 1,4-naphthoquinone and benzo[*b*]thiophene-1,1-dioxide as dienophiles. *Aust. J. Chem.*, **30**, 1523–30.

Berglind, L. (1982). Determination of polycyclic aromatic hydrocarbons in industrial discharge and other aqueous effluents. *Rep. Nord. PAH Proj.* **16**, 16p.

Berthou, F., Gourmelun, Y., Dreano, Y. and Friocourt, M. P. (1981). Application of gas chromatography on glass capillary columns to the analysis of hydrocarbon pollutants from the Amoco Cadiz oil spill. *J. Chromatogr.*, **203**, 279–92.

Berthou, F. and Vignier, V. (1986). Analysis and fate of dibenzothiophene derivatives in the marine environment. 3rd Workshop on the chemistry and analysis of hydrocarbons, Final Programmes and Abstracts, p. 188, Lausanne.

Bhide, S. V. and Jogdeo, P. S. (1974). Synthesis of heterocyclic steroids. *India A.E.C.*, *Bhabha At. Res. Cent. Barc.*, **764**, 96–100.

Bhide, S. V., Murdia, U. S. and Nair J. (1984). Polycyclic aromatic hydrocarbon profiles of pyrolyzed tobacco products commonly used in India. *Cancer Lett.*, **24**, 89–94.

Bieri, R. H. and Stamoudis, V. C. (1977). The fate of petroleum hydrocarbons from a No. 2 fuel oil spill in a seminatural estuarine environment. In '*Fate and Effects of Petroleum Hydrocarbons in Marine Ecosystems and Organisms*' (D. A. Wolfe, ed.), pp. 332–44. New York, Pergamon Press.

Bieri, R. H., Stamoudis, V. C. and Cueman, M. K. (1977). Chemical investigations of two experimental oil spills in an estuarine ecosystem, pp. 511–16. *Proc. 1977 Oil Spill Conf.* (*Prevention, Behaviour, Control, Cleanup*), Washington, D.C., American Petrol. Inst.

Bimber, R. M., Bluestone, H. and Rosen, O. (1964). Methanothianaphthene compounds. US Pat. 3,130,199 Apr. 21, 1964 (see C. A. **61**: 3073g (1964)).

Bingham, E. and Horton, A. W. (1966). Environmental carcinogenesis: Experimental observations related to occupational cancer. In '*Advances in Biology of Skin Vol. VII. Carcinogenesis*' (W. Montagna, ed.), pp. 183–93. Oxford, New York, Pergamon Press.

Birch, S. F. (1953). Sulfur compounds in petroleum. *J. Inst. Petroleum*, **39**, 185–205.

Birch, A. and Crombie, D. A. (1971). The abnormal Hinsberg condensation of acenaphthenequinone. *Chem. Ind.*, 177.

Birch, S. F., Hunter, N. J. and McAllan, D. T. (1956). Preparation and physical properties of sulfur compounds related to petroleum. VI. Endo-4,7-methano-cis-2-thiahydrindan and endo-4,7-ethano-cis-2-thiahydrindan. *J. Org. Chem.*, **21**, 970–4.

Birch, S. F., Cullum, T. V., Dean, R. A. and Redford, D. G. (1959). Sulfur compounds in the kerosine boiling range of middle east distillates. *Tetrahedron*, **7**, 311–18.

Bjørseth, A. (1978). Analysis of polycyclic aromatic hydrocarbons in environmental samples by glass capillary gas chromatography. *Carcinogen. Compr. Surv.*, **3**, 75–83.

Bjørseth, A. (ed.) (1983). *Handbook of Polycyclic Aromatic Hydrocarbons*, vol. I, 727 pp. New York, Marcel Dekker, Inc.

Bjørseth, A. and Lunde, G. (1977). Analysis of the polycyclic aromatic hydrocarbons content of airborne particulate pollutants in a Soderberg paste plant. *J. Am. Ind. Hyg. Assoc.*, **38**, 224–8.

Bjørseth, A. and Ramdahl, T. (eds.) (1986). *Handbook of Polycyclic Aromatic Hydrocarbons*, vol. II. 432 pp. New York, Marcel Dekker, Inc.

Bjørseth, A. Bjørseth, O. and Fjelstad, P. E. (1978a). Polycyclic aromatic hydrocarbons in the work atmosphere. II. Determination in a coke plant. *Scand. J. Work. Environ. Health*, **4**, 224–436.

Bjørseth, A., Bjørseth, O. and Fjelstad, P. E. (1978b). Polycyclic aromatic hydrocarbons in the work atmosphere. I. Determination in an aluminium reduction plant. *Scand. J. Work. Environ. Health*, **4**, 212–223.

Bjørseth, O., Krohn, C., Tøgersen, S. and Fjelstad, P. E. (1980). The working environment in the aluminium industry. Sampling for polynuclear aromatics by an alumina fluidized-bed sampler. *Electrochim. Acta*, **25**, 117–24.

Bjørseth, A. Bjørseth, O. and Fjelstad, P. E. (1981). Polycyclic aromatic hydrocarbons in the work atmosphere. Determination of area-specific concentrations and job-specific exposure in a vertical pin Soderberg aluminium plant. *Scand. J. Work. Environ. Health*, **7**, 223–32.

Blackburn, E. V., Cholerton, T. J. and Timmons, C. J. (1972). Longrange coupling in the proton nuclear magnetic resonance spectra of benzothiophene and benzofuran analogs. *J. Chem. Soc., Perkin Trans.*, **2**, 101–3.

Blatt, H., Brophy, J. J., Coleman, L. J. and Tairych, W. J. (1976). Reaction of diarylcarbinols and diarylolefins with thionyl chloride. *Austr. J. Chem.*, **29**, 883–90.

Blümer, G. P., Gundermann, K. D. and Zander, M. (1977). Aluminiumchloride-catalyzed skeleton rearrangements of dinaphtho[2,1-b:1',2'-d]thiophene. *Chem. Ber.*, **110**, 269–72.

Boehm, P. D., Barak, J. E., Fiest, D. L. and Elskus, A. A. (1982). A chemical investigation of the transport and fate of petroleum hydrocarbons in littoral and benthic environments: the Tsesis oil spill. *Mar. Environ. Res.*, **6**, 157–88.

Bohonos, N., Chou, T. W. and Spanggord, R. J. (1977). Some observations on biodegradation of pollutants in aquatic systems. *Jpn. J. Antibist.*, **30** (suppl.), 275–85.

Bordwell, F. G., McKellin, W. H. and Babcock, D. (1951). Benzothiophene chemistry. V. The pyrolysis of benzothiophene-1-dioxide. *J. Chem. Soc.*, **73**, 5566–8.

Borwitzky, H. and Schomburg, G. (1979). Separation and identification of polynuclear aromatic compounds in coal tar by using glass capillary chromatography-mass spectrometry. *J. Chromatogr.*, **170**, 99–124.

Borwitzky, H., Henneberg, D., Schomburg, G., Sauerland, H. D. and Zander, M. (1977). High-temperature coal-tars. The use of a capillary gas chromatography/mass spectrometry combination on high temperature coal tars. *Erdöl Kohle, Erdgas Petrochem.*, **30**, 370.

Boswell, D. E., Brennan, J. A., Laudis, P. S. and Rodewald, P. G. (1968). The nitrobenzo[*b*]thiophenes. *J. Heterocycl. Chem.*, **5**, 69.

Brass, K. and Köhler, L. (1922). Dibenzothianthrendichinon und Dinaphthothiophen-dichinon. (Umwandlung des Dithiin-Rings in den Thiophen-Ring). *Chem. Ber.*, **55**, 2543–68. .

Brodskii, E. S., Parfenova, M. A., Lukashenko, I. M., Kabanov, S. P., Petrov, A. A., Kupriyanov, S. E. and Lyapina, N. K. (1977). Analysis of hydrocarbons and heteroatomic compounds of the 360–410° fraction of western surgut. *Neftek khim.*, **17**, 616–20.

Brody, S. S. and Chaney, J. E. (1966). Flame photometric detector. The application of a specific detector for phosphorus and sulfur compounds – sensitive to subnanogram quantities. *J. Gas Chromatogr.*, **4**, 42.

Brune, H. and Deutsch-Wenzel, R. (1986). Unpublished results.

Buchenauer, H. (1971). Effect of phenanthrene and xanthene derivatives on fusarium- and verticillium-wilt of tomato. *Phytopathol. Z.*, **72**, 291–304.

Buchert, H., Bihler, S. and Ballschmiter, K. (1982). Studies of the global baseline pollution. VII. High-resolution gas chromatography of persistent chlorohydrocarbons (PCH) and polyaromatic hydrocarbons (PAH) in polluted and unpolluted lake sediments. *Fres. Z. Anal. Chem.*, **313**, 1–20.

Bugakova, L. P. and Rozantsev, E. G. (1964). Thioxanthones. Sintez i Issled. Effektivn. Stabilizatorov dlya Polimern. *Materialov., Sb. Voronezh.*, 211–18.

Buquet, A., Couture, A., Lablache-Combier, A. and Pollet, A. (1981). Photoreactivity of hexatrienyl heterocyclic systems. 2- or 3-arylbenzo[*b*]thiophene. *Tetrahedron*, **37**, 75–81.

Burchill, P., Herod, A. A. and James, R. G. (1978). A comparison of some chromatographic methods for estimation of polynuclear aromatic hydrocarbons in pollutants. In '*Carcinogenesis, vol. 3: Polynuclear aromatic hydrocarbons*' (P. W. Jones and R. I. Freudenthal, eds.), pp. 35–45. New York, Raven Press.

Burchill, P., Herod, A. A. and Pritchard, E. (1982*a*). Identification of sulfur heterocycles in coal tar and pitch. *J. Chromatogr.*, **242**, 51–64.

Burchill, P., Herod, A. A. and Pritchard, E. (1982*b*). Determination of nitrogen-sulfur mixed heteroatomic compounds and sulfur heterocycles in an anthracene oil. *J. Chromatogr.*, **242**, 65–76.

Burchill, P., Herod, A. A., Mahon, J. P. and Pritchard, J. E. (1983). The class separation of nitrogen compounds in coal tars by liquid chromatography on a polar bonded-phase silica. *J. Chromatogr.*, **281**, 109–24.

Burnett, C. H., Adams, D. F. and Farwell, S. O. (1978). Relative FDD responses for a systematic group of sulfur-containing compounds. *J. Chromatogr. Sci.*, **16**, 68–73.

Buu-Hoi, N. P. and Hoan, Ng (1948). Études dans la série du thiophène. I. Cétones dérivées du 2,5-diméthylthiophène(2,5-thioxene) et certaines de leurs réactions. *Rec. Trav. Chim. Pays-Bas*, **67**, 309–27.

Buu-Hoi, N. P. and Hoan, Ng (1949). The thiophene series. II. Some acids and ketones of the thiophene series and their derivatives. *Rec. Trav. Chim. Pay-Bas*, **68**, 5–33.

Buu-Hoi, N. P., Croisy, A. and Jacquignon, P. (1969). Thiophene derivatives. XVII. Preparation and structure of some benzo[*b*]thiophene aldehydes. *J. Chem. Soc.*, **C1969**, 339–40.

Caddy, B., Martin-Smith, M., Norris, R. K., Reid, S. T. and Stenhell, S. (1968). Proton magnetic resonance spectra of some benzo[*b*]thiophenes. An investigation of substituent effects in a heteroaromatic system. *Austr. J. Chem.*, **21**, 1853–66.

Cagniant, P., Cagniant, D. and Faller, P. (1961). Condensed sulfur heterocycles. XIII. Friedel-Crafts reaction with the thiochromans, synthesis of 5,6-benzothiochroman and of 6,7-benzothiochroman. *Bull. Soc. Chim. France*, 1560–7.

Cagniant, P. and Kirsch, G. (1975). Application of the method for thiophene heterocycle synthesis using sodium sulfide to the preparations of sulfur analogs of polycyclic aromatic hydrocarbons. *C.R. Hebd. Séances Acad. Sci. Sér. C*, **281**, 393–5.

Cagniant, P., Cagniant, D. and Faller, P. (1964a). Condensed sulfur-containing heterocycles. XXIII. Substitution of 6,7-benzo- and 4,5-benzothianaphthenes alkylated in the 3- and 2,3-positions. *Bull. Soc. Chim. France*, 1756–64.

Cagniant, P., Jecko, G. and Cagniant, D. (1964b). Condensed sulfur-containing heterocyclics. XXV. Semiaromatic tricyclic sulfides with a naphthalene nucleus. *Bull. Soc. Chim. France*, 2217–20.

Cagniant, P., Jecko, G. and Cagniant, D. (1966). Condensed sulfur-heterocycles. XXVIII. 3,4-dihydro-1*H*-naphtho[1,2-*c*]thiopyran and its derivatives. *Bull. Soc. Chim. France*, 236–40.

Cagniant, P., Briola, M. M. and Kirsch, G. (1977). New route to naphtho[2,3-*b*]thiophene and its derivatives; synthesis of two biheterocyclic analogs of benz[*a*]anthracene. *C.R. Hebd. Séances Acad. Sci. Sér. C*, **285**, 21–4.

Calder, J. A. and Boehm, P. D. (1979). The Chemistry of AMOCO CADIZ oil in the Aber Wrac'h(France) Amoco Cadiz: Consequences pollut. accd. hydrocarbures. *Actes Colloqu. Inst.* 1979 (publ. 1981), pp. 149–58.

Campaigne, E. E. and Cline, T. E. (1956). A new synthesis of thiophenes and condensed thiophenes by ring closure of disulfides. *J. Org. Chem.*, **21**, 39–44.

Campaigne, E. and Heaton, B. G. (1962). Novel disulfide ring closure. *Chem. Ind. (London)*, 96–7.

Campaigne, E. and Heaton, B. G. (1964). Sulfur heterocycles from the ring closure of bis(arylalkyl)disulfides. *J. Org. Chem.*, **29**, 2372–8.

Campaigne, E. and Knapp, D. R. (1970). Benzo[*b*]thiophene derivatives. XIV. Derivatives of naphtho[1,8-*bc*]thiophene. *J. Heterocycl. Chem.*, **7**, 107–15.

Campaigne, E. and Osborn, S. W. (1968). Preparation and ultraviolet absorption spectra of the isomeric naphthobenzothiophenes and naphthobenzofurans. *J. Heterocycl. Chem.*, **5**, 655–61.

Campaigne, E., Ashby, J. and Osborne, S. W. (1969). Methyl substituted benzo[*b*]naphtho[2,3-*d*]thiophenes. *J. Heterocycl. Chem.*, **6**, 885–9.

Campaigne, E., Ashby, J. and Bulbenko, G. F. (1970). Synthesis of the C-10,11 sulfur isosteres of cholanthrene and 3-methylcholanthrene. *J. Heterocycl. Chem.*, **7**, 1175–7.

Campbell, A. D. and Keen, A. R. (1964). Methyl-substituted 9-thia-1,2-benzofluorenes. *J. Chem. Soc.*, 1637–40.

Carruthers, W. (1953), 6,7-Benzothianaphthene. *J. Chem. Soc.*, 4186–7.

Carruthers, W. (1955). 1,8-Dimethylbenzothiophene in a Kuwait mineral oil fraction. *Nature*, **176**, 790–1.

Carruthers, W. (1963). Some reactions of naphtho[2,3-*b*]thiophene. *J. Chem. Soc.*, 4477–83.

Carruthers, W. and Crowder, J. R. (1957). Ultraviolet absorption spectra of some condensed thiophene derivates. *J. Chem. Soc.*, 1932–3.

Carruthers, W. and Douglas, A. G. (1957). The constituents of high-boiling petroleum distillates. Part IV. Some polycyclic aromatic hydrocarbons in a Kuwait oil. *J. Chem. Soc.*, 278–81.

Carruthers, W. and Douglas, A. G. (1959). Constituents of high boiling petroleum distillates. V. Some condensed thiophene derivatives in a Kuwait oil. *J. Chem. Soc.*, 2813–21.

Carruthers, W. and Douglas, A. G. (1964). Constituents of high-boiling petroleum distillates. Part IX. 3,4,6,7-tetramethyldibenzothiophene in a Kuwait oil. *J. Chem. Soc.*, 4077–8.

Carruthers, W. and Stewart, H. N. M. (1965*a*). Photocyclization of thiophene analogs of stilbenes. *Tetrahedron Lett.*, 301–2.

Carruthers, W. and Stewart, H. N. M. (1965*b*). Synthesis of methyl derivatives of naphtho[2,1-*b*]thiophene and 11-thiabenzo[*a*]fluorene by photocyclization of stilbene isosters. *J. Chem. Soc.*, 6221–7.

Carruthers, W. and Stewart, H. N. M. (1967). Constitutents of high boiling petroleum distillates. XI. Methylhomologs of chrysene and 11-thiabenzo[*a*]fluorene in a Kuwait oil. *J. Chem. Soc. C*, 560–2.

Carruthers, W., Douglas, A. G. and Hill, J. (1962). Synthesis of naphtho[2,3-*b*]thiophene. *J. Chem. Soc.*, 704–8.

Castex, H., Boult, R., Junguin, J. and Lepinasse, M. (1983). Analysis of kerosines and middle distillates by medium-resolution mass spectrometry. *Rev. Inst. Fr. Petr.*, **38**, 523–32.

Castle, R. N., Iwao, M., Tominaga, Y., Pratap, T., Tedjamulia, M. and Lee, M. L. (1983). The synthesis of potentially mutagenic polycyclic aromatic thiophenes and their methyl derivatives via the Wadsworth-Emmons reaction followed by photocyclization. In '*Polynuclear Aromatic Hydrocarbons*' (M. Cooke and A. J. Dennis, eds.), pp. 269–81. Columbus/Ohio, Battelle Press.

Castle, R. N., Tedjamulia, M. L., Tominaga, Y., Pratap, R., Sugiura, M., Kudo, H., Lee, M. L., Iwao, M., Thompson, R. D., Martin, G. E., Gampe, R. T., Musmar, M. J. Wilcott, R. M., Smith, S. L., Layton, W. J., Hurd, R. E. and Johnson, L. F. (1984). The synthesis and properties of polycyclic aromatic thiophenes and related heterocycles occurring in coal-derived products. *J. Heterocycl. Chem.*, **21**, Supplement Lectures in Heterocycl. Chem., **7**, 1–52.

Caullet, C., Salaun, M. and Hebert, M. (1967). Identification of a product obtained by the electrochemical reduction of 2-acetylthiophene in an acid medium in a water-tetrahydrofuran mixture. *C.R. Acad. Sci., Paris, Ser. C*, **264**, 228–31.

Cava, M. P. and Mangold, D. (1964). 1,2-Diphenylphenanthro[1]cyclobutadiene: A highly unstable condensed aromatic cyclobutadiene. *Tetrahedr. Lett.*, 1751–4.

Cava, M. P. and Muth, K. (1960). Condensed cyclobutane aromatic compounds. IX. Benzocyclobutenol and benzocyclobutenone. *J. Am. Chem. Soc.*, **82**, 652–4.

Cava, M. P. and VanMeter, J. P. (1962). Synthesis of some stabilized 2,3-naphthoquinoid systems. *J. Am. Chem. Soc.*, **84**, 2008–9.

Cava, M. P. and VanMeter, J. P. (1969). Condensed cyclobutane aromatic compounds. XXX. Synthesis of some unusual 2,3-naphthoquinoid heterocycles. A synthetic route to derivatives of naphtho[2,3-*b*]biphenylene and anthra[*b*]cyclobutene. *J. Org. Chem.*, **34**, 538–45.

Cava, M. P., Pollack, N. M., Mamer, O. A. and Mitchell, M. J. (1971). Synthetic route to benzo[*c*]thiophene and naphtho[*c*]thiophenes. *J. Org. Chem.*, **36**, 3932–7.

Chapiro, E. and Gach, P. (1933). Biphenylene sulfide and its derivatives. Belgian Pat. 390,439 (C.A. 27: 2696 (1933)).

Chapman, N. B., Ewing, D. F., Scrowston, R. M. and Westwood, R. (1968). The proton magnetic resonance spectra of some benzo[*b*]thiophene derivatives. *J. Chem. Soc. C*, 764–9.

Chapman, N. B., Hughes, C. G. and Scrowston, R. M. (1970). Thieno-[2,3-*b*][1]benzothiophene and thieno[3,2-*b*][1]thiophene. I. Preparation. *J. Chem. Soc. C*, 2431–5.

Chapman, N. B., Hughes, C. G. and Scrowston, R. M. (1971*a*). Thieno-[2,3-*b*][1]benzothiophene and thieno[3,2-*b*][1]thiophene. III. Substitution reactions of derivatives with substituents in the thiophene ring. *J. Chem. Soc. C*, 1308–13.

Chapman, N. B., Hughes, C. G. and Scrowston, R. M. (1971*b*). Thieno[2,3-*b*][1]benzothiophene. II. Substitution reaction. *J. Chem. Soc. C*, 463–8.

Cherry, W. H., Davies, W., Ennis, B. C. and Porter, Q. N. (1967). The base-catalyzed skeletal rearrangement of a thianaphthofluorene derivative. *Austr. J. Chem.*, **20**, 313–20.

Chiang, L. Y. and Meinwald, J. (1981). Peri-bridged naphthalenes. V. Improved synthesis of 1-thiaphenalene. *J. Org. Chem.*, **46**, 4060–2.

Chiu, K. S., Walsh, P. M., Beer, J. M. and Biemann, K. (1983). Polynuclear aromatic compounds in fluidized bed combustion of bituminous coal, subbituminous coal, and oil shale. In '*Polynuclear Aromatic Hydrocarbons*' (M. Cooke and A. J. Dennis, eds.) (publ. 1983), pp. 319–39. Columbus/Ohio, Battelle Press.

Choudhury, D. R. and Bush, B. (1981). Gas chromatography/mass spectrometric characterization of polynuclear aromatic hydrocarbons in particulate diesel emissions. *ACS Symp. Ser.*, **149**, 357–68.

Clar, E. (1964). *Polycyclic Hydrocarbons*. 2 vols., 487 and 487 pp. Academic Press/London-New York and Springer-Verlag/Berlin-Göttingen-Heidelberg.

Clar, E. (1972). *The Aromatic Sextet*. J. Wiley, London.

Clarke, A. and Law, R. (1981). Aliphatic and aromatic hydrocarbons in benthic invertebrates from two sites in antarctica. *Mar. Pollut. Bull.*, **12**, 10–14.

Clarke, K., Rawson, G. and Scrowston, R. M. (1969*a*). Substitution reactions of naphtho[2,1-*b*]thiophene. II. Influence of substituents in the thiophene ring. *J. Chem. Soc. C*, 1274–9.

Clarke, K., Rawson, G. and Scrowston, R. M. (1969*b*). Substitution reactions of naphtho[2,1-*b*]thiophene. *J. Chem. Soc. C*, 537–40.

Clarke, K., Gregory, D. N. and Scrowston, R. M. (1973). Naphtho[1,2-*b*]thiophene. I. Preparation and electrophilic substitution. *J. Chem. Soc., Perkin Trans.*, **1**, 2956–60.

Clement, L. E., Stekoll, M. S. and Shaew, D. G. (1980). Accumulation, fractionation and release of oil by the intertidal clam *Macoma balthica*. *Mar. Biol. (Berlin)*, **57**, 41–50.

Clugston, D. M., George, A. E., Montgomery, D. S., Smiley, G. T. and Sawatzky, H. (1972). Sulfur compounds in oils from western Canada tar belt. *Can. Mines Br. Res. Rep.*, **279**, 16 pp.

Clugston, D. M., George, A. E., Montgomery, D. S., Smiley G. T. and Sawatzky, H. (1974). Sulfur compounds in oils from western Canada tar belt. *Am. Chem. Soc., Div. Fuel Chem., Prepr.* **19**, 202–17.

Clugston, D. M., George, A. E., Montgomery, D. S., Smiley, G. T. and Sawatzky, H. (1976). Sulfur compounds in oils from the western Canada tar belt. *Adv. Chem. Ser.*, **151**, 11–27.

Collin, J. E. (1963). The resistance of some organic compounds of aromatic character to electron impact and to radiation. *Bull. Soc. Chim. Belges*, **72**, 38–49.

Colmsjö, A. L. and Östman, C. E. (1982). Shpol'skii spectra of polycyclic aromatic compounds in samples from carbon black and soil. In '*Polynuclear Aromatic Hydrocarbons*' (M. Cooke, A. J. Dennis and G. L. Fisher, eds.), pp. 201–10. Columbus/Ohio, Battelle Press.

Colmsjö, A. L., Zebühr, Y. U. and Östman, C. E. (1982). Shpol'skii effect in the analysis of sulfur-containing heterocyclic aromatic compounds. *Anal. Chem.*, **54**, 1673–7.

Colmsjö, A. L., Zebühr, Y. U. and Östman, C. E. (1984). The utility of Shpol'skii fluorescence in the identification of polynuclear aromatic compounds containing condensed thiophene rings. *Chem. Scr.*, **24**, 95–9.

Colmsjö, A. L., Zebühr, Y. Z. and Östman, C. E. (1985). A method for the synthesis of bay-region sulfur substituted polyaromatic hydrocarbons. In: '*Polynuclear Aromatic Hydrocarbons: A Decade of Progress*' (M. Cooke, A. J. Dennis, eds.), pp. 135–45. Columbus/Ohio, Battelle-Press.

Commoner, B. (1977). Carcinogens in the environment. *Chem. Tech.*, 76–82.

Cook, C. C. and Sutcliffe, F. K. (1968*a*). Dyes from 1-oxa and 1-thiaphenalene. *Chimica,* Suppl. 135–9.

Cook, C. C. and Sutcliffe, F. K. (1968*b*). The nitration of 1-thiaphenalene. *J. Chem. Soc.,* 957–60.

Corvers, A., van Mil, J. H., Sap, M. M. E. and Buck, H. M. (1977). Synthesis of thiophene containing steroid-like molecules via olefinic cyclization reactions. *Rec. Trav. Chim. Pays-Bas,* **96,** 18–22.

Cox, V. F. and Anderson, T. J. (1980). Pittsburgh Conference of Analytical Chemistry and Applied Spectroscopy. Abstract No. 208. Atlantic City New Jersey, March 1980.

Cox, A., Kemp, D. T., Lapouyade, T., De Mayo, P., Joussot-Dubien, J. and Bonneau, R. (1975). Thione photochemistry. Peri cyclization of some polycyclic aromatic thiones. *Can. J. Chem.,* **53,** 2386–93.

Crenshaw, R. R. and Luke, G. M. (1969). Synthesis of B-nor-6-thiaequilenin and related compounds. *Tetrahedron Lett.,* **52,** 4495–6.

Croisy, A., Jacquignon, P. and Perin, F. (1975). Unusual photocyclization of 1-benzothienyl-2-naphthylethylenes. *J. Chem. Soc., Chem. Commun.,* 106–7.

Croisy, A., Mispelter, J., Lhoste, J. M., Zajdela, F. and Jacquignon, P. (1984). Thiophene analogs of carcinogenic polycyclic hydrocarbons. Elbs pyrolysis of various aroylmethylbenzo[*b*]thiophenes. *J. Heterocycl. Chem.,* **21,** 353–9.

Croisy-Delcey, M., Ittah, Y. and Jerina, D. M. (1979). Synthesis of benzo[*c*]phenanthrene dihydrodiols. *Tetrahedron Lett.,* 2849.

Dacka, S. and Janczewski, M. (1980). Electrophilic substitution reactions of benzo[*b*]naphtho[2,1-*d*]thiophenes. *Pol. J. Chem.,* **54,** 863–4.

Dahlgren, T., Glans, I., Gronowitz, S., Davidson, A., Norden, B., Pedersen, P. B. and Thulstrup, E. W. (1979). Electronic spectra of dithieno analogs of phenanthrene. *Chem. Phys.,* **40,** 397–404.

Damsté, J. S. and de Leeuw, J. W. (1986). The origin and fate of isoprenoid C20 and C15 sulfur compounds in sediments and oils. *Int. J. Anal. Environ. Chem.,* in press.

Damsté, J. S., de Leeuw, J. W., Kock, A. C. and Schenck, P. A. (1986*a*). Generation of sulfur-containing compounds in recent sediments. 3rd Workshop on the chemistry and analysis of hydrocarbons. March 20–21, 1986 Lausanne.

Damsté, J. S., ten Haven, J. L., de Leeuw, J. W. and Schenck, P. A. (1986*b*). In *'Advances in Organic Geochemistry'* (D. Leythaeuser and J. Rullkötter, eds.). New York, Pergamon Press, in press.

Damsté, J. S., de Leeuw, J. W., Kock, A. C., de Zeeuw, M. A. and Schenck, P. A. (1987). The occurrence and identification of a series of organic sulphur compounds in oils and sediments extracts. I. A study of Rozel Point oil (USA). *Geochim. Cosmochim. Acta,* **51,** 2369–91.

Dann, O. and Kokorudz, M. (1958). Polynuclear thiophenes. V. Cyclization of aryl oxo sulfides to thianaphthenes. *Chem. Ber.,* **91,** 172–80.

Dannenberg, J. (1960). Carcinogenic activity of aromatic hydrocarbons and related compounds. *Z. Krebsforsch.,* **63,** 102–17.

DasGupta, N. K. and Birss, F. W. (1980). π-Electron structure of heterocyclic molecules containing sulfur. *Tetrahydron,* **36,** 2711–20.

Davies, W. and Porter, Q. N. (1956). Polymerization of thiophene derivatives. V. The self-condensation of 4,5- and 6,7-benzothianaphthene 1,1-dioxides. *J. Chem. Soc.,* 2609–14.

Davies, W. and Porter, Q. N. (1957*a*). Thianaphthene 1,1-dioxide as a dienophile. *J. Chem. Soc.,* 459–63.

Davies, W. and Porter, Q. N. (1957*b*). Polymerization of thiophene derivatives. VI. Some condensations of nitrothianaphthene 1,1-dioxides. *J. Chem. Soc.,* 826–31.

Davies, W. and Porter, Q. N. (1957*c*). Synthesis of condensed heterocyclic systems. I. Use of 2-vinylthiophene in the diene synthesis. *J. Chem. Soc.,* 4958–60.

Davies, W., Gamble, N. W., James, F. C. and Savige, W. E. (1952a). Communications to the EDITOR. The direct conversion of thiophene into dicyclic and tetracyclic derivatives. Chem. Ind., 804.

Davies, W., Gamble, N. W. and Savige, W. E. (1952b). The direct conversion of thionaphthene into derivatives of 9-thiafluorene. J. Chem. Soc., 4678–83.

Davies, W., Porter, Q. N. and Wilmshurst, J. R. (1957). Polymerization of thiophene derivatives. VII. The conversion of thianaphthene 1,1-thioxide into 1,10-benzothiaxanthene 5,5-oxide. J. Chem. Soc., 3360–70.

Davies, W., Ennis, B. C. and Porter, Q. N. (1968). The pyrolysis of 6a,11b-dihydro-7-thiabenzo[c]fluorene-7,7-dioxide and some of its derivatives. Austr. J. Chem., 21, 1571–9.

Dayagi, S., Goldberg, I. and Shmueli, U. (1970). Chemistry and structure of [1]benzothieno[2,3-b]benzothiophene. Tetrahedron, 26, 411–19.

Degani, I., Fochi, R. and Spunta, G. (1971). Heteroaromatic cations. XIV. Two new trinuclear heteroaromatic thiapyrylium cations, 1-thianthracenium and 2-thianthracenium. Ann. Chim., 61, 662–71.

Dehnen, W., Pitz, N. and Tomingas, R. (1977). The mutagenicity of air-borne particulate pollutants. Cancer Lett., 4, 5–12.

De Luca, G., Pizzabiocca, A. and Renzi, G. (1983). Reaction of diphenyl disulfide with 1,8-dehydronaphthalene. Tetrahedron Lett., 24, 821–4.

Depaus, R. (1979). Purification of commercial benzo[a]pyrene. Isolation and determination of major impurities. J. Chromatogr., 176, 337–47.

Derkosch, J. and Specht, I. (1962). Die IR-Spektroskopische Bestimmung des Substitutiontyps bei Thionaphthenen. Microchim. Acta, 55.

DeRoo, J. and Hodgson, D. W. (1978). Geochemical origin of organic sulfur compounds: thiophene derivatives from ethylbenzene and sulfur. Chem. Geol., 22, 71–8.

Desai, J. S. and Tilak, B. D. (1960). Thiophenes and thiapyrans. XXIII. Synthesis of dimercaptonaphthalenes and naphthalene-1,8-disulfide. J. Sci. Ind. Res. (India), 19B, 390–4.

Desai, J. S. and Tilak, B. D. (1961). Thiophenes and thiapyrans. XXV. Condensed thiophenes and thiapyrans from 1,5-, 1,4-, and 1,3-dimercaptonaphthalenes. J. Sci. Ind. Res. (India), 20B, 22–30.

Deutsche Gesellschaft für Mineralölwissenschaft und Kohlechemie e.V. DGMK (1983). Collaborative studies to determine polycyclic aromatic hydrocarbons (PHA). Ber.-DGMK 159; 19pp, Hamburg, FRG.

Dewar, P., Forrester, A. R. and Thompson, R. H. (1972). Persulfate oxidations. VIII. Oxidation of (arylthio)-, (arylsulfonyl)-, and (arylamino)acetic acids. J. Chem. Soc., Perkin Trans. 1, 2857–61.

Deward, M. J. S. and Trinajstic, N. (1970). Ground states of conjugated molecules. XX. SCF-MO treatment of compounds containing bivalent sulfur. J. Am. Chem. Soc., 92, 1543–9.

De Wit, J. Wynberg, J. (1973). Heterocyclic triptycenes. Synthesis and ultraviolet spectroscopy. Tetrahedron, 29, 1379–91.

Dillon, T. M., Neff, J. M. and Warner, J. S. (1978). Toxicity and sublethal effects of No. 2 fuel oil on the supralittoral isopod, Lygia exotica. Bull. Environ. Contam. Toxicol., 20, 320.

Dimitriev, M. T., Rastyannikov, E. G., Etlin, S. N. and Malysheva, A. G. (1984). Chromatographic mass spectrometric study of toxic substances adsorbed in dust. Gig. Sanit., 44–7.

Dopper, J. H. (1974). The synthesis and properties of some heterocirculenes. PhD Thesis, Univ. Groningen, V. R. B. Offsetdrukkerij, Groningen.

Dopper, J. H. and Wynberg, H. (1975). Synthesis and properties of some heterocirculenes. J. Org. Chem., 40, 1957–66.

Dopper, J. H., Oudman, D. and Wynberg, H. (1973). Use of thieno-[2,3-*b*]thiophene in the synthesis of heterohelicenes by double photocyclizations. *J. Am. Chem. Soc.*, **93**, 3692–8.

Dopper, J. H., Oudman, D. and Wynberg, H. (1975). Dehydrogenation of heterohelicenes by a Scholltype reaction. Dehydrohelicenes. *J. Org. Chem.*, **40**, 3398–401.

Douglas, A. G. and Mair, B. J. (1965). Sulfur in genesis of petroleum. *Science*, **147**, 499–501.

Dressler, M. (1983). Effect of detector temperature on flame photometric detector behaviour. *J. Chromatogr.*, **262**, 77–84.

Drozd, V. N., Pak, K. A. and Ustynyuk, Y. A. (1969*a*). Orienting action during nucleophilic attack on the benzene ring. III. Mechanism of the Smiles rearrangement of *o*-methyldiaryl sulfones; rearrangement of mesityl 6-tetralyl sulfones. *Zh. Org. Khim.*, **5**, 1446–53.

Drozd, V. N., Pak, K. A. and Ustynyuk, Y. A. (1969*b*). Mechanisms of Smiles rearrangement of *o*-methyl sulfones; rearrangement of naphthyl mesityl sulfones. *Zh. Org. Khim.*, **5**, 1267–74.

Drozd, V. N. and Pak, K. A. (1970). Mechanism of the Smiles rearrangement of *o*-methyl diaryl sulfones; effect of structural factors and reactions conditions on the mechanism of rearrangement. *Zh. Org. Khim.*, **6**, 818–25.

Drushel, H. V. and Miller, J. F. (1958). Polarographic estimation of thiophenes and aromatic sulfides in petroleum. *Anal. Chem.*, **30**, 1271–80.

Drushel, H. V. and Sommers, A. L. (1966). Combination of gas chromatography with fluorescence and phosphorescence in analysis of petroleum fractions II. *Anal. Chem.*, **38**, 10–19.

Drushel, H. V. and Sommers, A. L. (1967). Isolation and characterization of sulfur compounds in high-boiling petroleum fractions. *Anal. Chem.*, **39**, 1819–29.

DuVernet, R. B., Wennerstrom, O., Lawson, J., Otsubo, T. and Boekelheide, V. (1978). Bridged [18] annulenes. A study of the synthesis and properties of 12c,12d,12e,12f-tetrahydrobenzo[*ghi*]perylene and its analogs. *J. Am. Chem. Soc.*, **100**, 2457–64.

Eastmond, D. A., Booth, G. M. and Lee, M. L. (1984). Toxicity, accumulation, and elimination of polycyclic aromatic sulfur heterocycles in *Daphnia magna. Arch. Environ. Contam. Toxicol.*, **13**, 105–11.

Ebel, M., Legrand, L. and Lozac'h, N. (1963). Heterocyclic sulfur compounds. VIII. Sulfuration of isophorone. *Bull. Soc. Chim. France*, 161–6.

Edstrom, T. and Lewis, I. C. (1969). Chemical structure and graphitization: X-ray diffraction studies of graphites derived from polynuclear aromatics. *Carbon*, **7**, 85.

Eganhouse, R. P. and Kaplan, I. R. (1982). Extractable organic matter in municipal wastewaters. 2. Hydrocarbons: Molecular characterization. *Environ. Sci. Technol.*, **16**, 541–51.

El-Rayyes, N. R. and Al-Salman, N. A. (1975). Stobbs condensation with substituted succinic esters. I. Synthesis of benzothiophene derivatives. *J. Prakt. Chem.*, **317**, 552–60.

El'tsov, A. V., Shirokii, E. I. and Rogovik, V. I. (1982). Perylene chemistry. Photolysis of perylene 3,4,9,10-tetracarboxylic acid 1,12-sulfone. *Zh. Org. Khim.*, **18**, 168–77.

Etienne, A. (1947). 4,9-Diphenylthiophanthrene and ms-2-thienyl derivatives of anthracene. Photooxidation studies. *Bull. Soc. Chim. France*, 634–9.

Ewing, D. F. and Scrowston, R. M. (1971). NMR parameters of sulfur heterocycles. Solvent and concentration effects for thiophene and related systems. *Org. Magn. Resonance*, **3**, 405–16.

Ewing, D. F., Gregory, D. N. and Scrowston, R. M. (1974). NMR studies of sulfur heterocycles. II. Substituent effects in the thieno[2,3-*b*][1]benzothiophene and thieno[3,2-*b*][1]benzothiophene systems. *Org. Magn. Resonance*, **6**, 293–7.

238   *References*

Eyres, A. R. (1981). Polycyclic aromatic hydrocarbon contents of used metalworking oils. *Inst. Petr.* (Techn. Pap.), IP 81–002, 13pp.
Fabian, J., Mehlhorn, A. and Zahradnik, R. (1968). Semiempirical calculations on sulfur containing heterocycles. *J. Phys. Chem.*, **72**, 3975–85.
Faller, P. (1961a). Synthesis of a sulfur isostere of 3-methylcholanthrene. *Compt. Rend.*, **252**, 1034–6.
Faller, P. (1965). Synthesis of sulfur isosteres of cholanthrene. *Compt. Rend.*, **260**, 3686–7.
Faller, P. (1966a). Condensed sulfur heterocycles. XXXIII. Synthesis of sulfur isosteres of cholanthrene. *Bull. Soc. Chim. France*, 3667–74.
Faller, P. (1966b). Synthesis of sulfur isosteres of cholanthrene. *Compt. Rend. Sér. C*, **262**, 581–3.
Faller, P. (1967). Condensed sulfur heterocycles. XXXV. Nuclear magnetic resonance of sulfur analogs of cholanthrene and methylcholanthrene. *Bull. Soc. Chim. France*, 387–94.
Faller, P. (1968). Sulfur isosteres of benz[a]anthracene. *Compt. Rend. Sér. C*, **267**, 543–6.
Faller, P. and Cagniant, P. (1968). Condensed sulfur heterocycles. XXXVII. Sulfur isosteres of cholanthrene and of 4,5-dihydrocyclopenta(h,i)chrysene. *Bull. Soc. Chem. France*, 2985–7.
Fan, R. L., Dickstein, J. I. and Miller, S. I. (1982). Benzo[b]thiophene S-oxides and related compounds from the reactions of arylalkynes and antimony pentafluoride in sulfur dioxide. *J. Org. Chem.*, **47**, 2466–9.
Farbwerke Hoechst AG (1967). Anthraceno[2,1-m; 1,9-n; 9a,9-a]thioxanthene dyes. Fr. 1,470,793, Feb. 24, 1967; Ger. Appl. March 6,1965. 3pp.
Fedorak, P. M. and Westlake, D. W. S. (1983a). Effect of the dispersant Corexit 9527 on the microbial degradations of sulfur heterocycles in Prudhoe Bay oil. *Can. J. Microbiol.*, **29**, 623–727.
Fedorak, P. M. and Westlake, D. W. S. (1983b). Microbial degradation of organic sulfur compounds in Prudhoe Bay crude oil. *Can. J. Microbiol.*, **29**, 291–6.
Fedorak, P. M. and Westlake, D. W. S. (1984). Degradation of sulfur heterocycles in Prudhoe Bay crude oil by soil enrichments. *Water, Air, Soil Pollut.*, **31**, 223–30.
Fedotova, O. V., Kulikova, L. K., Shenderov, B. A., Kriven'ko, A. P., Karchenko, V. G. and Shub, G. M. (1977). Synthesis and antimicrobial activity of the salts of benzohydro(thia)chromylium and dibenzotetrahydro(thia)xanthylium and products of their reduction. *Khim. Farm. Zh.*, **11**, 72–6.
Fickentscher, K., Wittmann, R. and Roth, H. J. (1969). Farbreaktionen von 2,3-Dicyan-1,4-dithiaanthrachinon. 2. Mitteilung: Reaktion von 2,3-Dicyan-1,4-dithiaanthrachinon mit sekundären Aminen. *Arch. Pharm.*, **302**, 53–61.
Fields, E. K. and Meyerson, S. (1966). Formation of thiophene at high temperatures. *Chem. Commun.*, 708.
Fink, D. E. and Smith, L. E. (1936). Toxicity of certain organic compounds to culicine mosquito larvae. *J. Ec. Entomol.*, **29**, 804–12.
Finnerty, W. R., Shockley, K. and Attaway, H. (1983). Microbial desulfurization and denitrogenation of hydrocarbons. In '*Microb. Enhanced Oil Recovery*' (J. E. Zajic, D. C. G. Gooper, T. R. Jack, eds.), pp. 83–91. Tulsa/Oklahoma, PennWell Publ. Co.
Fitch, W. L. and Smith, D. H. (1979). Carbonaceous Part. Atmos. 14–24. Lawrence Berklea Lab. (Rep. J. LBL), LBL-9037.
Fitch, W. L., Everhardt, E. T. and Smith, D. H. (1978). Characterization of carbon black adsorbates and artifacts formed during extraction. *Anal. Chem.*, **50**, 2122–6.
Foght, J. M., Fedorak, P. M. and Westlake, D. W. S. (1983). Effect of the dispersant Corexit 9527 on the microbial degradation of sulfur heterocycles in Prudhoe Bay oil. *Can. J. Microl.*, **29**, 623–7.
Folkes, D. J. and Gramshaw, J. W. (1981). The flavor and volatiles of white bread crust. *Progr. Food Nutr. Sci.*, **5**, 369–76.

Folli, U., Larossi, D. and Taddei, F. (1974). 2*H*-naphtho[1,8-*bc*]thiophene and 2-methyl-2*H*-naphtho[1,8-*bc*]thiophene 1-oxides. Synthesis, configurational assignments and stereoselective interconversions. *J. Chem. Soc.*, Perkin Trans., **2**, 933–7.

Frederiksson, S. A. and Cedergreen, A. (1981). Effect of carrier flow geometry on the response of sulfur flame photometric detectors for gas chromatography. *Anal. Chem.*, **53**, 614–18.

Fredericks, E. M. and Harlow, G. A. (1964). Determination of mercaptans in sour natural gases by gas liquid chromatography and microcoulometric titration. *Anal. Chem.*, **36**, 263–6.

Friedel, R. A. and Orchin, M. (1951). *Ultraviolet Spectra of Aromatic Compounds*. John Wiley, New York.

Friocourt, M. P., Gourmelun, Y., Berthou, F., Cosson, R. and Marchand, M. (1981). Effects of AMOCO CADIZ on oyster population of northern Brittany (France). Chemical survey on pollution, purification and adaptation. Amoco Cadiz: Consequences Pollut. Accid. Hydrocarbures, Actes Coloqu. Int. 1979, 617–631.

Frycka, J. (1979). Contamination of some aromatic standards. *J. Chromatogr.*, **174**, 488–9.

Fukushima, D., Kim, Y. H., Iyanagi, T. and Oae, S. (1978). Enzymatic oxidation of disulfides and thiosulfinates by both rabbit liver microsomes and a reconstituted system with purified cytochrome P-450. *J. Biochem. (Tokyo)*, **83**, 1010–27.

Fukushima, S., Sumimoto, T., Miyata, H., Tanaka, R. and Kashimoto, T. (1983). Determination of organic contaminants in mussel by computerized GC-MS. *Osaka-furitsu Koshu Eisei Kenkyusho Kenkyu Hokoku, Shokohin Eisei Hen*, **14**, 29–40.

Gaertner, R. (1952). Reactions of 3-thianaphthenylmethylmagnesium chloride. *J. Am. Chem. Soc.*, **74**, 2185–8.

Gallegos, E. J. (1975). CHS$^+$ sulfur compound analysis by gas chromatography-mass spectrometry. *Anal. Chem.*, **47**, 1150–4.

Galloway, W. B., Lake, J. L., Phelps, D. K., Rogerson, P. F., Bowen, V. T., Farrington, J. W., Laseter, J. L., Lawler, G. C. et al. (1983). The mussel watch: Intercomparison of trace level constituent determinations. *Environ. Toxicol. Chem.*, **2**, 395–410.

Gal'pern, G. D., Karaulova, E. N., Numanov, I. U., Skobelina, A. I. and Chaiko, V. P. (1965). Isolation of sulfides from middle fractions of Khaudag and Kyzyl-Tumshuk crudes. *Neftekhimiya*, **5**, 747–52.

Gay, M. L., Belisle, A. A. and Patton, J. F. (1980). Quantification of petroleum-type hydrocarbons in avian tissue. *J. Chromatogr.*, **187**, 153–60.

Geering, E. J. (1966). Benzothiophene pesticides. U. S. Pat. 3,278,552.

Geering, F. J. (1969). Pesticidal benzothiophenes and benzothienobenzothiophenes. U. S. Pat. 3,433,874.

Geneste, P., Grimand, J., Olivé, J.-L. and Ung, S. N. (1975). Oxidation en sulfoxydes de benzo[*b*]thiophènes par l'hypochlorite de tertiobutyle. *Tetrahedron Lett.*, 2345–8.

Geneste, P., Olivé, J.-L. and Ung, S. N. (1977*a*). Reactivité de l'hypochlorite de tertiobutyle dans l'oxidation du benzothiophène. *J. Heterocycl. Chem.*, **14**, 449–54.

Geneste, P., Grimand, J., Olivé, J.-L. and Ung, S. N. (1977*b*). Oxidation en sulfoxydes de benzo[*b*]thiophènes monosubstitués. *Bull. Soc. Chim. France*, 271–5.

Geneste, P., Olivé, J.-L. and Ung, S. N. (1977*c*). Chloration et S-oxydation du benzo[*b*]thiophènes par l'hypochlorite de tertiobutyle. Mécanisme de la réaction. *J. Heterocycl. Chem.*, **14**, 953–6.

Gerasimenko, V. A., Kirilenko, A. V. and Nabivach, V. M. (1981). Capillary gas chromatography of aromatic compounds found in coal tar fractions. *J. Chromatogr.*, **208**, 9–16.

Ghaisas, V. V. and Tilak, B. D. (1955). Thiophene isosteres of carcinogenic hydrocarbons. III. 4,10-Dimethylthianaphtheno[6,5-*b*]thianaphthene and 6,12-dimethylbenzo[1,2-*b*:5,5-*b'*]bisthianaphthene. *J. Sci. Ind. Res. (India)*, **14B**, 11–13.

Ghaisas, V. V. and Tilak, B. D. (1957). Thiophenes and thiopyrans. XVI. Thianaphtheno[3,2-*b*]thianaphthene. *J. Sci. Ind. Res.* (*India*), **16B**, 345–8.

Giddings, J. M. (1979). Acute toxicity of selenastrum capricornutum of aromatic compounds from coal conversion. *Bull. Environ. Contam. Toxicol.*, **23**, 360–4.

Gilman, H. and Jacoby, A. L. (1938). Dibenzothiophene: Orientation and derivatives. *J. Org. Chem.*, **3**, 108–19.

Gjessing, E., Lygren, E., Berglind, I., Gulbrandsen, T. and Skaane, R. (1984). Effect of highway run off on lake water quality. *Sci. Total Environ.*, **33**, 245–7.

Glinzer, O., Severin, D., Beduerftig, C., Czogalla, C. D. and Puttins, U. (1983*a*). Mass spectrometry of sulfur compounds as model substances for crude oil analysis-bisanellated thiophenes. *Fresenius Z. Anal. Chem.*, **315**, 208–12.

Glinzer, O., Severin, D., Czogalla, C. D., Beduerftig, C. and Puttins, U. (1983*b*). Mass spectrometry of bisannulated thiophene S-oxides as model substances for oxidation products in crude oil. *Fresenius Z. Anal. Chem.*, **315**, 345–9.

Gogte, V. N. (1971). PMR spectra of some heteroatomic compounds containing hindered methylgroups. *Indian J. Chem.*, **9**, 121–4.

Gogte, V. N., Palkar, V. S. and Tilak, B. D. (1960). Synthesis of condensed thiophenes, biaryls, and bialkyls through aryllithium and alkyllithium derivatives. *Tetrahedron Lett.*, **6**, 30–4.

Gourier, J. and Canonne, P. (1970). Étude de la cycloalcoylation des (thiényl-2)-5-pentènes-1. *Can. J. Chem.*, **48**, 2587–95.

Gourier, J. and Canonne, P. (1973). Intramolecular cyclization of 1-(4-pentenyl)dibenzothiophenes and of 2,3-bis(2-methyl-4-pentenyl)dibenzothiophene. *Bull. Soc. Chim. France*, **11**, 3110–15.

Grahl-Nielsen, O., Staveland, J. T. and Wilhelmsen, S. (1978). Aromatic hydrocarbons in benthic organisms from coastal areas polluted by Iranian crude oil. *J. Fish. Res. Board Can.*, **35**, 615–23.

Grandolino, G. (1961). A linear benzobisthionaphthene. *Ann. Chim.* (*Rome*), **51**, 195.

Greinke, R. A. and Lewis, I. C. (1979*a*). Pyrolysis studies on model aromatic sulfur compounds. *Carbon*, **17**, 471–7.

Greinke, R. A. and Lewis, I. C. (1979*b*). A study of sulfur evolution during carbonization of thiophenes. *Carbon*, **14**, 415–16.

Grice, H. W., Yates, M. L. and David, D. J. (1970). Response characteristics of the melpar flame photometric detector. *J. Chromatogr. Sci.*, **8**, 90–4.

Grimmer, G. (1979). In '*Berichte 1/79 Luftqualitätkriterien für ausgewählte polycyclische aromatische Kohlenwasserstoffe*' (Umweltbundesamt, ed.). Erich Schmidt Verlag, Berlin.

Grimmer, G. (1982). Bilanzierung der krebserzeugenden Wirkung von Emissionen aus Kraftfahrzeugen und Kohleöfen mit carcinogen-spezifischen Testen. *Funkt. Biol. Med.*, **1**, 29–38.

Grimmer, G. (ed.) (1983). *Environmental Carcinogens: Polycyclic Aromatic Hydrocarbons*, 261 pp. Boca Raton/Florida, CRC Press.

Grimmer, G. and Böhnke, H. (1976). Anreicherung und gaschromatographische Profil-Analyse der polyclischen aromatischen Kohlenwasserstoffe in Schmieröl. *Chromatographia*, **9**, 30–40.

Grimmer, G. and Böhnke, H. (1978). Polyclische aromatische Kohlenwasserstoffe und Heterocyclen-Beziehung zum Reifegrad von Erdölen des Gifhorner Troges (Nordwestdeutschland). *Erdöl und Kohle*, **31**, 272–6.

Grimmer, G. and Glaser, A. (1975). Massenspektrometrische Untersuchungen von PAH aus Schmieröldestillatschnitten. EKEP-Synopse 75056. *Erdöl und Kohle-Erdgas-Petrochem.*, **28**, 570.

Grimmer, G. and Naujack, K.-W. (1979). Gaschromatographische Profilanalyse der polyclischen aromatischen Kohlenwasserstoffe im Wasser. *Vom Wasser*, **53**, 1–8.

Grimmer, G., Böhnke, H. and Borwitzki, H. (1978*a*). Gaschromatographische

Profilanalyse der polycyclischen aromatischen Kohlenwasserstoffe in Klärschlammproben. *Fresenius Z. Anal. Chem.*, **289**, 91–5.

Grimmer, G., Böhnke, H. and Glaser, A. (1978*b*). Investigation on the Carcinogenic Burden by Air Pollution in Man. XV. Polycyclic Aromatic Hydrocarbons in Automobile Exhaust Gas – An Inventory. *Zbl. Bakt. Hyg., I. Abt. Orig. B.*, **164**, 218–34.

Grimmer, G., Hilge, G. and Niemitz, W. (1980*a*). Vergleich der polycyclischen aromatischen Kohlenwasserstoff-Profile von Klärschlammproben aus 25 Kläranlagen. *Vom Wasser*, **54**, 255–72.

Grimmer, G., Naujack, K.-W. and Schneider, D. (1980*b*). Changes in PAH-profiles in different areas of a city during the year. In '*Polynuclear Aromatic Hydrocarbons: Chemistry and Biological effects*' (A. Bjørseth and A. J. Dennis, eds.). Columbus/Ohio, Battelle Press, pp. 107–25.

Grimmer, G., Jacob, J. and Naujack, K.-W. (1981*a*). Profile of the polycyclic aromatic hydrocarbons from lubricating oils. Inventory by GCGC/MS – PAH in environmental materials, Part I. *Fresenius Z. Anal. Chem.*, **306**, 347–55.

Grimmer, G., Jacob, J., Naujack, K.-W. and Dettbarn, G. (1981*b*). Profile of polycyclic aromatic hydrocarbons from used engine oil – Inventory GCGC/MS. – PAH in environmental materials, Part 2. *Fresenius Z. Anal. Chem.*, **309**, 13–19.

Grimmer, G., Schneider, D. and Dettbarn, G. (1981*c*). Pollution of different rivers in the Federal Republic of Germany by polycyclic aromatic hydrocarbons. *Vom Wasser*, **56**, 131–44.

Grimmer, G., Dettbarn, G., Brune, H., Deutsch-Wenzel, R. and Misfeld, J. (1982). Quantification of the carcinogenic effect of polycyclic aromatic hydrocarbons in used engine oil by topical application onto the skin of mice. *Int. Arch. Occup. Environ. Health*, **50**, 95–100.

Grimmer, G., Jacob, J. and Naujack, K.-W. (1983*a*). Profile of the polycyclic aromatic compounds from crude oils. Part 3. Inventory by GCGC/MS – PAH in environmental materials. *Fresenius Z. Anal. Chem.*, **314**, 29–36.

Grimmer, G., Jacob, J., Naujack, K.-W. and Dettbarn, G. (1983*b*). Determination of polycyclic compounds emitted from browncoal-fired residential stoves by gas chromatography/mass spectrometry. *Anal. Chem.*, **55**, 892–900.

Grimmer, G., Brune, H., Deutsch-Wenzel, R., Naujack, K.-W., Misfeld, J. and Timm, J. (1983*c*). On the contribution of polycyclic aromatic hydrocarbons to the carcinogenic impact of automobile exhaust condensate evaluated by local application onto the mouse skin. *Cancer Lett.*, **21**, 105–13.

Grimmer, G., Brune, H., Deutsch-Wenzel, R., Dettbarn, G. and Misfield, J. (1984). Contribution of polycyclic aromatic hydrocarbons to the carcinogenic impact of gasoline engine exhaust condensate evaluated by implantation into the lungs of rats. *J. Natl. Canc. Inst.*, **72**, 733–9.

Grimmer, G., Jacob, J., Dettbarn, G. and Naujack, K.-W. (1985). Determination of polycyclic aromatic hydrocarbons, azaarenes, and thiaarenes emitted from coal-fired residential furnaces by gas chromatography/mass spectrometry. *Fresenius Z. Anal. Chem.*, **322**, 596–602.

Grimmer, G., Jacob, J., Naujack, K.-W., Dettbarn, G., Brune, H., Deutsch-Wenzel, R., Misfeld, J. and Timm, J. (1986). Contribution of polycyclic aromatic compounds to the carcinogenicity of flue gas from hard-coal fired residential furnaces and characterization of arenes (PAH), azaarenes, oxaarenes, and thiaarenes. In '*Polynuclear Aromatic Hydrocarbons: Chemistry, Characterization and Carcinogenesis* (M. Cooke and A. J. Dennis, eds.), pp. 359–70. Columbus-Richland, Battelle Press.

Grob, R. L. (ed.) (1985). *Modern Practice of Gas Chromatography*, 897pp. New York, John Wiley & Sons.

Groen, M. B. and Wynberg, H. (1971). Optical properties of some heterohelicenes. Absolute configuration. *J. Am. Chem. Soc.*, **93**, 2797–809.

242   *References*

Groen, M. B., Schadenberg, H. and Wynberg, H. (1971). Synthesis and resolution of some heterohelicenes. *J. Org. Chem.*, **36**, 2797–809.
Gronowitz, S. and Dahlgren, T. (1977). Benzodithiophenes. A general method of synthesis. *Chem. Ser.*, **12**, 57–67.
Grünbauer, H. J. M. and Wegener, J. W. M. (1983). The relation between chemical structure and mutagenic activity of some polycyclic aromatic sulfur heterocycles. *Toxicol. Environ. Chem.*, **6**, 225–9.
Gruenhaus, H., Pailer, M. and Stof, S. (1976). Improved synthesis of indenothiophenes. Part III. Synthesis of indenothiophene-2-carboxylic acids. *J. Heterocycl. Chem.*, **13**, 1161–3.
Guerin, M. R., Epler, J. L., Griest, W. H., Clark, B. R. and Rao, T. K. (1978). Polycyclic aromatic hydrocarbons from fossil fuels conversion processes. In *'Carcinogenesis Vol. 3: Polynuclear Aromatic Hydrocarbons'* (P. W. Jones and R. I. Freudenthal, eds.), pp. 21–33. New York, Raven Press.
Güsten, H., Klasinc, L. and Volkert, O. (1969). Molecular orbitalation on 1,2-difuryl- and 1,2-dithienylethylenes and their cyclization products, the benzodifurans and benzodithiophenes. *Z. Naturforsch.*, **24B**, 12–15.
Gundermann, K. D. and Fuhrmann, K. D. (1978). Hydrogen sulfide cracking from organic sulfur compounds in hydrogenated coal extracts. *Compend. Dtsch. Ges. Mineralölwiss. Kohlechem.*, **78/79**, 1125–35.
Gundermann, K. D., Ansteeg, H. P. and Glitsch, A. (1983). Proceedings of the International Conference on Coal Science, 631p, Pittsburgh.
Gverdtsiteli, D. D. and Litvinov, V. P. (1970a). Series of condensed heteroatomic systems including a thiophene ring. 15. Preparation of and some reactions of benzo[b]naphtho[2,3-d]thiophene. *Izv. Akad. Nauk. SSR, Ser. Khim.*, **6**, 1340–4.
Gverdtsiteli, D. D. and Litvinov, V. P. (1970b). Thiophene-ring containing heterocyclic condensed systems. Synthesis of isomeric anthrabenzothiophenes. *Soobshch. Akad. Nauk. Gruz. SSR*, **58**, 333–6.
Gverdtsiteli, D. D. and Litvinov, V. P. (1970c). Structure of the products of cyclization and subsequent reduction of the o-(2-dibenzothenoyl)benzoic acid. *Soobshch. Akad. Nauk. Gruz. SSR*, **59**, 333–6.
Hansch, C., Schmidhalter, B., Reiter, F. and Saltonstall, W. (1956). Catalytic synthesis of heterocycles. VIII. Dehydrocyclization of o-ethylbenzenethiols to thianaphthenes. *J. Org. Chem.*, **21**, 265–70.
Hanson, R. L., Carpenter, R. L., Weisman, S. H. and Newton, G. J. (1977). Organic characterization of effluents from fluidized bed combustion of coals. *Ann. Rep. Inhalation Toxicol. Res. Inst.* (Lovelace Biomed. Environ. Res. Inst.), 1976–1977, pp. 235–42.
Hanson, R. L., Carpenter, R. L. and Newton, G. J. (1980). Chemical characterization of polynuclear aromatic hydrocarbons in airborne effluents from an experimental fluidized bed combustor. In *'Polynuclear Aromatic Hydrocarbons: Chemistry and Biological Effects* (A. Bjørseth and A. J. Dennis, eds.), pp. 599–616. Columbus/Ohio, Battelle Press.
Hanus, V. and Čermák, V. (1959). Note on the mass spectra of alkylthiophenes, and the structure of the ion $C_5H_5S^+$. *Coll. Czech. Chem. Commun.*, **24**, 1602–7.
Hart, H. and Sasaoka, M. (1978). Exocyclic benzenes. Synthesis and properties of benzo[1,2-c:3,4-c':5,6-c']thiophene, a tristhiahexaradialene. *J. Am. Chem. Soc.*, **100**, 4326–7.
Hartough, H. D. and Meisel, S. L. (1954). *Compounds with Condensed Thiophene Rings* (A. Weisburger, ed.). New York, J. Wiley (Interscience).
Hartwell, J. L. (1951). Survey of compounds tested for carcinogenic activity. U.S. Public Health Service.
Hasanen, E., Pohjola, V., Pyysalo, H. and Wickstrom, K. (1984). Polycyclic aromatic hydrocarbons in Finnish sauna air. *Sci. Total Environ.*, **37**, 223–31.

Hastings, S. H., Johnson, B. H. and Lumpkin, H. E. (1956). Analysis of the aromatic fraction of virgin gas oils by mass spectrometer. *Anal. Chem.*, **28**, 1243–7.

Hauptmann, S., Scholz, M. and Köhler, H. J. (1969). Synthesis and substitution reactions of acenaphtho[1,2-*b*]thiophene and 1-methylacenaphtho[1,2-*b*]pyrrole. *J. Prakt. Chem.*, **311** 614–20.

Hawthorne, D. G. and Porter, Q. N. (1966). Naphtho[1,8-*bc*]thiophenes. I. Syntheses. *Austr. J. Chem.*, **19**, 1909–25.

Hayatsu, R., Scot, R. G., Moore, L. P. and Studier, M. H. (1975). Aromatic units in coal. *Nature*, **257**, 378–80.

Heckman, R. C. (1959). Phosphorescence studies of some heterocyclic and related organic compounds. *J. Mol. Spectr.*, **2**, 27–41.

Heit, M. and Tan, Y. L. (1979). The concentrations of selected polynuclear aromatic hydrocarbons in the surface sediments of some fresh and marine waters of the United States. *Environ. Meas. Lab. Environ. Q.* (U.S. Dep. Energy), EML-353, I-3-I-39.

Herbes, S. E. and Risi, G.F. (1978). Metabolic alteration and excretion of anthracene by *Daphnia pulex. Bull. Environ. Contam. Toxicol.*, **19**, 147–55.

Herkstroeter, W. G. and Schultz, A. G. (1984). Direct observation of metastable intermediates in the photochemical ring closure of 2-naphthyl vinyl sulfides. *J. Am. Chem. Soc.*, **106**, 5553–9.

Herlan, A. (1974). Polycyclische aromatische Kohlenwasserstoffe in der Luft. Quantitative massenspektrometrische Bestimmung. *Erdöl, Kohle, Erdgas, Petrochem.*, **27**, 138–45.

Herlan, A. (1978). On the formation of polycyclic aromatics: Investigation of fuel oil and emissions by resolution mass-spectrometry. *Combustion and Flame*, **31**, 297–307.

Herlan, A. and Mayer, J. (1979). Polycyclische Aromaten in Verbrennungsgasen aus Öl- und Gasfeuerungen. *GWF Gas/Erdgas*, **120**, 82–9.

Herzschuh, R. and Paasivirta, J. (1983). Qualitative and quantitative determination of petroleum constituents in mussels and fishes of the Baltic Sea. *Instr. Anal. Toxicol. (Haupt. Vortr. Symp.)*, 201–10.

Hess, B. A. Jr. and Schaad, L. J. (1973). Hueckel molecular orbital π-resonance energies. Heterocycles containing divalent sulfur. *J. Am. Chem. Soc.*, **95**, 3907–12.

Hinsberg, O. (1910). Synthetische Versuche mit Thiodiglykolsäure. *Chem. Ber.*, **43**, 901–6.

Hites, R. A., Yu, M. L. and Thilly, W. G. (1981). Compounds associated with diesel exhaust particulates. In '*Chemical Analysis and Biological Fate: Polynuclear Aromatic Hydrocarbons*' (M. Cooke and A. J. Dennis, eds.), pp. 445–66. Columbus/Ohio, Battelle Press.

Ho, T. L. and Wong, C. M. (1975). Facile reduction of sulfoxides with sodium bis(2-methoxy)aluminium hydride. *Org. Prep. Proced. Int.*, **7**, 163–4.

Ho, T. Y., Rogers, M. A., Drushel, H. V. and Koons, C. B. (1975). Evolution of sulfur compounds in crude oils. *Am. Assoc. Petr. Geol. Bull.*, **58**, 2338–48.

Hoffman, E. J., Mills, G. L., Latimer, J. S. and Quinn, J. G. (1984). Urban runoff as a source of polycyclic aromatic hydrocarbons to coastal waters. *Environ. Sci. Technol.*, **18**, 580–7.

Holstein, W. and Severin, D. (1982). Characterization of a heavy coal liquification product by combined high-performance liquid chromatography/mass spectrometry. *Chromatographia*, **15**, 231–5.

Horner, C. J., Saris, L. E., Lakshmikantam and Cava, M. P. (1976). The formation of thiophenes by a base-catalyzed sulfoxide dehydration. *Tetrahedron Lett.*, 2581–4.

Horton, A. W. (1949). The mechanism of the reaction of hydrocarbons with sulfur. *J. Org. Chem.*, **14**, 761–70.

Horton, A. W., Burton, M. J., Tye, R. and Bingham, E. (1963). Composition versus carcinogenicity of distillate oils. *Am. Chem. Soc. Div. of Petrol Chemistry Preprints*, **8**, No. 4c, 59–63.

244   *References*

Horton, A. W., Bingham, E. L., Burton, M. J. G. and Tye, R. (1965). Carcinogenesis of the skin. III. The contribution of elemental sulfur and of organic compounds. *Cancer Res.*, **25**, 1759–63.

Howard, A. G. and Mills, G. A. (1983). Identification of polynuclear aromatic hydrocarbons in diesel particulate emissions. *Int. J. Environ. Anal. Chem.*, **14**, 43–53.

Hung, I. F. and Bernier, A. (1983). Polymer adsorbents in sampling and analysis of polycyclic aromatic hydrocarbons. *J. Environ. Health*, Part A, 445–54.

Hunt, D. F. and Shabanowitz, J. (1982). Determination of organosulfur compounds in hydrocarbon matrixes by collision activated dissociation mass spectrometry. *Anal. Chem.*, **54**, 574–8.

Hutchins, S. R. and Ward, C. H. (1984). A predicative laboratory study of trace organic contamination of groundwater: preliminary results. *J. Hydrol. (Amsterdam)*, **67**, 223–33.

International Agency for Research on Cancer (IARC) (1979). *Environmental Carcinogens Selected Methods of Analysis, vol. 3. Analysis of polycyclic aromatic hydrocarbons in environmental samples.* IARC Publ. No. 29 (Egan, H., Castegnaro, M., Bogovski, P., Kunte, H. and Walker, E. A., eds.), 240pp. Lyon.

Ibe, A., Nishijima, M., Saito, K., Kamimura, J., Ochiai, S., Nagayama, T., Ushiyama, H. and Naoi, Y. (1978). Hydrocarbons from petroleum in foods. III. Contents of hydrocarbons, 3,4-benzopyrene and organic sulfur compounds in shellfish from Tokyo Bay. *Tokyo Toritsu Eisei Kenkyusho Kenkyu Nempo*, **29**, 238–43.

Iddon, B. (1972). Benzo[c]thiophenes. *Adv. Heterocycl. Chem.*, **14**, 331–81.

Iddon, B. and Scrowston, R. M. (1970). Recent advances in the chemistry of benzo(b)thiophene. *Adv. Heterocycl. Chem.*, **11**, 177–381.

Iddon, B., Suschitzky, H. and Taylor, D. S. (1974). Condensed thiophene ring systems. XVII. New synthesis of 10H-indeno[1,2-b][1]benzothiophene. *J. Chem. Soc.*, Perkin Trans. 1, **21**, 2505–8.

Iglamova, N. A., Mazitova, F. N. and Brodskii, E. S. (1982). Mass-spectrometric study of petroleum sulfones. *Neftekhimiya*, **22**, 407–11.

Imanaka, M., Matsunaga, K., Saito, N. and Hata, H. (1980). Determination of pollutants in sediment. 6. Identification of the major peaks in the organosulfur compounds-containing fraction. *Okayama Ken Kankyo Hoken Senta Nempo*, **4**, 84–8.

Institute of Organic Synthesis. Academy of Sciences, Latvian S.S.R. (by M. G. Voronkov and V. Uridis (1966). Thianaphtheno[2,3-b]thianaphthene and its derivatives.

IUPAC – International Union of Pure and Applied Chemistry (1979). Nomenclature of Organic Chemistry. Sections A, B, C, D, E, F and H (S. P. Rigaudy and S. P. Klesney, eds.), 559pp. Pergamon Press.

Ismail, A. F. A. and El-Shafei, Z. M. (1957). Photodehydration photooxidation of some thermochromic ethylenes and related compounds. *J. Chem. Soc.*, 3393–6.

Iwai, I. and Ide, J. (1964). Acetylenic compounds. XXXVIII. The novel cyclization reaction of diacetylenic compounds to naphthalene derivatives involving prototropic rearrangement. *Chem. Pharm. Bull. (Tokyo)*, **12**, 1094–100.

Iwao, M., Lee, M. L. and Castle, R. N. (1980). Synthesis of phenanthro[b]thiophenes. *J. Heterocycl. Chem.*, **17**, 1259–64.

Jacob, G. and Cagniant, P. (1969). 6,7-Dihydro-8H-cyclopenta[6,7]naphtho[2,1-b]-thiophene and its 5-methyl derivative. *Compt. Rend. Acad. Sci. Paris Sér. C*, **268**, 194–6.

Jacob, G. and Cagniant, D. (1977). Synthesis of sulfur or oxygen-analogs of 6,7,8,12,13,14,16,17-octahydro-12-oxo-15H-cyclopenta[a]phenanthrene and some of their methylated derivatives. *Compt. Rend. Hebd. Séances Acad. Sci. Sér. C*, **284**, 373–5.

Jacob, J. (1986). Unpublished results.

Jacob, J. and Grimmer, G. (1979). Nomenclature and structure of polycyclic aromatic hydrocarbons. In '*Environmental Carcinogens Selected Methods of Analysis*, vol. 3'.

Analysis of polycyclic aromatic hydrocarbons in environmental samples. IARC Publ. No. 29, pp. 15–30. Lyon.

Jacob, J., Schmoldt, A., Raab, G., Hamann, M. and Grimmer, G. (1983). Induction of specific monooxygenases by isosteric heterocyclic compounds of benz[a]anthracene, benzo[c]phenanthrene and chrysene. *Cancer Lett.*, **20**, 341–8.

Jacob, J., Karcher, W., Grimmer, G., Schmoldt, A. and Hamann, M. (1986a). The influence of various monooxygenase inducers on rat liver microsomal chrysene oxidation. In *'Polynuclear Aromatic Hydrocarbons: Chemistry, Characterization and Carcinogenesis'* (M. Cooke and A. J. Dennis, eds.), pp. 417–26. Columbus/Ohio, Battelle Press.

Jacob, J., Schmoldt, A. and Grimmer, G. (1986b). The predominant role of S-oxidation in rat liver metabolism of thiaarenes. *Cancer Lett.*, **32**, 107–16.

Jacob, J., Mohtashamipur, E. and Norpoth, K. (1987a). Unpublished results.

Jacob, J., Schmoldt, A., Hamann, M., Raab, G. and Grimmer, G. (1987b). Monooxygenase induction by various xenobiotics and its influence on rat liver microsomal metabolism of chyrysene in comparison to benz[a]anthracene. *Cancer Lett.*, **34**, 91–102.

Jacquignon, P., Croisy, A., Ricci, A. and Balucani, D. (1973). Thiophene derivatives. XXII. Preparation of naphtho[2′,3′:4,5]-thieno[3,2-b][1]benzothiophene and some methyl homologs. *J. Chem. Soc.*, Perkin Trans., **1**, 734–5.

Jaeger, L. and Karrer, P. (1963). Dehydration of eschscholtzxanthin to rhodoxanthin. *Helv. Chim. Acta*, **46**, 687.

Jakubczyk, M. and Rabczuk, A. (1979). Removal of thiophene from naphthalene by column crystallization. *Koks, Smola, Gaz*, **24**, 156–8.

Jindal, S. L. and Tilak, B. D. (1969). Synthesis of sulfur heterocyclics. VII. Cationoid. *Indian J. Chem.*, **7**, 637–42.

Jogdeo, P. S. and Bhide, G. V. (1979). Total synthesis of heterocyclic steroids. Part II. Synthesis of +/-17-thia-3-methoxy-8, 14β-estra-1,3,5(10)-triene 17-dioxide. *Steroids*, **34**, 619–29.

Johansen, G. N. (1977). Use of a flame photometric detector with glass open tubular column, for analysis of sulfur compounds in petroleum products. *Chromatogr. Newsletter*, **5**, 37–9.

Jones, D. N., Helmy, E. and Edmonds, A. C. F. (1970). Steroidal sulfur compounds. VII. Pyrolysis and chiroptical properties of 3-alkylsulfinyl-5a-cholestanes. *J. Chem. Soc. C.*, 833–41.

Jones, D. W., Mattews, R. S. and Bartle, K. D. (1974). Indeterminateness from iterative analyses of four-spin NMR spectra with small δ_{AB}. Benzo[b]fluoranthene and dibenzothiophenes. *Spectrochim. Acta A.*, **30A**, 489–501.

Joyce, W. F. and Uden, P. C. (1983). Isolation of thiophenic compounds by argentation liquid chromatography. *Anal. Chem.*, **55**, 540–3.

Kaimai, T. and Matsunaga, A. (1978). Determination of sulfur compounds in high-boiling petroleum distillates by ligand-exchange thin-layer chromatography. *Anal. Chem.*, **50**, 268–70.

Kaishev, K. I., Iordanov, I. Z. and Anfreev, S. (1961). Usability of diesel oil from tulen petroleum in stationary engines. *Godishnik Khim.-Tekhnol. Inst.*, **8**, 135–49.

Kauralova, E. N., Gal'pern, G. D., Aristova, L. D., Bardina, T. A. and Korshunova, K. (1965). Chromatographic isolation of sulfoxides from oxidized distillates of sulfur-containing petroleums. *Neftekhimiya*, **5**, 753–9.

Karcher, W., Depaus, R., Van Eijk, J. and Jacob, J. (1979). Separation and identification of sulfur-containing polycyclic aromatic hydrocarbons (thiophene derivatives) from some PAH. In *'Polynuclear Aromatic Hydrocarbons'* (P. W. Jones and P. Leber, eds.), pp. 341–56. Ann Arbor/Michigan Ann Arbor Science.

Karcher, W., Nelen, A., Depaus, R., Van Eijk, J., Glaude, P. and Jacob, J. (1981). New results in the detection, identification and mutagenic testing of heterocyclic polycyclic aromatic hydrocarbons. In *'Chemical Analysis and Biological Fate: Polynuclear Aromatic Hydrocarbons* (M. Cooke and A. J. Dennis, eds.), pp. 317–27. Columbus/Ohio, Battelle Press.

Karcher, W., Fordham, R. J., Nelen, A., Depaus, R., Dubois, J. and Glaude, P. (1982). Molecular spectra of polycyclic aromatic hydrocarbons. In *'Polynuclear Aromatic Hydrocarbons: Physical and Biological Chemistry* (M. Cooke, A. J. Dennis, G. L. Fisher, eds.), pp. 405–16. Columbus/Ohio, Battelle Press.

Karcher, W., Fordham, R. J. and Jacob, J. (1983). The certification of polycyclic aromatic compounds, Part IV: BCR references materials Nos. 133, 134, 135, 136, 137, 138, 139 and 140. Comm. Eur. Communities EUR 1983, EUR 8497, 42 pp.

Karcher, W., Fordham, R. J., Dubois, J. J., Glaude, P. G. J. M. and Ligthart, J. A. M. (1985). *Spectral Atlas of Polycyclic Aromatic Compounds.* Dordrecht/Boston/Lancaster. D. Reidel Publishing Co., 818 pp.

Kargi, F. and Robinson, J. M. (1984). Microbial oxidation of dibenzothiophene by the thermophilic organism *Sulfolobus acidocaldarius*. *Biotechnol. Bioeng.*, **26**, 687–90.

Kaschani, D. T. (1983). Determination and recovery rates of polycyclic aromatic hydrocarbons (PAH) in samples with diesel soot content. *Staub-Reinhalt. Luft*, **43**, 72–4.

Katti, S. S., Westerman, D. W. B., Gates, B. C., Youngless, T. and Petrakis, T. (1984). Catalytic hydroprocessing of SRC-II heavy distillate fractions. 3. Hydrodesulfurization of the neutral oils. *Ind. Eng. Chem. Process. Des. Dev.*, **23**, 773–8.

Katz, M., Sakuma, T. and Tosine, H. (1978) (publ. 1980). Chromatographic and spectral analysis of polycyclic aromatic hydrocarbons in the air and water environments. *Environ. Sci. Res.*, 121–9.

Kazarova, V., Zhurovski, D. and Atanasov, K. (1979). Composition and quality of naphthalene produced in the by-product coke industry. *Khim. Ind. (Sofia)*, **51**, 309–11.

Kekin, N. A., Krupskii, K. N. and Gryzlov, A. V. (1978). Mass spectrometric analysis of by-product coke industry high-boiling products. *Zavod. Lab.*, **44**, 979–82.

Kemena, A., Norpoth, K. H. and Jacob, J. (1985) (publ. 1987). Differential induction of monooxygenase isoenzymes in mouse liver microsomes by polycyclic aromatic hydrocarbons. In: *'Polynuclear Aromatic Hydrocarbons: A Decade of Progress'* (M. Cooke and A. J. Dennis, eds.), pp. 449–60. Columbus-Richland, Battelle-Press.

Kennedy, R. J. and Stock, A. M. (1960). The oxidation of organic substances by potassium peroxymonosulfate. *J. Org. Chem.*, **25**, 1901–6.

Kharitonova, O. P. (1963). Absorption and luminescence spectra of thionaphthene in the near ultraviolet. *Opt. i Spectroskopya*, **1**, 77–83.

Kharchenko, V. G. and Krupina, T. I. (1967). Synthesis of hydrothioxanthenes. *Khim. Geterotsikl. Soedin*, 468–70.

Kipot, S. N., Rok, A. A. and Kekin, N. A. (1980). Mass-spectrometric method for the analysis of high-grade anthracene. *Koks Khim.*, 44–7.

Kira, S., Izumi, T. and Ogata, M. (1983). Detection of dibenzothiophene in mussel, *Mytilus edulis*, as a marker of pollution by organosulfur compounds in a marine environment. *Bull. Environ. Contam. Toxicol.*, **31**, 518–25.

Kishi, M. and Komeno, T. (1971). Thiosteroids. XXIX. Steroidal transannular 2a-, 5a-episulfides. 3. Synthesis of A-nor-3-thia- and A-nor-3-oxasteroids. *Tetrahedron*, **27**, 1527–43.

Klemm, L. H. (1982). Syntheses of tetracyclic and pentacyclic condensed thiophene systems. *Adv. Heterocycl. Chem.*, **32**, 127–232.

Klemm, L. H. and Hsin, W. (1976). The insertion and extrusion of heterosulfur bridges. III. A useful chemical-chromatographic separation procedure. *J. Heterocycl. Chem.*, **13**, 1245–7.

Klemm, L. H. and Karchesy, J. J. (1978). The insertion and extrusion of heterosulfur bridges. VIII. Dibenzothiophene from biphenyl and derivatives. *J. Heterocycl. Chem.*, **15**, 561–3.

Klemm. L. H. and Lawrence, R. F. (1979). The insertion and extrusion of heterosulfur bridges. X. Conversions in the triphenyleno[4,5-*bcd*]thiophene system. *J. Heterocycl. Chem.*, **16**, 599–601.

Klemm, L. H., McCoy, D. R. and Olson, D. R. (1970). Condensed thiophenes from sulfur bridging. I. Phenanthro[4,5-*bcd*]thiophene. *J. Heterocycl. Chem.*, **7**, 1347–52.

Klemm, L. H., Karchesy, J. J. and Lawrence, R. F. (1978). The insertion and extrusion of heterosulfur bridges. IX. Sulfur bridging in 2-phenylnaphthalene. *J. Heterocycl. Chem.*, **15**, 773–5.

Klemm, L. H., Karchesy, J. J. and McCoy, D. R. (1979*a*). Polycyclic thiophenes from the direct insertion of heterosulfur bridges into vinylarenes, biaryls, and angularly condensed arenes. *Phosphorous Sulfur*, **7**, 9–22.

Klemm, L. H., Lee, F. H. W. and Lawrence, R. F. (1979*b*). Comparative chromatographic adsorbabilities of some azines, thiols and thieno pyridines, their heteroatom oxides and other derivatives on silica gel. *J. Heterocycl. Chem.*, **16**, 73–9.

Kochkanyan, R. O., Baranov, S. N. and Belova, G. I. (1974). Dibenzo[*d,f*]isothionaphthene derivates. USSR Pat. 425,909 CA 81:49559 (1974).

Kodama, K., Nakatani, S., Umehara, K., Shimizu, K., Minoda, Y. and Yamada, K. (1970). Microbial conversion of petro-sulfur compounds. III. Isolation and identification of products from dibenzothiophene. *Agr. Biol. Chem.*, **34**, 1320–4.

Kodama. K., Umehara, K., Shimizu, K., Nakatani, S., Minoda, Y. and Yamada, K. (1973). Microbial conversion of petrosulfur compounds. IV. Identification of microbial products from dibenzothiophene and its proposed oxidation pathways. *Agr. Biol. Chem.*, **37**, 45–50.

Koehler, M., Genz, I., Babenzien, H. D., Eckardt, V. and Hieke, W. (1978). Microbial degradation of organic sulfur compounds. *Z. Allg. Mikrobiol.*, **18**, 67–8.

Koenst, W. M. B., Van-Bruynsvoort, J. L., Speckamp, W. N. and Huisman, H. (1970). Heterocyclic steroids. XVII. Anomalous spiro- and aromatized 6-thiaestrogens. *Tetrahedron Lett.*, **29**, 2527–30.

Konar, A. (1984). Nonclassical selenothiophenes. *Chem. Ser.*, **23**, 53–63.

Kong, R. C., Lee, M. L., Tominaga, Y., Pratap, R., Iwao, M., Castle, R. N. and Wise, S. A. (1982). Capillary column gas chromatographic resolution of isomeric polycyclic aromatic sulfur heterocycles in a coal liquid. *J. Chromatogr. Sci.*, **20**, 502–10.

Kong, R. C., Lee, M. L., Tominaga, Y., Pratap, R., Thompson, R. D. and Castle, R. N. (1984). Determination of sulfur heterocycles in selected synfuels. *Fuel*, **63**, 702–8.

Koshelev, V. I. and Plakidin, V. I. (1973). Reaction of diethyl thiodiglycolate with acenaphthene-quinone and structure of the resulting compounds. *Zh. Org. Khim'.*, **9**, 597–601.

Kossmehl, G., Beimling, P. and Manecke, G. (1983). Polyarylenealkenylenes and polyheteroarylenealkenylenes. 14. Syntheses and characterization of poly(thieno[2′,3′:1,2]benzo[4,5-*b*]thiophene-2,6-divinylenearylenevinylenes), poly(4,8-dimethoxythieno[2′,3′:1.2]benzo[4,5-*b*]thiophene-2,6-divinylenearylenevinylenes) and some model components. *Makromol. Chem.*, **184**, 627–50.

Kruber, O. (1927). Biphenylensulfid im Steinkohlenteer. *Chem. Ber.*, **53**, 1566–7.

Kruber, O. and Grigoleit, G. (1954). Über neue Stoffe des Steinkohlenpechs. *Chem. Ber.*, **87**, 1895–905.

Kruber, O. and Raeithel, A. (1953). Coal-tar anthracene oil constituents. *Chem. Ber.*, **86**, 366–71.

Kruber, O. and Raeithel, A. (1954). Zur Kenntnis des Steinkohlenteer-Anthracenöls. *Chem. Ber.*, **87**, 1469–78.

Kruber, O. and Rappen, L. (1940). Über das lin. – Dibenzothionaphthen im Steinkohlenteer. *Chem. Ber.*, **73**, 1184–6.

Kudo, H., Tedjamulia, M. L., Castle, R. N. and Lee, M. L. (1984). Angular polycyclic thiophenes containing two thiophene rings. *J. Heterocycl. Chem.*, **21**, 185–92.

Kudo, H., Castle, R. N. and Lee, M. L. (1985). Synthesis of monoamino- and monohydroxydibenzothiophenes. *J. Heterocycl. Chem.*, **22**, 215–18.

Kuei, J. C., Shelton, J. I., Castle, L. W., Kong, R. C., Richter, B. E., Bradshaw, J. S. and Lee, M. L. (1984). Polarizable biphenyl polysiloxane stationary phase for capillary column gas chromatography. *High Resolut. Chromatogr. Commun.*, **7**, 13–18.

Kumanova, B. and Vasileva, R. (1983). Determination of polyaromatic hydrocarbons (PAH's) in the air of the work zone in coke chemical production. *Khig. Zdraveopaz.*, **26**, 346–9.

Kuras, M., Kubelka, V., Vodicka, L. and Mostecky, I. (1982). Mass spectrometric analysis of sulfur compounds in the middle fractions of Romaskino petroleum. *Ropa Uhlic.*, **24**, 10–20.

Kuwabara, K., Nakamura, A. and Kashimoto, T. (1980). Effect of petroleum oil, pesticides, PCBs and other environmental contaminants on the hatchability of *Artemia salina* dry eggs. *Bull. Environ. Contam. Toxicol.*, **25**, 69–74.

Kveseth, K., Sortland, B. and Bokn, T. (1982). Polycyclic aromatic hydrocarbons in sewage, mussels and tap water. *Chemosphere*, **11**, 623–39.

Lamberton, A. H. and Paine, R. E. (1976). 2-(2-naphthyl)benzo[*b*]thiophene. Part IV. Further aspects of electrophilic substitution and ring closures to yield pentacyclic derivatives. *J. Chem. Soc.*, Perkin Trans. **1**, 683–7.

Landa, S. and Mrnkova, A. (1966). Hydrogenation of organic sulfur compounds in the presence of MoS_2 as catalyst. *Sb. Vys. Sk. Chem.-Technol. Praze, Technol. Paliv*, **11**, 5–34.

Lang, K. F. and Eigen, I. (1967). Im Steinkohlenteer nachgewiesene organische Verbindungen. *Fortschr. Chem. Forsch.*, **8**, 91–170.

Lapouyade, R. and DeMayo, P. (1972). Photochemical synthesis. 44. Photocyclization of aromatic thioketones. *Can. J. Chem.*, **50**, 4068–9.

Later, D. W., Lee, M. L., Bartle, K. D., Kong, C. R. and Vassilaros, D. L. (1981). Chemical class separation and characterization of organic compounds in synthetic fuels. *Anal. Chem.*, **53**, 1612–20.

Later, D. W., Wright, C. W., Loening, K. L. and Merritt, J. E. (1984). Systematic nomenclature of the nitrogen, oxygen, and sulfur functional polycyclic aromatic compounds. In: '*Polynuclear Aromatic Hydrocarbons: Chemistry, Characterization and Carcinogenesis*' (M. Cooke and A. J. Dennis, eds), pp. 451–71. Columbus-Richland, Battelle-Press.

Lawrence, G. W. (1971). Chemistry of 14*H*-dibenzo[*a,j*]xanthyl, 14*H*-dibenzo[*a,j*]-thioxanthyl, and 14*H*-dibenzo[*a,j*]thioxanthyl-7,7-dioxide systems. Avail. Univ. Microfilms, Ann Arbor. Mich., Order No. 72–15, 239 From Diss. Abstr. Int. B 1972, **32m**, 6301.

Lawson, J., DuVernet, R. and Boekelheide, V. (1973). Synthesis of a bridged [18]annulene. *J. Am. Chem. Soc.*, **93**, 956–7.

Lee, M. L. and Hites, R. A. (1976). Characterization of sulfur-containing polycyclic compounds in carbon blacks. *Anal. Chem.*, **48**, 1890–3.

Lee, M. L. and Wright, B. W. (1980). Capillary column gas chromatography of polycyclic aromatic compounds: A review. *J. Chromatogr. Sci.*, **18**, 345–58.

Lee, M. L., Prado, G. P., Howard, J. B. and Hites, R. A. (1977). Source identification of urban airborne polycyclic aromatic hydrocarbons by gas chromatographic mass spectrometry and high resolution mass spectrometry. *Biomed. Mass Spectrum.*, **4**, 182–6.

Lee, M. L., Willey, C., Castle, R. N. and White, C. M. (1980). Separation and identification of sulfur heterocycles in coal-derived products. In '*Polynuclear Aromatic Hydrocarbons: Chemical and Biological Effects*' (A. Bjørseth, A. J. Dennis eds), pp. 59–73. Columbus/Ohio, Battelle Press.

Lee, M. L., Novotny, M. V. and Bartle, K. D. (eds.) (1981). *Analytical Chemistry of Polycyclic Aromatic Compounds*, 462pp. New York, Academic Press.

Lee, M. L., Vassilaros, D. L. and Later, D. W. (1982). Capillary column gas chromatography of environmental polycyclic aromatic compounds. *Int. J. Environ. Anal. Chem.*, **11**, 251–62.

Lee, M. L., Kuei, J. C., Adams, N. W., Tarbet, B. J., Nishioka, M., Jones, B. A. and Bradshaw, J. S. (1984). Polarizable polysiloxane stationary phases for capillary column gas chromatography. *J. Chromatogr.*, **302**, 303–18.

Le Guillanton, G. (1966). Utilization of 2-cyclopentylidenecyclopentanone in the preparation of decahydro- and hexahydro-as-indacene derivatives. IV. Condensation of 1,1-cyclopentenyl with low reactivity dienophiles. *Bull. Soc. Chim. France*, 1702–6.

Lentz, R. W., Handlovits, C. E. and Smith, H. A. (1962). Phenylene sulfide polymers. III. The synthesis of linear polyphenylene sulfide. *J. Polymer. Sci.*, **58**, 351–67.

Litvinov, V. P., Ferapontov, V. A., Gverdtsiteli, D. D. and Ostapenko, E. G. (1973). Condensed heteroatomic systems including a thiophene ring. XXII. Gas-chromatograpic behaviour of polycondensed heteroatomic compounds in an isothermal system. *Khim. Geterotsikl. Soedin.*, 188–95.

Locati, G., Fantuzzi, A., Consonn, G., Ligotti, I. and Bonomi, G. (1979). *Am. Ind. Hyg. Assoc. J.*, **40**, 644–652.

Loening, K. T. and Merritt, J. E. (1983). Some aids for naming polycyclic aromatic hydrocarbons and their heterocyclic analogs. In '*Polynuclear Aromatic Hydrocarbons: Formation, Metabolism, and Measurement*' (M. Cooke and A. J. Dennis, eds.), pp. 819–43. Columbus/Ohio, Battelle Press.

Lohinska-Gasowska, A., Badora, K. and Muszynski, J. (1979). Sulfur compounds in heavy distillate from the Romashkino crude oil. *Nafta(Katowice)*, **35**, 384–8.

Lu, P. Y., Metcalf, R. L. and Carlson, E. M. (1978). Environmental fate of five radiolabeled coal conversion by-products evaluated in a laboratory ecosystem. *Environ. Health Persp.*, **24**, 201–8.

Lucas, H. J. and Kennedy, E. R. (1955). Iodobenzene dichloride. *Org. Synth. Coll.* Vol. III. 482–3.

Lucke, R. B., Later, D. W., Wright, C. W., Chess, E. K. and Weimer, W. C. (1985). Integrated multiple-stage chromatographic method for the separation and identification of polycyclic aromatic hydrocarbons in complex coal liquids. *Anal. Chem.*, **37**, 633–9.

Lüttringhaus, A. and Kolb, A. (1961). Thioaromatics. V. 9-Thiaphenanthrenium perchlorate. *Z. Naturforsch.*, **16b**, 762–3.

Lumpkin, H. E. (1964). Analysis of trinuclear aromatic petroleum fraction by high resolution mass spectrometry. *Anal. Chem.*, **36**, 2399–401.

Lunden, L., Ahling, B. and Edner, S. (1982). Emissions from incineration of combustible fractions of domestic wastes. *Inst. Vatten-Luft-vardsforsk.* Publ. B IVL B 674, 44pp.

Lyapina, N. K., Parfenova, M. A., Nikitina, T. S., Brodskii, E. S. and Ulendeeva, A. U. (1980a). Composition and structure of organosulfur compounds of a 410–450° distillate of western surgut petroleum. *Neftkhimiya*, **20**, 747–52.

Lyapina, N. K., Parfenova, M. A., Nikitina, T. S., Brodskii, E. S. and Ulendeeva, A. U. (1980b). Composition and structure of organosulfur compounds of a 360°–410° distillate of western surgut petroleum. *Neftkhimiya*, **20**, 619–24.

Lyapina, N. K., Parfenova, M. A., Nikitina, V. S., Vol'tsov, A. A. and Mel'nikova, L. A. (1982). Organosulfur compounds of sulfuric acid concentrates. *Khim. Tekhnol. Topl. Masel*, 27–31.

Lygren, E., Gjessing, E. and Berglind, L. (1984). Pollution transport from a high way. *Sci. Total. Environ.*, **33**, 147–59.

MacDowell, D. W. H. and Childers, R. L. (1962). 4-5-Diethylphenanthrene-9,10-dicarboxylic acid anhydride. *J. Org. Chem.*, **27**, 2630–1.

MacDowell, D. W. H. and Jeffries, A. T. (1970). Chemistry of indenothiophenes. II. 4H-Indeno[1,2-b]thiophene and 8H-indeno[1,2-c]thiophenes. *J. Org. Chem.*, **35**, 871–5.

MacDowell, D. W. H. and Maxwell, M. H. (1970). Thiophene analogs of phenanthrene. I. Benzo[1,2-*c*:3,4-*c'*]dithiophene. *J. Org. Chem.*, **35**, 799–801.

MacDowell, D. W. H. and Patrick, T. B. (1967*a*). The chemistry of indenothiophenes. I. 8*H*-Indeno[2,1-*b*]thiophene. *J. Org. Chem.*, **32**, 2441–5.

MacDowell, D. W. H. and Patrick, T. B. (1967*b*). 5*H*,7*H*-Bisindeno[2,3-*b*:3',2'-*d*]thiophene. *J. Heterocycl. Chem.*, **4**, 425–6.

MacDowell, D. W. H. and Wisowaty, J. C. (1972). Thiophene analogs of anthraquinone. *J. Org. Chem.*, **37**, 1712–17.

MacDowell, D. W. H., Jourdenais, R. A., Naylor, R. and Paulovicks, G. E. (1971). Synthesis and methalation of some phenalenothiophenes and a fused benzo derivative. *J. Org. Chem.*, **36**, 2683–9.

Mackie, P. R., Hardy, R., Whittle, K. J., Bruce, C. and McGill, A. S. (1980). The tissue hydrocarbon burden of mussels from various sites around the scottish coast. In 'Polynuclear Aromatic Hydrocarbons: Chemical Biological Effects' (A. Bjørseth, A. J. Dennis, eds.), pp. 379–93. Columbus/Ohio. Battelle Press.

Madison, J. J. and Roberts, R. M. (1958). Pyrolysis of aromatics and related heterocyclics. *Ind. Eng. Chem.*, **50**, 237–50.

Mallion, R. B. (1973). π-Electron ring current intensities in sulfur heterocyclic analogs of fluoranthene. *J. Chem. Soc.*, Perkin Trans., **2**, 235–7.

Manhas, M. S. and Rao, V. V. (1969). Synthesis of thieno- and furopyrimidinethiones. *J. Chem. Soc. C*, 1937–9.

Mark, V. (1962). 4,7-Methanoisobenzofurans and 4,7-methanoisobenzothiophenes. US pat. 3,256,299 (C.A. 65: P5444b).

Martin, G. E., Smith, S. L., Layton, W. J., Willcott, M. R. III, Iwao, M., Lee, M. L. and Castle, R. N. (1983). Assignment of the proton and carbon-13 NMR spectra of phenanthro[1,2-*b*]thiophene through the concerted application of two-dimensional NMR spectroscopic techniques. *J. Heterocycl. Chem.*, **20**, 1367–81.

Martin, R. L. and Grant, J. A. (1965*a*). Determination of sulfur-compound distributions in petroleum samples by gas chromatography with a coulometric detector. *Anal. Chem.*, **37**, 644–9.

Martin, R. L. and Grant, J. A. (1965*b*). Determination of thiophenic compounds by types in petroleum samples. *Anal. Chem.*, **37**, 649–57.

Marty, A. and Viallet, P. (1974). Active vibrational symmetry in the fluorescence and phosphorescence spectra of carbazol, dibenzofuran, and dibenzothiophene. *J. Photochem.*, **3**, 133–42.

Maruyama, K., Mitsui, K. and Otsuki, T. (1977). Photochemical synthesis of new sulfur-containing polycyclic aromatic compounds – anthra[2,1-*b*]thiophene. *Chem. Lett.*, **8**, 853–4.

Maruyama, K., Otsuki, T., Mitsui, K. and Tojo, M. (1980). Photochemical synthesis of heteroatom-containing polycyclic aromatic compounds. *J. Heterocycl.*, **17**, 695–700.

Masciantonio, P. S. and Walter, J. (1964). Pyrolysis of polycyclic compounds containing sulfur. In *Amer. Conf. on Coal Science*, p. 687. Pennsylvania State University.

Mattox, C. F. and Humenick, M. J. (1979). Organic groundwater contaminants from underground coal gasification. Proc. Underground Coal Convers. Symp., 5th, 281–94.

May, W. E., Wasik, S. P. and Freeman, D. W. (1978). Determination of the aqueous solubility of polynuclear aromatic hydrocarbons by a coupled column liquid chromatographic technique. *Anal. Chem.*, **50**, 175–9.

Mayer, F., Mombour, A., Lassmann, W., Werner, W., Landmann, P. and Schneider, E. (1931). Farbstoffstudien in der Thionaphtenreihe. *Liebigs Ann. Chem.*, **488**, 259–96.

Mayer, R. (1957). Pseudotropones of the type alpha- and gamma-pyrone, thia- and thiathiopyrone and the corresponding benzo-derivatives. 2,3:6,7-Dibenzotropo-1-thione. *Chem. Ber.*, **90**, 2362–9.

Mayer, R., Kleinert, J., Richter, S. and Gewald, K. (1962). Isonaphthene. *Ang. Chem.*, **74**, 118.

Mayer, R., Kleinert, H., Richter, S. and Gewald, K. (1963). Schwefelheterocyclen. XI. Isothionaphthen. *J. Prakt. Chem.*, **20**, 244–9.

McCall, E. B. (1953). 6,7,8,9-Tetrahydrodibenzothiophene and its associated compounds. *Brit. Pat.*, 701, 267.

McCarthy, L. V., Overton, E. B., Maberry, M. A., Antoine, S. A. and Laseter, J. L. (1981). Glass capillary gas chromatography with simultaneous flame ionization (FID) and Hall-element-specific (HECD) detection. *J. High Resolut. Chromatogr. Commun.*, **4**, 164–8.

McDonald, F. R. and Cook, G. L. (1967). Infrared vibrations of benzene rings in condensed thiophenes. U.S. Bur. Mines Rep. Invest. No. 6911, 25pp.

McFall, T., Booth, G. M., Lee, M. L., Tominaga, Y., Pratap, R., Tedjamulia, M. and Castle, R. N. (1984). Mutagenic activity of methyl-substituted tri- and tetracyclic aromatic sulfur heterocycles. *Mutat. Res.*, **135**, 97–103.

McKague, A. B. and Meier, H. P. (1984). Analysis of thianaphthene in commercial naphthalene. *J. Chromatogr.*, **299**, 487–8.

McKinnon, D. M. and Wong, J. Y. (1971). Preparation of some heterocyclic analogs of triptycene. *Can. J. Chem.*, **49**, 3178–84.

McNaught, A. D. (1976). The nomenclature of heterocycles. *Adv. Heterocycl. Chem.*, **20**, 175–319.

Melikadse, L. and Gverdtsiteli, D. D. (1975). Sulfur compounds of petroleum. *Izv. Akad. Nauk. Gruz. SSR, Ser. Khim.*, **1**, 49–53.

Mel'nikova, L. A., Karmanova, L. P., Lyapina, N. K. and Smarkalov, A. A. (1979). Study of organosulfur compounds of distillates of Yarega petroleum. *Neftekhimiya*, **19**, 273–7.

Mel'nikova, L. A., Lyapina, N. K. and Karmanova, L. P. (1980). Group structure composition of organo-sulfur compounds and hydrocarbons of a 200–236° distillate of Usinso petroleum. *Neftekhimiya*, **20**, 612–18.

Mel'nikova, L. A., Lyapina, N. K., Brodskii, E. S. and Karmanova, L. P. (1981). Organosulfur compounds and hydrocarbons of a 360–410° distillate of heavy Usinskaya petroleum. *Neftekhimiya*, **21**, 149–55.

Messerle, P. E. and Musina, T. K. (1976). Glass-reinforced plastics based on polyoxoarenes. *Otkrytiya, Izobret., Prom. Obraztsy, Tavarnye Znaki*, **58**, 62–3.

Meyerson, S. and Fields, E. K. (1968). Decomposition of dibenzothiophene and naphthothiophene under electron impact. *J. Org. Chem.*, **33**, 847–8.

Meyerson, S. and Vander Haar, R. W. (1962). Multiple charged organic ions in mass spectra. *J. Chem. Phys.*, **37**, 2458–62.

Mikes, F. and Boshart, G. (1978). Binaphthyl-2,2'-diyl hydrogen phosphate. A new chiral atropisomeric selector for the resolution of helicenes using high performance liquid chromatography. *J. Chem. Soc. Chem. Commun.*, 173–5.

Miki, Y. and Sugimoto, Y. (1983). Gas chromatographic analysis of hydrogenated anthracene oil. *Nippon Kagaku Kaishi*, 704–12.

Millar, I. T. and Wilson, K. V. (1964). Phenanthrene chemistry. Part III. 9,10-Phenanthraquinodimethane and 9,10-anthraquinodimethane. *J. Chem. Soc.*, 2121–7.

Mironov, D. G. and Shchekaturina, T. L. (1981). Accumulation of petroleum hydrocarbons in the Black Sea Crab *Eriphia verrucosa*. *Forskal. Biol. Nauki* (*Moscow*), 30–5.

Mitra, R. B. and Tilak, B. D. (1956a). Heterocyclic steroids. II. Synthesis of a thiophene analog of 3-deoxyestradiol. *J. Sci. Ind. Res.* (*India*), **15B**, 573–9.

Mitra, R. B. and Tilak, B. D. (1956b). Heterocyclic steroids. I. Synthesis of thiophene analog of 3-deoxyequilenin. *J. Sci. Ind. Res.* (*India*), **15B**, 497–505.

Mitra, R. B., Pandya, L. J. and Tilak, B. D. (1957). Thiophenes and thiopyrans. XVII:

Thieno[2,3-*b*]thianaphthene and thianaphtheno[2,3-*b*]thianaphthene. *J. Sci. Ind. Res. (India)*, **16B**, 348–54.

Mlochowski, J. and Skrzywan, B. (1969). Polycyclic sulfur compounds in coal tar (thionaphthene, dibenzothiophene, dibenzothionaphthenes). *Wiad. Chem.*, **23**, 259–79.

Moehnle, K., Krivan, V. and Grallath, E. (1984). Microtitrimetric determination of inorganic and organic sulfur in airborne dust. *Fresenius Z. Anal. Chem.*, **317**, 300–3.

Momicchioli, F. and Rastelli, A. (1970). Theoretical studies on the ultraviolet spectra of five-membered heterocycles. II. Systems isoelectronic with condensed aromatic hydrocarbons. *J. Chem. Soc. B*, 1353–8.

Moore, R. J. and Greensfelder, B. S. (1947). The catalytic synthesis of benzothiophene. *J. Am. Chem. Soc.*, **69**, 2008–9.

Morel, J. and Mollier, Y. (1965). Synthesis of some acenaphtheno[1,2-*b*]thiophenes. *Compt. Rend.*, **360**, 5300–1.

Mostecky, I. (1982). Application of mass spectrometric and chromatographic techniques for the analysis of sulfur compounds in petroleum fractions. *Sb. Vys. Sk. Chem.-Technol. Praze, Technol. Paliv*, **46**, 262–292.

Müller, E. and Beissner, C. (1972). Diin-reaktion mit Tris-(triphenylphosphin)-iridiumchlorid. *Chem. Ztg., App.*, **96**, 170.

Müller, E., Muhm, H. and Langer, E. (1971). Heteroacen- und Tetracen- chinonderivate aus Übergangsmetallkomplexen. XI. Mitteilung. *Chem. Ztg., App.*, **95**, 525–6.

Müller, E., Luppold, E. and Winter, W. (1975). Diyne reaction. XXXIV. Mono- and bis-heterocondensed benzoquinones. Benzofuro-, thiopheno-, selenopheno-, tellurophene-, pyrrolodibenzothiophenoquinones. *Chem. Ber.*, **108**, 237–43.

Muller, J. F. and Cagniant, P. (1968). Synthesis of benzo[*e*]naphtho[1,8-*bc*]thiopyran derivatives. *Compt. Rend. Acad. Sci. Paris Ser. C*, 1072–4.

Muller, D., Muller, J. F. and Cagniant, D. (1977). Synthesis of naphtho[1,2-*b*:8,7-*b'*]dithiophene. *J. Chem. Res.*, **12**, 328–9.

Munro, D. P. and Sharp, J. T. (1984). Electrocyclic aromatic substitution by the diazogroup. Part 5. The reaction of a-(2-arylthienyl)diazoalkanes. *J. Chem. Soc., Perkin Trans. 1*, 571–4.

Murayama, H. and Moriyama, N. (1982). Determination of sulfur-containing polycyclic aromatic hydrocarbons by FDP-GC and GC/MS. *Niigata-ken Kogai Kenkyusho Kenkyu Hokuku*, **6**, 93–5.

Murray, A. P., Gibbs, C. F. and Kavanagh, P. E. (1983). Estimation of total aromatic hydrocarbons in environmental samples by high pressure liquid chromatography. *Int. J. Environ. Anal. Chem.*, **16**, 167–95.

Murray, K. E., Shipton, J., Whitfield, F. B. and Last, J. H. (1976). The volatiles of off-flavored unblanched green peas (*Pisum sativium*). *J. Sci. Food Agric.*, **27**, 1093–107.

Murthy, T. S., Pandya, L. J. and Tilak, B. D. (1961). Thiophenes and thiapyrans. XXVI. Synthesis of condensed thiophenes from diaryls. *J. Sci. Ind. Res. (India)*, **20B**, 169–76.

Musmar, M. J., Gampe, R. T., Martin, G. E., Layton, W. J., Smith, S. L., Thompson, R. D., Iwao, M., Lee, M. L. and Castle, R. N. (1984). Combined application of auto-correlated(COSY) and homonuclear J-resolved two-dimensional NMR-spectra for the assignment of congested, non-first order spectra of polycyclic aromatic systems. Assignment of the proton NMR spectrum of benzo[2,3]phenanthro[4,5-*bcd*]thiophene and an investigation of long range proton-proton spin coupling constants. *J. Heterocycl. Chem.*, **21**, 225–33.

Nair, P. M. and Gogte, V. N. (1974). Proton chemical shifts in some condensed thiophenes. *Indian J. Chem.*, **12**, 589–96.

Nakamura, A. (1983). Studies on technology for environmental assessment. 2. Analysis and indexing on capillary column. *Osakafuritsu Koshu Eisei Kenkyusho Kenkyu Hokoku, Shokuhin Eisei Hen*, **14**, 69–73.

Nakamura, A. and Kashimoto, T. (1977). Contamination by organic sulfur compounds in marine products. *Shokuhin Eiseigaku Zasshi*, **18**, 252–9.

Nakamura, A. and Kashimoto, T. (1979a). Quantitation of sulfur containing oil compounds and polychlorinated biphenyls (PCBs) in sediments from waters of the Osaka Port area. *Arch. Environ. Contam. Toxicol.*, **8**, 563–71.

Nakamura, A. and Kashimoto, T. (1979b). Toxicological assessment of heavy oil and sulfur-containing oil components by various conventional biological tests. II. Studies on heavy oil components in food. *Shokuhin Eiseigaku Zasshi*, **20**, 161.

Nakamura, A., Kuwabara, K. and Kashimoto, T. (1979). Studies on crude oil components in food. 4. Uptake and discharge of sulfur containing oil compounds by shellfish. *Osaka-furitsu Koshu Eisei Kenkyusho Kenkyu Hokoku, Shokuhin Eisei Hen*, **10**, 137–40.

Nakasuji, K., Kubota, H., Kotani, T., Murata, I., Saito, G., Enoki, T., Imaeda, K., Inokuchi, H., Honda, M., Katayama, C. and Tanaka, J. (1986). Novel peri-condensed Weitz-type donors: Synthesis, physical properties and crystal structures of 3,10-dithiaperylene (DTPR), 1,6-dithiapyrene (DTPY), and some of their CT complexes. *J. Am. Chem. Soc.*, **108**, 3460–6.

Navivach, V. M., Gerasimenko, V. A., Ryabozad, A. S., Voitenko, B. I., Grumberg, L. R., Chernyshov, Y. A. and Shvarts, S. G. (1982). Gas-liquid chromatography study of the composition of impurities in by-product coke naphthalene. *Koks Khim.*, 37–40.

Nazarov, I. N., Gurvich, I. A. and Kuznetsova, A. I. (1953a). XXIII. Synthesis of sulfur analogs of steroidal compounds by diene condensation of cyclic γ-keto sulfones with bicyclic dienes. *Bull. Acad. Sci. U.S.S.R., Div. Chem. Sci.*, 1091–9.

Nazarov, I. N., Shmonina, L. I. and Torgov, I. V. (1953b). Synthesis of polycyclic compounds related to steroids. XXI. Condensation of 1-vinyl-9-methyl-1,6-hexahydronaphthalene with α,β-unsaturated cyclic ketones. Synthesis of steroid ketones with hydrogenated skeletons of cyclopentanophenanthrene and chrysene. *Bull. Acad. Sci. U.S.S.R., Div. Chem. Sci.*, 955–68.

Neff, J. M. (1979). *Polycyclic Aromatic Hydrocarbons in the Aquatic Environment: Sources, Fates and Biological Effects.* London Applied Science Publ. Ltd.

Neidlein, R. and Humburg, G. (1979). Heterocyclic 12π- and 14π-systems. VVIX. Reactivity in the 2-position nonsubstituted thiapseudophenalenones. *Chem. Ber.*, **112**, 349–54.

Nespoli, G. and Tiecco, M. (1966). Homolytic intramolecular arylation. II. Reaction of *o*-bromoaryl sulfides with Grignard salts and cobalt chloride. *Bol. Sci. Fac. Chim. Ind. Bologna, Suppl.*, **24**, 239–47.

Nesterenko, V. I., Alekseev, A. P. and Plyusnin, A. N. (1983). Composition of concentrates of petroleum heteroatomic compounds violated by complexing with titanium tetrachloride. *Neftekhimiya*, **23**, 604–9.

Newman, M. S. and Ihrman, K. G. (1958). The behaviour of *o*-aroylbenzoic acid types in acidic media. *J. Am. Chem. Soc.*, **80**, 3652–6.

Nicolaides, D. N. (1976). Synthesis of triphenyleno[2,3-*b*]thiophene derivatives. *Synthesis*, 675–7.

Nielsen, T. (1984). Characterization of polycyclic organic matter (POM) in flue gases from coal-fired power plants and in the atmosphere and investigation of their transformation in the atmosphere, Risø Nat. Lab. Rep. Risø-M 1984, Risø-M-2420, 113pp.

Nikitina, A. N., Gverdtsiteli, D. D., Romanova, O. A. and Litvinov, V. P. (1972). Condensed heteroatomic systems including a thiophene ring. XXI. Electronic adsorption and fluorescence spectra of condensed thiophene-containing systems. *Khim. Geterosikl. Soedin*, 925–32.

Nikolaeva, V. G., Zvereva, E. V. and Demicheva, M. A. (1959). Chemistry of organic sulfur compounds in petroleum and petroleum products. Proceedings of the 3rd Scientific Session, Ufa, June 3–8, 1957, Akad. Nauk SSSR, p. 135.

Nishioka, M., Bradshaw, J. S., Lee, M. L., Tominaga, Y., Tedjamulia, M. and Castle, R. N. (1985a). Capillary column gas chromatography of sulfur heterocycles in heavy oils and tars using a biphenylpolysiloxane stationary phase. *Anal. Chem.*, **57**, 309–12.

254   *References*

Nishioka, M., Smith, P. A., Booth, G. M., Lee, M. L., Kudo, H., Muchiri, D. R., Castle, R. N. and Klemm, L. H. (1985*b*). Determination of polycyclic aromatic compounds containing both sulfur and nitrogen heteroatoms in coal derived products. *Prep. Pap.-Am. Chem. Soc. Div. Fuel Chem.*, **30**, 93–8.

Nishioka, M., Lee, M. L., Kudo, H., Muchiri, D. R., Baldwin, L. J., Pakray, S., Stuart, J. G. and Castle, R. N. (1985*c*). Determination of hydroxylated thiophenic compounds in a coal liquid. *Anal. Chem.*, **57**, 1327–30.

Nishioka, M., Campbell, R. M., West, W. R., Smith, P. A., Booth, G. M. and Lee, M. L. (1985*d*). Determination of aminodibenzothiophenes in a coal liquid. *Anal. Chem.*, **57**, 1868–71.

Nishioka, M., Campbell, R. M., Lee, M. L. and Castle, R. N. (1986*a*). Isolation of sulfur heterocycles from petroleum- and coal-derived materials by ligand exchange chromatography. *Fuel*, **65**, 270–3.

Nishioka, M., Lee, M. L. and Castle, R. N. (1986*b*). Sulfur heterocycles in coal-derived products. Relation between structure and abundance. *Fuel*, **65**, 390–6.

Nishioka, M., Smith, P. A., Booth, G. M., Lee, M. L., Kudo, H., Muchiri, D. R., Castle, R. M. and Klemm, L. H. (1986*c*). Determination and mutagenic activity of nitrogen-containing thiophenic compounds in coal-derived products. *Fuel*, **65**, 711–14.

Norpoth, K., Kemena, A., Jacob, J. and Schuemann, C. (1984). The influence of 18 environmentally relevant polycyclic aromatic hydrocarbons and Clophen A 50 as liver monooxygenase inducers on the mutagenic activity of benz[*a*]anthracene in the Ames test. *Carcinogenesis*, **5**, 747–52.

Numan, H. and Wynberg, H. (1975). Methano-bridged heterohelicenes. *Tetrahedron Lett.*, **13**, 1097–100.

Numan, H., Helder, R. and Wynberg, H. (1976). The resolution of heterohelicenes. A facile method using HPLC (high pressure liquid chromatography). (Preliminary communication.) *Rec. Trav. Chim. Pays-Bas*, **95**, 211–12.

Numanov, I. U. (1977). Structural-group composition of organosulfur compounds in petroleum from Khandag deposit. *Dokl. Akad. Nauk Tadzh. SSR*, **20**, 23–6.

Nuzzi, M. and Casalini, A. (1978). Condensed thiophenic structures in the residue of a Kuwait crude oil having asphaltenes removed by n-pentane. *Riv. Combust.*, **32**, 295–303.

Obolentsev, R. D., Netupskaya, S. V., Gladkova, L. K., Bukharov, V. G. and Mashkina, A. V. (1956). Synthesis of sulfur compounds related to petroleum constituents. *Khim. Sera-Org. Soedin. Soderzh. Neft i. Nefteprod. Akad. Nauk. S.S.S.R., Bashkir. Filial, Materialy Vtoroi Sessin*, 87–94.

O'Brien, S. and Smith, D. C. C. (1963). Synthesis of heterocyclic analogs of phenalene (perinaphthene) containing one hetero atom. *J. Chem. Soc.*, 2907–17.

O'Donnell, G. (1951). Separating asphalt into its chemical constituents. *Anal. Chem.*, **23**, 894–8.

Oehme, M. (1982). Schwefelnachweisende Detektoren. In '*Gas-Chromatographische Detektoren*' (F. Oehme, ed.), pp. 83–4. Heidelberg, Dr Alfred Hüthig Verlag.

Ogata, M. and Fujisawa, K. (1980). Transfer of organic sulfur compounds in petroleum from crude oil suspension or polluted chlorella to rotifer. *Igaku to Seibutsugaku*, **101**, 197–201.

Ogata, M. and Fujisawa, K. (1983). Fate of benzo[*b*]thiophene and dibenzothiophene in the rat liver. *Igaku to Seibutsugaku*, **106**, 77–80.

Ogata, M. and Hasegawa, T. (1982). The effects of benzothiophene and dibenzothiophene on the mitochondrial membrane of the goldfish. *Igaku to Seibutsugaku*, **104**, 247–50.

Ogata, M. and Miyake, Y. (1978). Identification of organic sulfur compounds transferred to fish from petroleum suspension. *Acta Med. Okayama*, **32**, 419–25.

Ogata, M. and Miyake, Y. (1979). Identification of organic sulfur compounds transferred to fish from petroleum suspension by mass chromatography. *Water Res.*, **13**, 1179–85.

Ogata, M. and Miyake, Y (1980). Gas chromatography combined with mass spectrometry for the identification of organic sulfur compounds in shellfish and fish. *J. Chromatogr. Sci.*, **18**, 594–605.

Ogata, M. and Miyake, Y. (1981). Identification of organic sulfur compounds and polycyclic hydrocarbons transferred to shellfish from petroleum suspension by capillary gas chromatography. *Water Res.*, **15**, 257–66.

Ogata, M., Miyake, Y. and Yamasaki, Y. (1979). Identification of substances transferred to fish or shellfish from petroleum suspension. *Water Res.*, **13**, 613–18.

Ogata, M., Miyake, Y., Fujisawa, K. and Yoshida, Y. (1980a). Accumulation and dissipation of organosulfur compounds in short-necked slam and eel. *Bull. Environ. Contam. Toxicol.*, **25**, 130–5.

Ogata, M., Miyake, Y. and Fujisawa, K. (1980b). Transfer to goldfish of organic sulfur compounds in petroleum. *Igaku to Seibutsugaku*, **101**, 103–8.

Ogata, M., Fujisawa, K. and Miyake, Y. (1981a). Transfer to hillifish of organic sulfur compounds in crude oil suspension and oil contaminated rotifer. *Igaku to Seibutsugaku*, **103**, 457–61.

Ogata, M., Fujisawa, K. and Miyake, Y. (1981b). Transfer of organic sulfur compounds in petroleum from crude oil suspension to the mussel. *Igaku to Seibutsugaku*, **103**, 243–7.

Ohmura, H., Karakasa, T., Satsumabyashi, S. and Motoki, S. (1982). The reaction of 2-benzylidenetetralin-1-thione-S-oxide with a aroyl nitrile or styrene. *Bull. Chem. Soc. Jpn.*, **55**, 333–4.

Olufsen, B. (1980). Polynuclear aromatic hydrocarbons in Norwegian drinking water resources. In '*Polynuclear Aromatic Hydrocarbons: Chemistry and Biological Effects*' (A. Bjørseth and A. J. Dennis, eds.), pp. 333–43. Columbus/Ohio, Battelle Press.

Orr, W. L. (1966). Separation of alkyl sulfides by liquid–liquid chromatography on stationary phases containing mercuric acetate. *Anal. Chem.*, **38**, 1558–62.

Orr, W. L. (1967). Aqueous zinc chloride as a stationary phase for liquid–liquid chromatography of organic sulfides. *Anal. Chem.*, **39**, 1163–4.

Oshima, S., Fuji, K. and Nakai, M. (1966). Mass-spectrometric investigation of petroleum. IX. Mass-spectrometric analysis of aromatic hydrocarbons and sulfur compounds. *Shitsuryo Bunseki*, **14**, 209–14.

Oudot, J., Fusey, P., van Praet, M., Feral, J. P. and Gaill, F. (1981). Hydrocarbon weathering in seashore invertebrates and sediments over a two-year period following the Amoco Cadiz oil spill: influence of microbial metabolism. *Environ. Pollut.*, Ser. A 26.

Ozdemir, H. I. (1971). Qualitative determination of sulfur compounds in Turkish coals. *Istanbul Tek. Univ. Bull.*, **24**, 28–52.

Paasivirta, J., Herzschuh, R., Lahtipera, M., Pellinen, J. and Sinkkonen, S. (1981). Oil residues in Baltic sediment, mussel and fish. I. Development of the analysis method. *Chemosphere*, **10**, 919–28.

Pai, S. R. and Ranadive, K. J. (1965). Biological testing of analogs of 3,4-benzopyrene. *Indian J. Med. Res.*, **53**, 638–44.

Pailer, M. and Berner-Fenz, L. (1973). Boroheterocyclics. *Monatsh. Chem.*, **104**, 339–51.

Pailer, M. and Gruenhaus, H. (1974). Synthesis of indenothiophenes. *Monatsh. Chem.*, **105**, 1362–73.

Pailer, M. and Romberger, E. (1961). Boroheterocycles. *Monatsh. Chem.*, **92**, 677–83.

Pailer, M., Gruenhaus, H. and Stof, S. (1976). Synthesis of indenothiophenes II. *Monatsh. Chem.*, **107**, 521–30.

Pandya, L. J. and Tilak, B. D. (1958). Synthesis of aryl ω-dimethoxyethyl sulfides. Synthesis of thieno[2,3-*b*:5,4-*b*']dithiophene, and thieno[3,4-*b*]pyrene. *Chem. Ind. (London)*, 981–2.

Pandya, L. J. and Tilak, B. D. (1959a). Thiophenes and thiopyrans. XXI. A new synthesis of aryl ω-dimethoxyethyl sulfides and synthesis of thieno[2,3-b:5,4-b']dithiophene and thieno[3,4-b]pyrene. *J. Sci. Ind. Res. (India)*, **18B**, 371–6.

Pandya, L. J. and Tilak, B. D. (1959b). Thiophenes and thiopyrans. XX. Synthesis of condensed thiophenes from biaryls. *J. Sci. Ind. Res. (India)*, **18B**, 198–202.

Paramonov, V. D., Mostoslavskii, M. A. and Shevshuk, I. N. (1978). Effect of naphthalene fragment annelation on the absorption spectrum and quantum yield of photoisomerization of perinaphthoindigo. *Zh. Fiz. Khim.*, **52**, 2676–7.

Paresh, C. D. and Chaudhury, D. N. (1951). Indigoid dyes. XII. Phenanthrothiophene-indigos. *J. Indian Chem. Soc.*, **28**, 169–74.

Parfenova, M. A., Lyapina, N. K., Nikitina, T. S. and Smarkalor, A. A. (1977). Organosulfur compounds of a Samotlor, petroleum (190–360°) distillate. *Neftekhimiya*, **17**, 315–20.

Parham, W. E. and Gadsby, B. (1960). Synthesis of thienothianaphthene derivatives by ring formation with sulfur. *J. Org. Chem.*, **25**, 234–6.

Parkanyi, C. and Herndon, W. C. (1978). Bond length and bond orders in π-electron heterocycles. *Phosphorus Sulfur*, **4**, 1–7.

Patterson, J. A., Conary, R. E., McCleary, R. F., Culnane, C. H., Ruidisch, L. E. and Holder, C. B. (1959). Thianaphthene and homologs from hydrocarbons and hydrogen sulfide. *World Petrol. Congr. Proc. 5th*, **4**, 309.

Patterson, P. L. (1978). Comparison of quenching effects in single- and dual-flame photometric detectors. *Anal. Chem.*, **30**, 345–8.

Patterson, P. L., Howe, R. L. and Abu-Shumays, A. (1978). Dual-flame photometric detector for sulfur and phosphorus compounds in gas chromatograph effluents. *Anal. Chem.*, **50**, 339–44.

Payzant, J. D., Montgomery, D. S. and Strauss, O. P. (1983). Novel terpenoid sulfoxides and sulfides in petroleum. *Tetrahedron Lett.*, **24**, 651–4.

Peaden, P. A., Lee, M. L., Hirata, Y. and Novotny, M. (1980). High performance liquid chromatographic separation of high-molecular weight polycyclic aromatic compounds in carbon black. *Anal. Chem.*, **52**, 2268–71.

Peake, E. and Parker, K. (1980). Polycyclic aromatic hydrocarbons and the mutagenicity of used crankcase oils. In 'Polynuclear Aromatic Hydrocarbons: Chemistry and Biological Effects' (A. Bjørseth and A. J. Dennis, eds.), pp. 1025–39. Columbus/Ohio, Battelle-Press.

Pearlman, R. S., Yalkowsky, S. H. and Banerjee, S. (1984). Water solubilities of polynuclear aromatic and heteroaromatic compounds. *J. Phys. Chem. Ref. Data*, **13**, 555–62.

Pelroy, R. A., Stewart, D. L., Tominaga, Y., Iwao, M., Castle, R. N. and Lee, M. L. (1983). Microbial mutagenicity of 3- and 4-ring polycyclic aromatic sulfur heterocycles. *Mutat. Res.*, **117**, 31–40.

Pelz, K. and Protiva, M. (1963). 3,4-Benzothiaxanthenes. Czech. Pat. 113,256 (Cl.C.07c) Jan. 15, 1965 Appl. Jan. 30, 1963, 4 pp.

Peters, A. T. and Tenny, B. A. (1977). 1,4-Dihydroxyanthraquinone-2-thio ethers. Dyes for synthetic polymer fibers. *J. Soc. Dyers Colour*, **93**, 373–8.

Pillai, G. N., Murthy, T. S. and Tilak, B. D. (1963). Thiophene isosteres of carcinogenic hydrocarbons. IV. Synthesis of 2,3:7,8- and 2,3:5,6-dibenzothiophanthrenes and 6,12-dimethylbenzo[1,2-b:5,4-b']dithionaphthene. *Indian J. Chem.*, **1**, 112–15.

Pitts, J. N., Grosjean, D., Mischke, T., Simmon, V. F. and Poole, D. (1977). Mutagenic activity of airborne particulate organic pollutants. *Toxicol. Lett.*, **1**, 65–70.

Platt, J. R. (1964). *Systematics of the Electronic Spectra of Conjugated Molecules*. J. Wiley, New York.

Poirier, M. A. and Das, S. B. (1984). Characterization of polynuclear aromatic hydrocarbons in bitumen, heavy oil fractions boiling above 350° by GC–MS. *Fuel*, **63**, 361–7.

Poirier, M. A. and Smiley, G. T. (1984). A novel method for separation and identification of sulfur compounds in naphthenes (30–200°) and middle distillate (200–350°) fractions of Lloydminster heavy oil by GC/MS. *J. Chromatogr. Sci.*, **22**, 304–9.

Poirier, Y. and Lozac'h, N. (1966). Heterocyclic sulfur-compounds. XXII. Sulfuration of 2-alkyl-1-indanones and 2-arylmethylene-1-indanones. *Bull. Soc. Chim. France*, 1062–8.

Popl, M., Stejskal, M. and Mostecky, J. (1975). Determination of polycyclic aromatic hydrocarbons in white petroleum products. *Anal. Chem.*, **47**, 1947–50.

Porter, Q. N. (1967). Mass-spectrometric studies. I. Benzo[*b*]thiophene some alkyl and aryl derivatives, and the 1,1-dioxide and 2,3-dihydro-1,1-dioxide. *Austr. J. Chem.*, **20**, 103–16.

Potolovskii, L. A., Polyakova, A. A., Katrenko, T. I., Bessonova, R. N., Fufaer, A. A., Kogan, L. O. and Semanyuk, R. N. (1977). Composition and structure of compounds of basic oil DS-14 produced from a mixture of Siberian petroleum. *Khim. Tekhnol. Topl. Masel*, 22–5.

Pratap, R., Lee, M. L. and Castle, R. N. (1981*a*). Synthesis of triphenyleno[*b*]thiophenes. *J. Heterocycl. Chem.*, **18**, 1457–9.

Pratap, R., Tominaga, Y., Lee, M. L. and Castle, R. N. (1981*b*). Synthesis of pyreno[*b*]thiophenes. *J. Heterocycl. Chem.*, **18**, 973–5.

Pratap, R., Castle, R. N. and Lee, M. L. (1982*a*). Synthesis of benzo[1,2]phenaleno[*bc*]thiophenes. *J. Heterocycl. Chem.*, **19**, 439–41.

Pratap, R., Lee, M. L. and Castle, R. N. (1982*b*). Synthesis of benzo[*b*]phenanthro[*d*]thiophenes. *J. Heterocycl. Chem.*, **19**, 219–20.

Prinzler, H. W. (1964). Beiträge zur Analytik der schwefelhaltigen Inhaltsstoffe von Erdölprodukten. Charakterisierung sulfidischer Strukturen. *Z. Chem.*, **4**, 374–7.

Proksch, E. (1966). Gas-chromatographic analysis of VOEST anthracene oil. *Oesterr. Chemiker-Ztg.*, **67**, 105–12.

Rabindran, K. and Tilak, B. D. (1951*a*). A new synthesis of dibenzothiophene. *Curr. Sci. (India)*, **20**, 207.

Rabindran, K. and Tilak, B. D. (1951*b*). An improved method for the cyclization of aryl-2,2-dimethoxyethyl sulfide. *Curr. Sci. (India)*, 205–6.

Rabindran, K. and Tilak, B. D. (1953*a*). Thiophenes and thiapyrans. IX. Studies in the dehydrogenation of 1,2,3,4-tetrahydrodibenzothiophene. *Proc. Indian. Acad. Sci.*, **37A**, 557–63.

Rabindran, K. and Tilak, B. D. (1953*b*). Thiophenes and thiapyrans. X. 1,2-Benzo-9-thiafluorene and 3,4-benzo-9-thiafluorene. *Proc. Indian Acad. Sci.*, **37A**, 564–70.

Rabindran, K. and Tilak, B. D. (1953*c*). Thiophenes and thiapyrans. XI. A new route to polycyclic thiophenes. *Proc. Indian Acad. Sci.*, **38A**, 271–6.

Ranadive, K. J. and Mashelkar, B. N. (1972). In vitro studies on chemical carcinogenesis. *Indian J. Cancer*, **9**, 121–31.

Ranadive, K. J., Mohile, S. V. and Gangal, S. G. (1963). Cytological studies on in vitro testing of chemical carcinogens. *Nucleus (Calcutta)*, **6**, 17–30.

Rao, D. S. and Tilak, B. D. (1954). Thiophenes and thiapyrans. XIII. Synthesis of benzodithiophenes and benzodithionaphthenes. *J. Sci. Ind. Res. (India)*, **13B**, 829–34.

Rao, D. S. and Tilak, B. D. (1957). Thiophenes and thiapyrans. XV. Benzo[1,2-*b*:4,3-*b'*]dithiophene and benzo[1,2-*b*:4,5-*b'*]dithiophene. *J. Sci. Ind. Res. (India)*, **16B**, 65–8.

Rao, D. S. and Tilak, B. D. (1958). Thiophenes and thiopyrans. XVIII. Benzo[2,1-*b*:4,3-*b'*]dithiophene and benzodithionaphthenes. *J. Sci. Ind. Res. (India)*, **17B**, 260–6.

Ratajzak, E. A., Ahland, E., Grimmer, G. and Dettbarn, G. (1982). PAH and S-PAC-Emissionen aus Heizölverdampferöfen. EKEP Synopse 8245. *Erdöl und Kohle-Erdgas-Petrochemie*, **35**, 530.

Ray, S. and Frei, R. W. (1972). Separation of polynuclear aza-heterocyclics by high-speed liquid chromatography on a chemically bonded stationary phase. *J. Chromatogr.*, **71**, 451–7.

Rebbert, R. E., Chesler, S. N., Guenther, F. R. and Parris, M. R. (1984). Liquid chromatography-gas chromatography procedure to determine the concentration of dibenzothiophene in a crude oil matrix. *J. Chromatogr.*, **284**, 211–17.

Reid, W. K., Mead, W. L. and Bowen, K. M. (1966). Combination of high resolution and low ionizing voltages in the determination of hydrocarbons and sulfur compound types in petroleum fractions using mass spectrometry. *Adv. Masspectrometr.*, **3**, 731–45.

Reinecke, M. G. and Ballard, H. H. (1979). Heterotriptycenes from a five-membered heterocyclic diazonium carboxylate. *Tetrahydron Lett.*, 4981–2.

Ricci, A., Balucani, D., Rossi, C. and Croisy, A. (1969). New heterocyclic systems. III. Heterocycles containing a fused thiophene ring. *Boll. Sci. Fac. Chim. Ind. Bologna*, **27**, 279–87.

Ricci, A., Balucani, D. and Bettelli, M. (1971). Synthesis and properties of the thieno[3,2-b]benzo[b]thiophenes. *Gazz. Chim. Ital.*, **101**, 774–86.

Ricci, A., Balucani, D. and Berado, B. (1972). Unexpected synthesis of benzo[b]thieno[3,2-b]benzo[b]thiophenes. *C.R. Acad. Sci. Ser. C.*, **273**, 139–42.

Riepe, W. and Zander, M. (1979). The mass spectrometric fragmentation behavior of thiophene benzologs. *Org. Mass. Spectrom.*, **14**, 455–6.

Rogovik, V. I. (1970). Derivatives of perylene-3,4,9,10-tetracarboxylic acid containing substituents in the perylene ring. *Otkrytiya, Izobret., Prom. Obraztsy, Tovarnye Znaki*, **47**, 38.

Rogovik, V. I. (1974). Chemistry of perylene. Preparation of thienoperylenetetracarboxylic acid and thienoperylene. *Zh. Org. Khim.*, **10**, 1072–5.

Royer, R., Demerseman, P., Lechartier, J.-P. and Cheutin, A. (1962). Benzo[b]thiophene. III. Synthesis of hydroxylated diphenylalkanes from anisyl derivatives of benzo[b]thiophene. *J. Org. Chem.*, **27**, 3808–14.

Saint-Ruf, G., Buu-Hoi, N. G. and Jacquignon, P. (1959). Cyclodehydration of arylidene-α-tetralones derived from fluorene, dibenzofuran, dibenzothiophene. *J. Chem. Soc.*, 3237–41.

Sandin, R. B. and Fieser, L. F. (1940). Synthesis of 9,10-dimethyl-1,2-benzanthracene and of a thiophene isolog. *J. Am. Chem. Soc.*, **62**, 3098–105.

Sasaki, T., Hayakawa, K. and Nishida, S. (1982). Photochemistry of organosulfur compounds. Part 4. Photochemical ring closure of α,α-1-bisulfenylated carbonyl compounds. Stereoselective formation of cis-dihydrobenzothiophenes. *Tetrahedron*, **38**, 75–83.

Sastry, G. R. N. and Tilak, B. D. (1961). Thiophenes and thiopyrans. XXVII. A new route to polycyclic thiophenes. *J. Sci. Ind. Res.*, **20B**, 286–9.

Sato, Y., Kunieda, N. and Kinoshita, M. (1974). Oxidation of sulfides to sulfoxides with N-bromo-ε-caprolactam. *Mem. Fac. Eng., Osaka City Univ.*, **15**, 101–3.

Sauter, F. and Dzerovicz, A. (1969). Chemistry of sulfur-containing heterocycles. IV. 6H-Benzo[b]indeno[1,2-d]thiophene and 10H-benzo[b]indeno[1,2-d]thiophene. *Monatsh. Chem.*, **100**, 913–15.

Sawicki, E., Stanley, T. W. and Elbert, W. C. (1964). Quenchofluorometric analysis for fluoranthenic hydrocarbons. *Talanta*, **11**, 1431–9.

Schenck, G. O. and Krauch, C. H. (1963). Sulfones by photosensitized oxygen transfer to sulfoxides. *Chem. Ber.*, **96**, 517–19.

Schmid, E. R., Bachlechner, G., Varmuza, K. and Klus, H. (1985). Determination of polycyclic aromatic hydrocarbons, polycyclic aromatic sulfur and oxygen heterocycles in cigarette smoke condensate. *Fresenius Z. Anal. Chem.*, **322**, 213–19.

Schmidt, W., Grimmer, G., Jacob, J. and Dettbarn, G. (1986). Polycyclic aromatic hydrocarbons and thiaarenes in the emission from hard-coal combustion. *Toxicol. Environ. Chem.*, **13**, 1–16.

Schmidt, W., Grimmer, G., Jacob, J., Dettbarn, G. and Naujack, K.-W. (1987). Polycyclic aromatic hydrocarbons with mass number 300 and 302 in hard-coal flue gas condensate. *Fresenius Z. Anal. Chem.*, **326**, 401–3.

Schoenberg, A. and Sidky, M. M. (1974). Photochemical reactions. XXIII. Photocyclization of 9-benzylidenexanthenes and 9-benzylidenethioxanthenes. *Chem. Ber.*, **107**, 1207–12.

Scholz, M. and Heidrich, D. (1967). Molecular orbital calculations for heterocyclics. V.H.M.O. (Hueckel M.O.) models of new heterocyclic systems derived from acenaphthylene or fluoranthene. *Z. Chem.*, **7**, 349–51.

Scholz, M., Walzel, E. and Hofmann, H. J. (1973). MO calculations of heterocycles. IX. π-electron structure and uv spectra of [1,2-*b*]- and [1,2-*c*]fused acenaphthothiophene and N-methylacenaphthopyrrole. *J. Prakt. Chem.*, **315**, 1105–12.

Schroeder, H. E. and Weinmayer, V. (1952). The synthesis of thiophanthraquinones from thenoyl and thenylbenzoic acids. *J. Am. Chem. Soc.*, **74**, 4357–61.

Schultz, A. G. (1974). Heteroatom-directed photoarylation. A new method for introduction of angular carbon–carbon bonds. *J. Org. Chem.*, **39**, 3185–6.

Schultz, A. G. and DeTar, M. B. (1976). Thiocarbonyl ylides. Photogeneration, rearrangement, and cycloaddition reactions. *J. Am. Chem. Soc.*, **98**, 3564–72.

Schultz, A. G., Fu, W. Y., Lucci, R. D., Kurr, B. G., Lo, K. M. and Boxer, M. (1978). Heteroatom directed photoarylation. Synthetic potential of the heteroatom sulfur. *J. Am. Chem. Soc.*, **100**, 2140–9.

Schultz, R. V., Jorgenson, J. W., Maskarinec, M. P., Novotny, M. and Todd, L. J. (1979). Characterization of polynuclear aromatic and aliphatic hydrocarbon fractions of solvent-refined coal by glass capillary gas chromatography/mass spectrometry. *Fuel*, **58**, 783–9.

Schuyer, J., Blom, L. and Van Krevelen, D. W. (1953). Molar refraction of condensed aromatic compounds. *Trans. Faraday Soc.*, **49**, 1391–401.

Scrowston, R. M. (1981). Recent advances in the chemistry of benzo[*b*]thiophene. *Adv. Heterocycl. Chem.*, **29**, 172–249.

Sergienko, S. R., Perchenko, V. N. and Mikhnovskaya, A. A. (1960). The effect of the structure of organic compounds on the rates of oxidation and of catalytic hydrogenation. *Khim. Sera. Azotorg. Soedin., Soderzh. Neftyakh Neft.*, **3**, 353–61.

Serth, R. W. and Hughes, T. W. (1980). Polycyclic organic matter (POM) and trace element contents of carbon black vent gas. *Environ. Sci. Technol.*, **14**, 298–301.

Sharanin, Y. A. and Promonenkov, V. K. (1980). 2'-Aminoandrost-2-eno[2,3-*b*]thiophenes. *Khim. Geterotsikl. Soedin.*, 1564–5.

Sharkey, A. G. (1976). Mass spectrometric analysis of process streams for coalderived fuels. In '*Carcinogenesis*', vol. 1 (R. Freudenthal and P. W. Jones, eds.), pp. 341–7. New York, Raven Press.

Shenbor, M. I. and Tsaberyabyi, A. T. (1969). Synthesis and some transformations of 4-fluoranthenethiol. *Izv. Vyssh. Ucheb. Zaved. Khim. Khim. Tekhnol.*, **12**, 1379–80.

Shevchuk, I. N. and Paramonov, V. D. (1976). Pyreno[3,4-*bc*]thiopyran-3-one. *Otkrytiya, Izobret., Prom. Obraztsy, Tovarnye Znaki*, **53**, 76–7.

Shields, J. E., Remy, D. E. and Bornstein, J. (1975). Phenanthro[9,10-*c*]thiophene. Synthesis and reactions. *J. Org. Chem.*, **40**, 477–9.

Shiro, M., Nakai, H., Okada, T. and Terasawa, T. (1982). ($\pm$)-3-Methoxy-17aα-acetoxy-16-thia-D-homoestra-1,3,5(10), 8-tetraene. *Cryst. Struct. Commun.*, **11**, 423–6.

Showiman, S. S., Al-Najjar, I. A. and Amin, H. B. (1982). Carbon-13-NMR spectra of benzo[*b*]thiophene and 1-(X-benzo[*b*]thienyl)-ethylacetate derivatives. *Org. Magn. Reson.*, **20**, 105–12.

Shultz, J. L., Freidel, R. A. and Sharkey, A. G., jr. (1965). Analysis of coal tar pitch by mass spectrometry. *Fuel*, **44**, 55–61.

Sidorenko, T. N., Terent'eva, G. A., Andrienko, O. S., Savinykh, Y. V. and Aksenov, V. S. (1983*a*). Synthesis and chemical reactions in isomeric naphtho[*b*]thiophenes. *Khim. Geterotsikl. Soedin*, 192–6.

Sidorenko, T. N., Terent'eva, G. A. and Aksenov, V. S. (1983*b*). Preparation of phenanthro[9,10-*b*]thiophene and properties of its derivatives. *Khim. Geterotsikl. Soedin.*, 197–9.

Silva, S., Russo, S. and Scotti, I. A. (1982). Carbon black pollution: environmental effects and related health problems. *Ann. Fac. Agrar.*, **22**, 131–141.

Skramstad, J. (1969). Cyclopentathiophenes. II. Synthesis of 4*H*-cyclopenta[*c*]thiophene. *Acta Chem. Scand.*, **23**, 703–5.

Smith, R. W., Games, D. E. and Noel, S. F. (1983). LC/MS of polynuclear aromatic and heterocyclic compounds. *Int. J. Mass. Spectrometr. Ion Phys.*, **48**, 327–30.

Snook, M. E. (1978). Nitrogen analogues of polynuclear aromatic hydrocarbons in tobacco smoke. In '*Carcinogenesis, vol. 3: Polynuclear Aromatic Hydrocarbons*' (P. W. Jones and R. I. Freudenthal, eds.), pp. 203–215. New York, Raven Press.

Snook, M. E., Severson, R. F., Higman, H. C., Arrendale, R. F. and Chortyk, O. T. (1979). Methods for characterization of complex mixtures of polynuclear aromatic hydrocarbons. In '*Polynuclear Aromatic Hydrocarbon. 3rd Int. Sympos. on Chemistry and Biology – Carcinogenesis and Mutagenesis*' (P. W. Jones and P. Leber, eds.), pp. 231–60. Ann Arbor, Ann Arbor Science.

Speight, J. G. and Pancirov, R. J. (1983). Some aspects of the structure of petroleum asphaltenes. *Prepr.-Am. Chem. Soc., Div. Pet. Chem.*, **28**, 1319–32.

Spietschka, E. and Landler, J. (1971). Benzothiaxanthene derivatives Ger. Offen. 2,134,518, 25 Jan. 1973, Appl. p21 34 518.6, 10 July 1971, 8pp.

Spietschka, E. and Landler, J. (1972). Benzothiaxanthenes. Ger. Offen 2,134,517, 14 Dec. 1972, Appl. p21 34 517.5-42, 10 Jul. 1971, 4pp.

Spitzer, T. and Dannecker, W. (1984). Clean-up of polynuclear aromatic hydrocarbons and 3-ring azaarenes and their GC-analysis on whisker-walled open tubular columns. *J. High Resol. Chromatogr. Chromatogr. Commun.*, **7**, 301–5.

Sporstol, S., Gjos, N., Lichtenthaler, R. G., Gustavsen, K. O., Urdal, K., Oreld, F. and Skei, J. (1983). Source identification of aromatic hydrocarbons in sediments using GC/MS. *Environ. Sci. Technol.*, **17**, 282–6.

Stacy, G. W., Papa, A. J., Villaescusa, F. W. and Ray, S. C. (1964). A tautomeric nitrile-thiol iminothiolactone system. *J. Org. Chem.*, **29**, 607–12.

Stadelhofer, J. W. and Gerhards, R. (1981). Carbon-13-NMR study on hydroaromatic compounds in anthracene oil. *Fuel*, **60**, 367–8.

Steinkopf, W. (1935). Studien in der Thiophenreihe. XXIX. Über das Flavophen. *Liebigs Ann. Chem.*, **519**, 297–300.

Stenberg, U. R. and Alsberg, T. E. (1981). Vacuum sublimation and solvent extraction of polycyclic aromatic compounds adsorbed on carbonaceous materials. *Anal. Chem.*, **53**, 2067–72.

Stille, J. K. and Foster, R. T. (1963). Some reactions involving 9,10-phenanthroquinodimethane as an intermediate. *J. Org. Chem.*, **28**, 2708.

Stulen, G. and Visser, G. J. (1969). Crystal structure of heterohelicene. *J. Chem. Soc. D.*, 965.

Sugiura, M., Tedjamulia, M. L., Tominaga, Y., Castle, R. N. and Lee, M. L. (1983). The synthesis of the monomethylbenzo[2,3]phenanthro[4,5-*bcd*]thiophenes. *J. Heterocycl. Chem.*, **30**, 1453–9.

Sun, S. (1983). GC-MS analysis of aliphatic and polycyclic aromatic hydrocarbons in airborne particulates. *Huanjing Kexue*, **4**, 22–6.

Szumuszkovicz, J. and Modest, E. J. (1950). Condensation of thienylcycloalkenes with maleic anhydride. *J. Am. Chem. Soc.*, **72**, 571–7.

Taits, S. Z., Zaretskii, M. I., Podilyak, V. G., Golub, V. B., Chatov, E. M. and Usyshkina, I. V. (1984). Separation of valuable heterocyclic compounds from crude benzene and coal tar. *Koks Khim.*, 30–3.

Takahashi, T., Kim, Y. H., Fukushima, D., Fujimori, K., Oae, S. and Iyanagi T. (1978). Structure-dependent reactivity in the oxygenation of thiane analogs by a cytochrome P-450 reconstituted enzyme system. *Heterocycles*, **10**, 229–35.

Takata, T., Yamazaki, M., Fujimori, K., Kim, Y. H., Iyanagi, T. and Oae, S. (1983). Enzymic oxygenation of sulfides with cytochrome P-450 from rabbit liver. Stereochemistry of sulfoxide formation. *Bull. Chem. Soc. Jpn.*, **56**, 2300–10.

Takeda, K. and Komeno, T. (1964) (publ. 1965). Intramolecular condensation of some 6-acetylthiosteroids. Hormonal steroids. Proc. Intern. Congr. Hormonal Steroids 1st, 1964, pp. 109–16.

Talcott, R. and Wei, E. (1977). Brief communication: Airborne mutagens bioassayed in *Salmonella typhimurium*. *J. Natl. Canc. Inst.*, **58**, 449–51.

Tan, Y. L. (1979). Rapid simple sample preparation technique for analyzing polynuclear aromatic hydrocarbons in sediments by gas chromatography-mass spectrometry. *J. Chromatogr.*, **176**, 319–27.

Tatsumi, K., Kitamura, D. and Yamada, H. (1983). Sulfoxide reductase activity of liver aldehyde oxidase. *Biochim. Biophys. Acta*, **747**, 86–92.

Taylor, W. F. and Wallace, T. J. (1968). Kinetics of the self-condensation of benzo[b]thiophene-1,1-dioxide. *Tetrahedron*, **24**, 5081–7.

Taylor, W. F., Kellher, J. M. and Wallace, T. J. (1968). Pyrolytic decomposition of 6a,11b-dihydronaphtho[2,1-b]benzo[d]thiophene-7,7-dioxide. *Chem. Ind.*, **20**, 651–2.

Teal, J. M., Burns, K. and Farrington, J. (1978). Analysis of aromatic hydrocarbons in intertidal sediments resulting from two spills of No. 2 fuel oil in Buzzards Bay, Massachusetts. *J. Fish. Res. Board Can.*, **35**, 510–20.

Tedjamulia, M. L., Tominaga, Y., Castle, R. N. and Lee, M. L. (1983a). The synthesis of phenanthro[4,5-bcd]thiophenes. *J. Heterocycl. Chem.*, **20**, 1149–52.

Tedjamulia, M. L., Tominaga, Y., Castle, R. N. and Lee, M. L. (1983b) The synthesis of dinaphthothiophenes. *J. Heterocycl. Chem.*, **20**, 1143–8.

Tedjamulia, M. L., Tominaga, Y., Castle, R. N. and Lee, M. L. (1983c). The synthesis of benzo[b]phenanthro[d]thiophenes and anthra[b]benzo[d]thiophenes. *J. Heterocycl. Chem.*, **20**, 861–6.

Tedjamulia, M. L., Kudo, H. and Castle, R. N. (1984). Angular polycyclic thiophenes containing two thiophene rings. Part II. *J. Heterocycl. Chem.*, **21**, 321–5.

Ten Haven, H. L., de Leeuw, J. W., Damsté, J. S., Schenck, P. A., Palmer, S. E. and Zumberge, J. E. (1986). In '*Lacustrine Petroleum Source Rocks*' (K. Kelts, A. J. Fleet and M. Talbot, eds.). Blackwell, London.

Teplitskaya, T. A., Melikadze, L. A., Akhobadze, R. N. and Utkina, L. F. (1981). Sensitivity of determining benzothiophenes in aromatic fractions of petroleum by quasilinear luminescence spectra. *Soobshch. Akad., Nauk Gruz. SSR*, **102**, 357–60.

Teranishi, K., Hamada, K. and Watanabe, W. (1978). Mutagenicity in *Salmonella typhimurium* mutants of the benzene soluble organic fractions. *Mutation Res.*, **56**, 273–80.

Thompson, C. J., Coleman, H. J., Hopkins, R. L. and Rall, H. T. (1964). Identification of alkyl cycloalkyl sulfides in petroleum. *J. Chem. Eng. Data*, **9**, 293–6.

Thompson, R. D., Iwao, M., Lee, M. L. and Castle, R. N. (1981). Synthesis of benzo[3,2]phenanthro[4,5-bcd]thiophene and chryseno[4,5-bcd]thiophene. *J. Heterocycl. Chem.*, **18**, 981–4.

Tiecco, M. (1968). Aromatization by homolytic arylation. *Corsi-Semin. Chim.*, **10**, 56–7.

Tiecco, M., de Luca, G., Martelli, G. and Spagnolo, P. (1970). Photochemical cyclization of some iodophenyl- and iodothienyl(thienyl)ethylenes. *J. Chem. Org. Soc.*, 2504–8.

Tilak, B. D. (1951a). Thiophenes and thiapyrans from naphthalenethiols. *Proc. Indian Acad. Sci.*, **33A**, 71–7.

Tilak, B. D. (1951b). S-isosteres of carcinogenic hydrocarbons. *Proc. Indian Acad. Sci.*, **33A**, 131–41.

Tilak, B. D. (1960). Carcinogenesis by thiophene isosteres of polycyclic hydrocarbons. Synthesis of condensed thiophenes. *Tetrahedron*, **9**, 76–95.

Tilak, B. D., Gogte, V. N. and Jindal, S. L. (1969). Synthesis of sulfur heterocyclics. IX. NMR spectra of polycyclic sulfur compounds. *Indian J. Chem.*, **7**, 741–3.

Tokiwa, H., Morita, K., Takeyoshi, H. and Ohnishi, Y. (1977). Detection of mutagenic activity in particulate air pollutants. *Mutation Res.*, **48**, 237–48.

Tominaga, Y., Lee, M. L. and Castle, R. N. (1981a). Synthesis of benzo[b]naphtho[d]thiophenes. *J. Heterocycl. Chem.*, **18**, 967–72.

Tominaga, Y., Lee, M. L. and Castle, R. N. (1981b). Synthesis of phenaleno[1,9-bc]thiophenes. *J. Heterocycl. Chem.*, **18**, 977–9.

Tominaga, Y., Castle, R. N. and Lee, M. L. (1982a). Synthesis of benzo[4,5]phenaleno[1,9-bc]-thiophene and benzo[4,5]phenaleno[9,1-bc]thiophene. *J. Heterocycl. Chem.*, **19**, 1125–30.

Tominaga, Y., Pratap, R., Castle, R. N. and Lee, M. L. (1982b). The synthesis of all the monomethyl isomers of benzo[b]naphtho[2,1-d]thiophene. *J. Heterocycl. Chem.*, **19**, 859–63.

Tominaga, Y., Pratap. R., Castle, R. N. and Lee, M. L. (1982c). The synthesis of all the monomethyl isomers of benzo[b]naphtho[1,2-d]thiophene. *J. Heterocycl. Chem.*, **19**, 871–7.

Tominaga, Y., Tedjamulia, M. L., Castle, R. N. and Lee, M. L. (1983). Synthesis of all of the monomethyl isomers of naphtho[2,1-b]thiophene. *J. Heterocycl. Chem.*, **20**, 487–90.

Tong, H. Y. and Karasek, F. W. (1984). Quantitation of polycyclic aromatic hydrocarbons in diesel exhaust particulate matter by high-performance liquid chromatography fractionation and high-resolution gas chromatography. *Anal. Chem.*, **56**, 2129–34.

Tong, H. Y., Shore, D. L., Karasek, F. W., Helland, P. and Jellum, E. (1984). Identification of organic compounds obtained from incineration of municipal waste by high-performance liquid chromatographic fractionation and gas chromatography-mass spectrometry. *J. Chromatogr.*, **285**, 423–41.

Trinajstic, N. and Hinchliffe, A. (1968). Molecular orbital calculations for the benzothiophenes and naphthothiophenes. *Z. Phys. Chem.*, **59**, 271–81.

Trost, B. M. and Curran, D. P. (1981). Chemoselective oxidation of sulfides to sulfones with potassium hydrogen persulfate. *Tetrahedron Lett.*, **22**, 1287–90.

Tschunkur, E. and Himmer, E. (1934). Biphenylene sulfide. German Pat. 579,917; (C.A. **28**: 1053 (1934)).

Utkina, L. F., Akhobadze, R. N. and Teplitskaya, T. A. (1976a). Quasilinear spectra of anthra[2,3-b]benzo[d]thiophene at 77°K. *Soobshch. Akad. Nauk Gruz SSR*, **82**, 373–6.

Utkina, L. F., Akhobadze, R. N. and Teplitskaya, T. A. (1976b). Electronic absorption of naphthobenzothiophenes. *Soobshch. Akad. Nauk Gruz SSR*, **82**, 605–8.

VanderMeulen, J. H. (1981). Contamination of marine population by hydrocarbons: Note of synthesis. In '*AMOCO CADIZ: Fates and Effects of the Oil Spill*', p. 563. Brest Cedex, France Centre National pour L'Exploitation des Océans.

Van Graas, G., de Leeuw, J. W., Schenck, P. A. and Haverkamp, J. (1981). Kerogen of Toarcian shales of the Paris basin. A study of its maturation by flash pyrolysis technique. *Geochim. Cosmochim. Acta*, **45**, 2465–74.

Van Hes, R., Skolnik, S., Pandit, K. and Huisman, H. O. (1968). Polynuclear heterocyclic systems. V. Heterocycles related to steroids and C-nor steroids. *Rec. Trav. Chim. Pays-Bas*, **87**, 151–60.

Van Zyl, G., Bredeweg, C. J., Rynbrandt, R. H. and Neckers, D. C. (1966). A study of the substitution reactions of benzo[b]thiophene and its derivatives. *Can. J. Chem.*, **44**, 2283–9.

Vassilaros, D. L., Eastmond, D. A., West, W. R., Booth, G. M. and Lee, M. L. (1982a). Determination and bioconcentration of polycyclic aromatic sulfur heterocycles in aquatic biota. In '*Polynuclear Aromatic Hydrocarbons*' (M. Cooke, A. J. Dennis, G. L. Fisher, eds.), pp. 845–7. Columbus/Ohio, Battelle Press.

Vassilaros, D. L., Stoker, P. W., Booth, G. M. and Lee, M. L. (1982b). Capillary gas chromatographic determination of polycyclic aromatic compounds in vertebrate fish tissue. *Anal. Chem.*, **54**, 106–12.

Vassilaros, D. L., Kong, R. C., Later, D. W. and Lee, M. L. (1982c). Linear retention index system for polycyclic aromatic compounds. Critical evaluation and additional indices. *J. Chromatogr.*, **252**, 1–20.

Vial, M., Jarosz, J., Martin-Bouyer, M. and Paturel, L. (1986). Emission spectrum of dibenzothiophene in Shpol'skii matrix at 10 K. *J. Photochem.*, **33**, 67–79.

Vignier, V., Berthou, F., Dreano, Y. and Floch, H. H. (1985). Dibenzothiophene sulphoxidation: a new and fast high-performance liquid chromatographic assay of mixed-function oxidation. *Xenobiotica*, **15**, 991–9.

Vingiello, F. A. and Henson, P. D. (1966). New benzo[b]thiophene derivatives of anthracene and benz[a]anthracene. *J. Org. Chem.*, **31**, 1357–9.

Vo-dingh, T. and Martinez, P. R. (1981). Direct determination of selected polynuclear aromatic hydrocarbons in a coal liquification product by synchronus luminescence technique. *Anal. Chem. Acta*, **125**, 13–19.

Vogh, J. W. and Dooley, J. E. (1975). Separation of organic sulfides from aromatic concentrates by ligand exchange chromatography. *Anal. Chem.*, **47**, 816–21.

Vol'tsov, A. A. and Lyapina, N. K. (1980). Organosulfur compounds of condensates from Orenburg and Sovkhozneusk deposits. *Khim. Teknol. Topl. Masel*, 37–40.

Voronkov, M. G. and Faitel'son, F. D. (1967). Reaction of sulfur with organic compounds. XII. Synthesis of dibenzothiophene, di- and tetramethylthianthrenes and their sulfones. *Khim. Geterotsikl. Soedin*, **2**, 1079–84.

Voronkov, M. G. and Khokhlova, L. N. (1974). Reaction of sulfur with organic compounds. XXIII. Reaction of sulfur with o-halotoluenes and some of their eso and exo derivatives. *Zh. Org. Khim.*, **10**, 811–16.

Voronkov, M. G. and Pereferkovich, A. N. (1969). Formation of sulfur-containing heterocycles. *Ang. Chem. Int. Ed. Engl.*, **8**, 272–3.

Voronkov, M. G. and Udre, V. (1968). Reactions of sulfur with organic compounds. XVI. Effect of sulfur on exo-halo derivatives of 1,1-diphenylethane, and 1,2,2-triphenylethane. *Khim. Geterotsikl. Soedin*, **1**, 43–8.

Voronkov, M. G. and Udre, V. E. (1972). Reaction of sulfur with aralkyl halides. *Khim. Seraorg. Soedin., Soderzh. Neftyakh Nefteprod.*, **9**, 233–9.

Voronkov, M. G., Deryagina, E. N., Khokhlova, L. G. and Ivanova, G. M. (1977). High-temperature organic synthesis. IV. Reaction of thiophenol with halogen derivatives of benzene and its substituents. *Zh. Org. Khim.*, **13**, 2575–84.

Voronkov, M. G., Deryagina, E. N., Shagun, L. G. and Vitovskii, V. Y. (1983). High-temperature organic synthesis. XXII. Thermal transformations of exo-chloro-substituted derivatives of toluene. *Zh. Org. Khim.*, **19**, 1079–84.

Walsh, P. M., Chiu, K. S., Beer, J. M. and Biermann, K. (1983). Polycyclic aromatic compounds in fluidized bed combustion of coal. *Prepr. Pap.-Am. Chem. Soc., Div. Fuel Chem.*, **28**, 251–64.

Waravdekar, S. S. and Ranadive, K. J. (1957). Biological testing of sulfur isosters of carcinogenic hydrocarbons. *J. Natl. Cancer Inst.*, **18**, 555–63.

Warner, J. S. (1975). Determination of sulfur-containing petroleum products in marines samples. Proc. Conf. Prev. Control Oil Pollut., 97–101.

Watanabe, Y., Iyanagi, T. and Oae, S. (1981a). Kinetic study on enzymatic S-oxygenation promoted by a reconstituted system with purified cytochrome P-450. *Tetrahedron Lett.*, **21**, 3685–8.

Watanabe, Y., Numata, T., Iyanagi, T. and Oae, S. (1981b). Enzymatic oxidation of alkyl sulfides by cytochrome P-450 and hydroxyl radical. *Bull. Chem. Soc. Jpn.*, **54**, 1163–70.

Watkins, C. H. and DeRossett, A. J. (1957). Hydrogen use high for some stocks. *Petrol. Refiner*, **36**, 201–4.

Weissgerber, R. and Kruber, O. (1920). Über das Thionaphthen im Steinkohlenteer. *Chem. Ber.*, **53**, 1551–65.

Weissgerber, R. and Moehrle, E. (1921). The sulfur in heavy coal-tar oils. *Brennstoff-Chem.*, **2**, 1.

Wenzel, B. and Aiken, R. L. (1979). Thiophenic sulfur distribution in petroleum fractions by gas chromatography with a flame photometric detector. *Rec. Trav. Chim.*, **68**, 509–19.

Werner, E. G. G. (1949). Synthesis of benzothiophenes. *Rec. Trav. Chim.*, **68**, 509–19.

West, W. R., Smith, P. A., Stoker, P. W., Booth, G. M., Smith-Oliver, T., Butterworth, B. E. and Lee, M. L. (1985). Analysis and genotoxicity of a PAC-polluted river sediment. In *'Polynuclear Aromatic Hydrocarbons: Mechanisms, Methods and Metabolism'* (M. Cooke and A. J. Dennis, eds.), pp. 1395–411. Columbus/Ohio, Battelle Press.

West, W. R., Wise, S. A., Campbell, R. M., Bartle, K. D. and Lee, M. L. (1986). The analysis of polycyclic aromatic hydrocarbon minerals Curtisite and Idrialite by high resolution gas and liquid chromatographic techniques. In *'Polynuclear Aromatic Hydrocarbons: Chemistry, Characterization and Carcinogenesis'* (M. Cooke and A. J. Dennis, eds.), pp. 995–1009. Columbus/Ohio, Battelle Press.

White, C. M. and Lee, M. L. (1980). Identification and geochemical significance of some aromatic components of coal. *Geochim. Cosmochim. Geochim. Cosmochim. Acta*, **44**, 1825–32.

Wiersema, A. K. and Gronowitz, S. (1970). Thiophene analogs of fluorene. IV. Unusual behaviour of a cyclopentadithiophenone in the reaction with dienophiles. *Acta Chem. Scand.*, **24**, 2653–5.

Wijmenga, S. S., Numan, H. and Vos, A. (1978). The crystal and molecular structure of the heterohelicene 1-tert-butylbenzo[*d*]naphtho[1,2-*d'*]benzo[1,2-*b*:4,3-*b'*]dithiophene at 110 K. *Acta Crystallogr.*, Sect. B, **B34**, 846–9.

Wilder, P. and Feliu-Otero, L. A. (1965). The 2-thia-1,2-dihydro- and tetrahydrodicyclopentadienes. *J. Org. Chem.*, **30**, 2560–4.

Wilder, P. and Gratz, R. F. (1970). Synthesis and nuclear magnetic resonance spectra of some disubstituted derivatives of 2-methyl-6-thiatricyclo[3,2,1,1^{3,8}] nonane. *J. Org. Chem.*, **35**, 3295–9.

Willey, C., Pelroy, R. A. and Stewart, D. L. (1981a). Comparative analysis of polycyclic aromatic sulfur heterocycles isolated from four shale oils. In *'Polynuclear Aromatic Hydrocarbons: Physical and Biological Chemistry'* (M. Cooke, A. J. Dennis and G. L. Fisher, eds.), pp. 907–17. Columbus/Ohio, Batelle Press.

Willey, C., Iwao, M., Castle, R. N. and Lee, M. L. (1981b). Determination of sulfur heterocycles in coal liquids and shale oils. *Anal. Chem.*, **53**, 400–7.

Wilputte, R. and Martin, R. H. (1956). Synthesis of carcinogenic compounds. XV. Polybenzo-9-thiafluorenes and 4,5-thianaphthenedicarboxylic acid anhydride. *Bull. Soc. Chim. Belg.*, **65**, 874–98.

Wilson, B. W., Pelroy, R. A., Mahlum, D. D., Frazier, M. E., Later, D. W. and Wright, C. W. (1984). Comparative chemical composition and biological activity of single- and two-stage coal liquefaction process stream. *Fuel*, **63**, 46–55.

Winters, K. and Parker, P. L. (1977). Water-soluble components of crude oils, fuel oils, and used crank-case oils. *API Publ.* 1977, 4284 (Proc. Oil Spill Conf.), pp. 579–581.

Wise, S. A. (1983). High-performance liquid chromatography for the determination of polycyclic aromatic hydrocarbons. In *'Handbook of Polycyclic Hydrocarbons'* (A. Bjørseth, ed.), pp. 183–256. New York, Marcel Dekker, Inc.

Wise, S. A. and May, W. E. (1983). Effect of C_{18}-surface coverage on selectivity in reversed-phase liquid chromatography of polycyclic aromatic hydrocarbons. *Anal. Chem.*, **55**, 1479–85.

Wise, S. A., Bonnet, W. J. and May, W. E. (1980). Normal and reversed phase liquid chromatographic separation of polycyclic aromatic hydrocarbons. In '*Polynuclear Aromatic Hydrocarbons: Chemistry and Biological Effects*' (A. Bjørseth and A. J. Dennis, eds.), pp. 791–806. Columbus/Ohio, Battelle Press.

Wise, S. A., Campbell, R. M., May, W. E., Lee, M. L. and Castle, R. M. (1983). Normal and reversed phase liquid chromatographic separations of polycyclic aromatic sulfur heterocycles. In '*Polynuclear Aromatic Hydrocarbons*' (M. Cooke and A. J. Dennis, eds.), pp. 1247–66. Columbus/Ohio, Battelle Press.

Wise, S. A., Campbell, R. M., West, W. R., Lee, M. L. and Bartle, K. D. (1986). Characterization of polycyclic aromatic hydrocarbon minerals curtisite, idrialite, and pendletonite using liquid chromatography, gas chromatography, mass spectrometry and nuclear magnetic resonance. *Chem. Geol.*, **54**, 339–57.

Wofford, H. W. and Neff, J. M. (1978). Structure–activity relations of organic pollutants: comparative toxicity of fluorene, dibenzofuran, dibenzothiophene and carbazole to estuarine crustaceans and fish. Unpubl. results (ref. in: Neff (1979) '*Polycyclic Aromatic Hydrocarbons in the Aquatic Environment*'. Appl. Science Publ. Ltd., London).

Wolff, M. E. and Zanati, G. (1970a). Thia steroids. II. 2-Thia-A-nor-2-thia-α-nor-5α-pregnan-20-one. *J. Med. Chem.*, **13**, 563.

Wolff, M. E. and Zanati, G. (1970b). Preparation and androgenic activity of novel heterocyclic steroids. *Experientia*, **26**, 1115–16.

Wolff, M. E., Zanati, G., Shanmugasundarum, G., Gupte, S. and Aadahl, G. (1970). Thia steroids. III. Derivatives of 2-thia-A-nor-5α-androstan-17β-ol as probes of steroid–receptor interactions. *J. Med. Chem.*, **13**, 531–4.

Wood, K. V., Cooks, R. G., Laugal, J. A. and Benkeser, R. A. (1985). Combination of chemical reduction of tandem mass spectrometry for the characterization of sulfur-containing fuel constituents. *Anal. Chem.*, **57**, 691–4.

Wulf, K., Unna, P. J. and Willers, M. (1963). Experimental investigations on the photodynamic action of bituminous coal tar constituents. *Hautarzt*, **14**, 292–7.

Wudl, F., Haddon, R. C., Zellers, E. T. and Bramwell, F. B. (1979). 3,4:3′,4′-Bibenzo[b]thiophene. *J. Org. Chem.*, **44**, 2491–3.

Wynberg, H. and Groen, M. B. (1968). Synthesis, resolution, and optical rotatory dispersion of a hexa- and a heptaheterohelicene. *J. Am. Chem. Soc.*, **90**, 5339–41.

Wynberg, H. and Groen, M. B. (1969). Racemization of two hexaheterohelicenes. *J. Chem. Soc. D.*, 964–5.

Wynberg, H. and Klunder, A. J. H. (1969). Synthesis of some bicycloheterenes. *Rec. Trav. Chim. Pays-Bas*, **88**, 328–33.

Wynberg, H., Van Driel, H., Kellogg, R. M. and Buter, J. (1967). The photochemistry of thiophenes. IV. Observations on the scope of arylthiophene rearrangements. *J. Am. Chem. Soc.*, **89**, 3487–94.

Wynberg, H., De Wit, J. and Sinnige, H. J. M. (1970). Synthesis of an asymmetric heterotriptycene. *J. Org. Chem.*, **35**, 711–15.

Yamada, K., Minoda, Y., Kodama, K., Nakatani, S. and Akasaki, T. (1968). Microbial conversion of petrosulfur compounds. I. Isolation and identification of dibenzothiophene-utilizing bacteria. *Agr. Biol. Chem.*, **32**, 840–5.

York Research Corp. (1979). Analyzing organics in air emissions. *Environ. Sci. Technol.*, **13**, 1340–2.

Yu, L. M. and Hites, R. A. (1981). Identification of organic compounds on diesel engine soot. *Anal. Chem.*, **53**, 951–4.

Zahradnik, R. and Parkanyi, C. (1965). A molecular orbital (M.O.) study of naphthothiophenes, naphthobenzothiophenes and phenanthrobenzothiophenes. *Collection Czech. Chem. Commun.*, **30**, 195–207.

Zander, M. (1976). Phosphorescence properties of dibenzocarbazoles and structural analogs of dinaphthothiophenes. *Z. Naturforsch.*, **31A**, 677–8.

Zander, M. (1977). Benzogenous Diels-Alder syntheses using bis-(benzo[*b*]thienylene). *Chem.-Ztg.*, **101**, 507–8.

Zander, M. and Franke, W. H. (1973). Synthesis of tetrabenzo[*a,c,h,j*]thianthrene, diphenanthro[9,10-*b*:9′,10′-*d*]thiophene, and dibenzo[2,3:10,11]perylo[1,12-*bcd*]thiophene from phenanthrene. *Chem. Ber.*, **106**, 2752–4.

Zander, M., Jacob, J. and Lee, M. L. (1987). Empirical quantitative relationship between molecular structure and phosphorescence transition energy of polycyclic aromatic thiophenes. *Z. Naturforsch.*, **42a**, 735–8.

Zeller, K. P. and Petersen, H. (1975). Photochemical production of dibenzofurans and dibenzothiophens. *Synthesis*, 532–3.

Zherdeva, S. Y., Zheltov, A. Y., Kozik, T. A. and Stepanov, B. I. (1980). Study of products of the reduction of stilbene-2,2′-disulfonyl chloride by hydroiodic acid. *Zh. Org. Khim.*, **16**, 425–9.

Index